VOLUME 1
IN A SERIES ON

FOODS, NUTRITION AND DENTAL HEALTH

Editors: John J. Hefferren, Ph.D.
Director, Research Institute of American Dental Association Health Foundation

Henry M. Koehler, M.S.
Research Institute of the American Dental Association Health Foundation

SPONSORED BY
RESEARCH INSTITUTE OF THE AMERICAN DENTAL ASSOCIATION HEALTH FOUNDATION

PATHOTOX PUBLISHERS, INC.
2405 Bond Street
Park Forest South, Illinois 60466
U.S.A.

PATHOTOX PUBLISHERS, INC.
2405 Bond Street, Park Forest South, Illinois 60466

Library of Congress Catalog Card Number:80-84606
ISBN 0-930376-21-8 (Volume 1)
ISBN 0-930376-27-7 (Set)

Printed in The United States of America

TABLE OF CONTENTS

SECTION A: CARIOGENICITY OF FOODS, BEVERAGES, CONFECTIONS AND CHEWING GUM

SECTION A:

CARIOGENICITY OF FOODS, BEVERAGES CONFECTIONS AND CHEWING GUM

I. INTRODUCTION

WELCOME

C. Gordon Watson, D.D.S.*

Ladies and gentlemen, it is a pleasure to welcome you to this Workshop on behalf of the officers and trustees of the American Dental Association.

We have been aware of many of the problems of caries and disease of oral structures. We know many things can be done about them, but there is little interest. As a profession, however, we are vitally concerned with dental health, and the participants in the Workshop have responded to this challenge—people from food science, related academic areas, manufacturers of products which contribute to the dental health challenge, National Institute of Dental Research, US Department of Agriculture and, of course, the American Dental Association and our Health Foundation. Together, we can accomplish a great deal for the good of the dental health of our constituents.

It has been said that "Good men will eventually do the right thing after exhausting all other alternatives." I think we have exhausted all the other alternatives on this subject and it's time to do the right thing right now.

AIMS OF THE WORKSHOP

John J. Hefferren, Ph.D.

I, too, welcome you and, because you have come, I assume you also welcome this opportunity.

I would like each of you to respond to the various subjects under consideration from your own vantage point. No one knows your vantage point better than you do. Some people think they know it, but that is a large assumption and one that all too frequently is wrong.

We have three broad charges to consider regarding the cariogencity of foods:

1. Can they be ranked according to cariogenicity?
2. Given the food as it has been delivered for a number of years, can its cariogenicity—that characteristic of that food item—be altered? I am speaking of food in the traditional sense, be it baby or adult, soft drinks, confections of one sort or another, and chewing gum.
3. How do you go about measuring the cariogenicity of foods? I am sure there are a number of ways to do it. I am sure that most, if not all, of you have measured it in one way or another. How does your method compare with that of others who are doing the same thing?

---

*Dr. Watson is executive director of the American Dental Association.

II. FOOD AS FOOD

Philip White, Sc.D., Chairman

THE FUNCTION OF FOOD

Robert E. Smith, Ph.D.

As you can see by the agenda, I have been assigned to discuss the function of food. Obviously, it is difficult to bring anything new to this topic, but let us review what we think we know about food and its use.

On the surface at least, food has many uses. Dr. Madeline Leininger has summarized some of these uses, as follows:

> First and foremost, food is used universally to provide body energy and to satisfy man's hunger. Apart from this basic function, food is used to initiate and maintain interpersonal relationships with friends, kinsmen, and strangers. Food is used for the expression of socio-religious ideas. Food is used to establish social status, social prestige, and for special individual and group achievements. Food is used to help man cope with his psychological stresses and needs. Food is used to reward and to punish or influence the behavior of others. Food is used to influence the political and economic status of a group. Finally, food is used to detect, treat and prevent social, physical and cultural behavior deviations and illness manifestations.

No one will quarrel with the premise that food is the most acceptable vehicle to provide needed nutrients. Our bodies are uniquely equipped to ingest, digest and assimilate the nutrients contained in food. By definition, these nutrients are those chemicals in food that feed our biochemistry or alter our physiology in such a manner as to affect the bio-availability of required nutrients. To go one step further, nutrition is the science that interprets the relationship of food to the functioning of the living organism. Because man has no inborn or natural instinctive urges to keep him on the safe side of malnutrition, it is essential that nutritional needs be addressed in foods and food selection, and, because of this, nutrition and the nutrionist have a right to their claim on the function of foods.

In addressing the majority of the foregoing uses of food, it is obvious that food selection beyond basic hunger needs is the result of the sum of a person's culture and traditions, desires and emotions, character and experiences. For most of us, food consumption does not occur just to meet nutritional needs. Even worse, food over-consumption may even be harmful. It is essential, therefore, that we consider two major functions of food: (1) food must function as a nutrient conveyor, and (2) food must function as a social instrument.

---

*Affiliations of all participants are described in the "List of Persons Attending" included in the Appendix.

The final use of food mentioned above comes closest to summarizing the newest use of food, i.e.: "Food is used to detect, treat and prevent social, physical and cultural behavior deviations and illness manifestations." Even if we remove the effects of nutrition on social, behavioral and illness manifestations, and the preachings of Adele Davis and others certainly hit hard on this subject, it still leaves a great deal of responsibility on the function of food to prevent all other social and physiological ills; so much so that to describe this function adequately, one should perhaps, borrow the medical term 'therapeutic." This leads us to a revised description of the function of food as: (1) a nutrient conveyor, (2) a social instrument, and (3) a therapeutic device.

Having briefly described the function of food, and we might just as easily admit the fact that foods—especially prepared foods—are easily amenable to alteration, we might now address how we realize the achievable functions of foods. This is generally accomplished through the efforts of food professionals, and I would like to use this introduction to bridge the gap between what is food and how we manipulate it.

We start with the classical crop geneticist. He is willing and able to breed into virtually all growing foods, production yields, disease resistance, nutrient increases and energy efficiency. But for the most part, he feels his contribution is via greater food production, and most of his efforts are concentrated here. Thus, at least total calories are assured.

To the classical nutritionist, food is the input to nutrition. He perceives food to be functional only when it meets the nutrient requirements of the consumer. This, as you know, is a difficult objective, as no single food satisfies all the needs for some 42 known essential nutrients. The nutritionist, therefore, rationalizes that many foods of certain types must be eaten during the course of a day, and if a sufficient variety is available, nutritional needs will be met. Where there is danger of normal foodstuffs not meeting these needs, the nutritionist demands nutrient fortification of certain foods. His major long-term objective is to provide all the needed nutrients in proportion to energy content, so that optimal nutrient balance is assured.

To the classical food development scientist, food is functional only when it is highly acceptable and readily eaten. In the process of eating food, man eats many chemicals which are not nutrients. The non-nutrient chemicals primarily function in two ways. One obvious function is to impart the color, flavor, and texture by which these chemicals give food its organoleptic characteristics. The much less obvious function which non-nutrient chemicals exert is on the physiology of the organism. The classical food scientist thus manipulates the first type of non-nutrient chemicals until he achieves his goal, i.e., he extrudes; expands; dries; puffs; cooks; steams; freezes; adds enzymes, colors, antioxidants, emulsifiers, preservatives, flavors, fillers, stabilizers, etc., and then packs the food in the most attractive container he can afford. If the foodstuff is accepted by the consumer—and is repurchased—his goals, for the most part, have been met.

But are these individual efforts enough to guarantee optimization of food function? No, and recent experience so indicates. During the last decade, there has been emerging a type of scientist who is not easily classified; for the sake of differentiation let us call him the responsible food scientist. He is the individual who would like all foods to be highly acceptable, to provide all necessary nutrients in proper balance, to contain no harmful or allegedly harmful chemicals, and to relieve undesirable maladies wherever possible. He is cognizant of the second type of non-nutrient chemicals and their function in our foods, i.e., those that affect physiology. This type of chemical or nutrient participates in a way distinct from that of being an essential nutrient or imparting a chemical reaction. For example, the presence of fat in the stomach increases the length of time food remains in the stomach; fiber in foods increases the bulk of the diet and can stimulate the rate of passage of digesting food through the gastrointestinal tract, with obvious health effects. Our food scientist is concerned because oxalates, phytates, and even fiber may bind various mineral nutrients, such as calcium and iron, so tenaciously that their bioavailability may be diminished dramatically. He worries that some plant foods contain some chemicals with pharmacological properties, even though the quantity present is usually so small that it is innocuous. This scientist is increasingly concerned about chemicals in food which can influence body chemistry or function but which are not nutrients. Unfortunately, most of the things he worries about have not been studied extensively, and these chemicals represent a significant gray area in food science knowledge. This frustrates such a food scientist.

Beyond these considerations, this type of scientist also advocates that foods should contain certain added chemicals to improve the quality of life, if possible. In this, he addresses the last food function, that of food being a therapeutic device.

Thus, he is able to come to us today and not only ask us whether sugar in foods is harmful, but in the event that it might be, he asks us if we can add phosphates to circumvent or neutralize possible dental caries problems. He can ask if highly saturated fat-containing foods are harmful, and then demand that polyunsaturated fats be added to such foods. He can ask whether foods containing salt contribute to hypertension and, based on only the remotest possibility, demand that we manufacture foods with less salt. This individual can ask if food colors cause hyperactivity in children, then without conclusive results ask why it is necessary to color food at all. The examples are limitless. This kind of food scientist is essential to our determination of what is the real function of food, and he needs a lot of help from others. He needs the help of the toxicologist, the physician, the biostatistician, the physical chemist, the physiologist, the epidemiologist, and virtually every "ologist" imaginable. Fortunately, this type of scientist may be a geneticist, nutritionist, or a food technologist, and he may even, surprisingly, look like you or me.

It is obvious to me that we all want to be this kind of responsible food scientist, and our presence here attests to this desire. For some time now, I have felt that the food industry and the dental profession should be working more closely together. I sincerely hope that the American Dental Association can play a prominent ròle in forging this relationship.

EVOLUTION OF FOOD

Ray G. Kelly

The term food evokes various associations: pleasure, nutrition, sociability, variety, world shortage, and many others. But a term seldom associated with food is *change*—particularly with regard to the foods we eat. To examine the assumption that foods don't change, I would like to look at our society in 1900 and as it is today, to compare the foods we ate then with those we eat now and to consider the reasons for the changes that have taken place.

Going back to 1900, fairly recent in terms of civilization and of food, what was our soceity like? The typical family lived on a farm, farmers actually comprising 42% of the total population. The farmer worked from dawn to dusk at hard physical labor, six days each week. The farm wife also worked long and strenuous hours, mostly in the kitchen, but also raising vegetables, gathering eggs, sewing, cleaning, and dealing with a host of other work. The three children had chores before and after school and helped in the field and kitchen during ths summer. The family worked hard, and when the work was done, most activity centered around such relaxation as reading, church socials, or a square dance.

The family ate three hearty meals each day, with the mid-day meal often being the largest. Foods were simple and varied with what was available in season. Meats, dairy and cereal products were widely available. Food preparation was very time-consuming as everything was prepared from scratch. Food storage was limited because most foods were prepared from a few basic ingredients and products requiring refrigerated storage were limited to those which could be stored in the ice box. Between-meal eating was very limited and usually consisted of biscuits or pie or other leftovers. Candy and cookies were rare treats.

The farm wife—and the city mother—shopped in small stores with a limited selection. Many foods were stored in bulk barrels, kegs, and bags to be measured individually by the store owner at the shopper's discretion.

For contrast, let's take a look at the family today. The percent of our population on farms has dropped from 42% to 4.8%, while the population has tripled from 76 to 220 million. Tom Typical, the father, works in an office and his main physical activity consists of walking down the hall to get a cup of coffee. His wife, Mary, probably also works, in any of a wide variety of occupations, but with one thing in common with her husband: a low level of physical labor. Both parents work a standard 37.5 hour week and are home by 5 o'clock, shortly after the kids come home from school.

In many families, this is the first time during the day that the family has been together and often they will be together for only a brief time. Tonight, Tom and Tom Jr. race off to a Little League game. Daughter Sally has a club meeting at the high school, and mother has to shop for the weekend camping trip before going to her macrame class. Clearly, the affluence and diversity of our society has increased leisure time greatly and has enormously expanded the scope of activities available. The increasingly mental and decreasingly physical nature of work has created the need for physical forms of relaxation.

But when do these people eat? Tom Typical overslept this morning and had a Danish pastry and cup of coffee from the pastry cart in the office. He ate lunch in the company cafeteria and had a candy bar with soda pop at mid-afternoon. He and Tom Jr. ate at McDonald's on the way to the Little League game.

Mary Typical, the mother, ate a scrambled egg with a piece of toast and orange juice and coffee for breakfast while she called to the kids to get up and get ready for school. She left cold cereal and milk on the table for them as she went to work. She carried a bologna sandwich for lunch and ate it at her desk with a soft drink from the vending machine. For dinner she fixed a frozen pizza in the microwave oven for herself and her daughter.

For breakfast Tom Jr. toasted a pastry while he gathered his books and gym bag. He ate it on the school bus and had lunch in the school cafeteria. After school he had a peanut butter sandwich and a glass of milk for a snack.

Daughter Sally didn't even pass through the kitchen in the morning and the cereal and milk stayed on the table all day. She bought two doughnuts at the shop across the street from the high school and skipped lunch because she thought she should go on a diet; however, she did have a soft drink to quench her thirst. The diet must have worked because after school some boys asked Sally and her girlfriend to stop for a hamburger on the way home, which they did, complete with french fries and milkshake.

When the family once again gathered at home at about 9 o'clock, they prepared popcorn and had beer or soda.

So what has happened to food consumption in 77 years?

Lunch has long ago disappeared as a family occasion and breakfast is rapidly following. The family more often than not eats dinner together, but frequently in a restaurant, or at home with carry-out food from a restaurant. In fact, 36% of all food expenditures today are in restaurants.

In the last 77 years, food technology has permitted new lifestyles and a higher standard of living. These new lifestyles and a desire for higher standards of living have forced changes in our basic food supply system. The more obvious advances, such as the popularity of canning, mechanical refrigeration, freezing, freeze-drying and greatly improved transportation have made foods available the year round to the average citizen which, in 1900, were only available seasonally to the very wealthy.

Our prosperity and unparalleled wealth have made more activities accessible to us and forced greater flexibility on eating patterns, together with a diminishing concern for the traditional three-square-meals-a-day nutrition.

We are all familiar with the new families of convenience foods brought into being by today's lifestyles and affluence. We have mixes; frozen, freeze-dried, and semi-moist foods; now retort pouches, and perhaps soon, irradiated foods.

A discussion of baking may give us some perspective on the changes which have occurred. In 1900, mother baked bread and rolls in the kitchen. Gradually she began to buy bread in the store and occasionally to bake rolls at home. Today, Mary Typical can go to the store and buy baked bread or rolls, "brown'n serve," or even refrigerated dough. Or she can buy a mix from which she can make bread, biscuits, rolls, pancakes, waffles, corn bread, and even scones.

From a nutritional standpoint, what has occurred in this century?

The average calories consumed have dropped from 3,530 to 3,300 per day, less than the decrease in physical activity. As a result, we have a population which is overweight and suffering resultant heart problems and circulatory disorders. The calories we get from fats have increased from 32% to 41% of our total, but the animal fat portion remained level at 27%. Protein still provides 12% of our calories, but here the animal source has increased from 6% to 8%. Carbohydrates as a calorie source have decreased from 56% to 47% as a result of the cereal products decline, but sugar consumption has increased to 50% of the total because of the increased percentages of sugar in foods and the popularity of soft drinks.

During this century some additives have been put in our foods which are significant in relation to our health but are not accepted by and are actually unknown to many younger persons. In 1924, iodine was added to salt, and virtually eliminated goiter in the United States. In the 1930's, vitamin D in milk greatly reduced the incidence of rickets. In the 1940's, thiamine, riboflavin, niacin and iron were added to bread and flour. Thus it is interesting and relevant to note these precedents for widespread food additives to combat disease.

Another group of food additives, one that has received considerable publicity lately, preserve foods during the extended period required to get from food manufacturer to the dinner table. These include antioxidants and mold and bacteria retardants.

Some additives make foods more appealing, modifying flavor, color, and texture. These additives usually accomplish a function which is not possible naturally, or is achievable only to a limited degree.

The fourth major function of food additives is to provide popular foods at lower cost, placing them within the reach of more families. Artificial flavors are perhaps the most common example of this type of additive.

Thus, it is clear that the eating habits of the nation have changed and will continue to change. In the eyes of many, nutritional practices are declining in quality. Paradoxically, some nutritional trends are emerging which can definitely benefit our health.

People are weight conscious. The beautiful people are thin, and in 1976 36% of the population reported they had been on a diet within the last year. This percentage is increasing yearly; 41% of the population report they buy one or more foods for health purposes, including low-calorie soft drinks, skim milk, sugar substitutes, low-fat cottage cheese, yogurt, low-calorie salad dressings, low-fat ice cream, dietetic canned fruit, low-calorie prepared entrees, and now even low-calorie beer.

In fact, this concern for health has spawned a whole new classification of foods with purportedly superior properties to natural products. We have egg-like and meat-like products which have been formulated to eliminate cholesterol from the diet. We have sugarless candy and chewing gum. We have high-fiber breads and cereals to increase roughage. We have salt-free and low-salt products.

Where is the world of food going? It's difficult to predict. But given knowledge and a choice of options, many consumers will make an informed choice of the foods they consume.

However, in our zeal, let's not forget what food is all about. People eat food because they are hungry and it's enjoyable. People don't eat foods which taste like they are good for you. When foods can be made to taste good, people have shown increasingly that they will buy them for health considerations.

DISCUSSION

Dr. White: The function of this first session is to get things on record so that the more detailed discussion of dental caries can go forward on a firm basis.

Dr. Kent Stewart: You discussed the evolution of food in the last 77 years. What happened to the evolution of public health in the United States over that same period?

Dr. White: One problem we have, of course, is that the recording of the kinds of disease problems that we are having now was not well advanced 75 years ago. The classification of morbidity and mortality has itself been changing. It is very difficult to know, for example, what the heart disease rate was in those days, or even much about cancer. People 75 years ago died of dyspepsia. Clearly, what information we do have suggests that we have gotten out of the period of classical vitamin deficiencies which earlier were major problems. We have gotten into more subtle aspects of the problem—iron deficiency anemia, other anemias that are more common.

I would question whether dental caries is any worse today. We simply know more about the relationship between nutrition and disease and consequently tend to think that our food supply and our eating habits are so bad that this relationship must be direct. Today's sophisticated techniques may be uncovering information that existed 50 to 75 years ago, but methods were not available to look for it.

Dr. Smith: Dr. White is exactly right that we are recording the diseases and talking among ourselves about them far more than in the past. We came through a period in which cancer and heart disease were our biggest concerns; they still are. They are the major killers in this country. But there is an interesting fact learned from talking to people concerned with the fitness program: they are having some difficulty with control situations in which the controls are not developing heart problems as they did in the past. We may be seeing a downward trend in some of these major killers. If the question is: Are we having more problems with our food today than we did in 1900?, the answer may be no; however, I'll leave that to further discussion.

Dr. Bollenback: In the last figures that Dr. Kelly showed about food content, I would like to call attention to the fact that the 23.5% sugar is not sugar. That consists of sugars: 3% of the 24% is lactose which is found in milk; 3% are sugars found in fruits and vegetables, and in the remaining 18%, about two-thirds is sucrose or what most of us recognize as sugar, and the other 6% is composed of corn sweeteners. People should recognize this; it is misinformation that has been started in the past year and should be corrected.

Mr. Khan: There has been an undertone that we are to make some changes in our food supply. We need to watch because the zone between the therapeutic and the nutritive uses of food is a very narrow one and it's a zone seeded with mines. I think these explosive charges have been placed there by regulatory agencies, by the public, by public health agencies, and by others. We will be considering food and its alleged role in caries promotion. I think we ought to agree at least that food does have a therapeutic use; the absence of food causes illness. At the very least, we can all agree that the proper food intake, whatever proper means, is indeed a prophylactic measure for it does prevent many possible disorders. In considering modification of foods, we in the food industry are in a legitimate area of activity. We only have to determine now how to make those modifications, for whom we make those modifications, and how we are going to do it. That should be simple. The famous Karen Ann Quinlan case has shown that we can maintain life artificially through intravenous feeding of nutrients.

Luckily most of us sustain life by the oral route. Unfortunately, the oral route always requires at least some rudimentary knowledge of what is good and what is not good, what is needed and what is not needed, and, above all, it requires will power to refrain from the excesses of too much or too little. As a representative of the food industry, I admit that we try constantly to bring our wares to the attention of the potential buyer, and that we use all of the foregoing causes to motivate a purchase. Throughout the country, demands are being made for changes in our food supply. To make those changes requires a basic realization which has already been pointed out—that is, the change in a single food supply, a single food source, is fairly meaningless. There has to be a change in the entire food supply; any of the changes that people desire, that public health officials desire, must be brought to the attention of the public through advertising, through labeling, and so forth, and finally that changes in foods ultimately lead to changes in diet. We in the food industry do not control diets. We control only foods. It is individuals who ultimately make diets.

FUNCTION OF FOOD CONSTITUENTS

F.M. Clydesdale, Ph.D.

Food constituents play a valuable if not vital role in the maintenance of a varied, nutritious, acceptable, and accessible diet for the consumer. Too often such constituents are dismissed as being frivolous adjuncts to an otherwise nutritious diet. This is simply not true; it is a view that promotes disorder and misunderstanding not only among the public but among health professionals as well.

It is a rather unfortunate truth that most consumers do not eat for scientific, nutritionally sound reasons. In fact, the realities of food purchase surveys as well as food habits point to other parameters in terms of the dietary choices of the public. These other parameters are not frivolous, but very real, practical, and important considerations. Most consumers view cost, quality, acceptability, availability, convenience, and safety as vital reasons for purchasing and using food. Much of this is subconscious but nonetheless real. Who can deny the importance of cost in an uncertain economic time? At this time of mistrust, who would argue the importance of safety? The psychological values in our society imply a demand for good sensory qualities leading to increased acceptability. At this time of struggling for individual rights and the role of women in our society, who would argue the importance of convenience which liberates the cook from the kitchen?

It is essential that consumers and public health educators be aware of this view of nutrition within the total framework in which food and feeding technology is to be understood and utilized. It must be remembered that, no matter how nutritious or noncariogenic a food, it will not be eaten unless it satisfies the realities of food purchasing and food habits. All else is useless unless the food manufactured is available, is purchased, is safe and is eaten.

Unfortunately, many choose to ignore these realities and make the broad assumption that people can be educated to eat solely for nutrition or for the prevention of dental caries. This is a uni-dimensional view of education in the extreme and ultimately will result in confusion and negativism, leading to a diet which may in fact be less nutritious in totality.

Food constituents as such, when used in a rational sense with the appropriate motivation, can satisfy some of the realities of food purchasing while satisfying public health demands. However, in viewing food constituents, care must be taken in dismissing food constituents as being present solely in manufactured foods for dubious reasons. To illustrate this point, it might be advantageous to look briefly at a food constituent, its role and concentration in food.

Sugars are a group of compounds which play an extremely important role as food constituents. Also they are fermentable substrates and therefore, like other fermentable substrates, are involved in the etiology of dental caries. The word "sugars" should be stressed because too often overzealous educators mean all sugars, but imply or speak directly only about sucrose.

Before recommending the abolition of sugars from the diet, the realities of such food constituents should be considered. (1) They provide a safe, economic, and pleasurable form of calories. Admittedly, caloric input and the lack of calories are not a problem in the United States. However, considering a whole-world view and a larger focus, it seems rather shortsighted to suggest that we ban or prohibit the sale of a safe, economical and pleasurable form of calories. (2) They provide a safe and effective form of preservation. This point should be stressed because too often the preservative action of sugars in general and sucrose in particular is forgotten. The preservative effect of sugars is based primarily on the well known phenomenon of decreased vapor pressure resulting from the presence of solutes and described by Raoult's law. This results in a decreased water activity (A_w), which may be defined as a measure of unbound, free water in a system, available to support biological and chemical reactions. Water activity, not absolute water content, is what bacteria, enzymes, and chemical reactions depend on at the microenvironmental level in food materials.

Dried foods and in particular intermediate moisture foods (IM) owe their availability and keeping qualities to such a method of preservation.

Intermediate moisture or semi-moist foods, in one form or another, have been important items of diet for a long time. Generally they contain moderate levels of moisture, of the order of 20 to 50% by weight, which is less than is normally present in natural fruits, vegetables, or meats and more moisture than is left in conventionally dehydrated products. But in addition, IM foods have dissolved in this moisture concentrations of solutes sufficient to decrease water activity below that required to support microbial growth. As a consequence, IM foods do not require refrigeration to prevent microbial deterioration. In the past, there have been various kinds of IM foods: natural IM products such as honey; manufactured confectionery products high in sugar: jellies, jams, and bakery items such as fruit cakes; and partially dried products including figs, dates, jerky, pemmican, pepperoni, and the like. Sweetened condensed milk with a sugar level of about 63% based on the water content also could be considered as IM food. In all of these products, preservation is partially from high osmotic pressure associated with the high concentration of solutes; in some, additional preservative effect is contributed by salt, acid and other specific solutes.

Thus, if "sugars" or sucrose were to be used as some kind of "marker" for nutritional adequacy or dental health, there would be a tremendous number of foods removed from the market. At times I find it difficult to accept sweeping generalizations which recommend that a cereal product of 30 to 50% sugar (which means in effect a serving of cereal in a bowl containing approximately the same amount of sugar as one tablespoon of jelly, one tablespoon of pancake syrup, or two canned peach halves served with two tablespoons of the fruit syrup) be banned from the marketplace while a sticky product like dried fruit at 70% sugar is blithely ignored.

In a consideration of the availability of food, it might be of interest to view the case 200 years ago. "Apples were the most popular fruit because of their keeping qualitites and cider potential...peaches, pears and plums were also grown... frequently these fruits were left to rot or fed to hogs after daily needs were met, as preservation required pound for pound of sugar it was costly."[1] It seems to be as absurd to use sugars as "markers" as it is to advertise "natural" jam, jellies and preserves as "free from preservatives" when in reality they contain 55% sugars which are present as preservatives.

As scientists and educators, it is essential that we make recommendations to the public to improve not only its dental health but its total nutritional well-being. However, as scientists we also have an obligation to view food constituents both in the natural and formulated state in their totality. It is the uni-dimensional approach to view a constituent solely on the basis of "one-effect." This is counterproductive and negative. As Dr. Bibby has pointed out so well, "Foods cause dental caries," not a particular food ingredient. There is ample evidence to support this comment when the cariogenicity of different foods is reviewed. It is not a direct function of sugar content, nor acid content, nor starch content. Obviously, sugars are involved. However, the rational educational approach would seem to be to find out which foods are most cariogenic and then make recommendations for new, less cariogenic foods. The approach of removing all sugars from the diet is rather irrational when one considers that fruits owe 70% of their total calories to sugars. As well, the removal of both refined starches and sugars would reduce our caloric intake by about 50% and I cannot believe that anyone would recommend that we replace this with fat or protein.

Immoderation is the general key which opens the door to poor health Added to immoderation may be the role of certain foods, rather than particular food ingredients in the case of dental caries.

Immoderation by the consuming public should not be answered by immoderation from scientists and educators. A moderate, well balanced, scientific viewpoint which considers all the realities of food purchasing and food habits must be taken if we are to succeed in educating the public to a better, healthier way of life.

REFERENCE

1. Weigley, E.S. Food in the days of the Declaration of Independence. J. Amer. Dietetics Assoc. 45:35-40, 1964.

DISCUSSION

Dr. White: The function of the discussion is not to review other public health problems or personal nutritional problems related to food. Our job now is to be sure that we have provided an adequate foundation about food composition and the evolution of food uses to provide a proper basis for the forthcoming discussion.

Dr. Dwevide: We talk about what is good and what is not good, but one point that is missing most of the time is the basic element in connection with the major diet which must be emphasized — we overeat. This "over" is the basic problem. It is really not important whether we eat polyunsaturated fats or saturated fats; if these fats are used in right proportion and in right amounts, there is no problem. I hoped someone might shed some light on why there is lack of communication between industry, scientific bodies, and the consumer. Why this particular message is not conveyed to the consumer — that he is overeating. The public should also understand nutritional principles a little better. I believe that probably only 10% of consumers understand what low calorie really means.

Dr. Smith: I take exception to your statement that few people are cognizant of obesity. Every time we survey the population, we find that a very large proportion of the female population, in particular, are terribly cognizant of the problem of overweight. A high proportion of these people are on diets. That is not to say that they know what to do, but they certainly are aware of being overweight. Earlier, I tried to give some of the reasons why people eat food and yet don't think about nutrition when they are doing it. That is the key to the problem. How can we handle that? We can't just go to the food industry and tell them to advertise "do not eat food." What we have to be able to do is tailor our foodstuffs to this new kind of lifestyle and be cognizant of the number of calories that we do put in many of these foods. I feel that we must offer alternatives; by that I mean low calorie alternatives. People should not feel that they are suffering if they choose a low caloric intake. There are many problems involved in that kind of approach because we have to come up with something that will be a substitute on the lower calorie level. At the moment we are not doing very well in the chemical additives that we attempted to find, so that we can have satiety and acceptance and still have lower calories. It becomes a difficult problem; I hope we don't solve it all by fiber.

Dr. White: I doubt that we have adequate knowledge about the amounts of the macronutrients needed simply to maintain health and not cause any adverse effects.

Dr. Boggs: I would like to build on what Dr. Smith said. I think the data were presented to us in terms of overeating. The physiological drive for calories in the last 77 years has only gone down 200 calories, and yet our lifestyles have changed dramatically. What has happened is that the physiological regulators are the same as they have been for the last 100 years or for the lifetime of man, but emotion and other things are starting to overplay this. I am sure you have seen people sit in front of the television and eat peanuts and drink various things. Whether you can superimpose on that, and whether you can intercept that is a very difficult problem. We may not be able to control those other factors which are emotional or psychological; how many people who are overweight are also suffering from some type of psychological problem or stress? I think that we are moving now into an arena where we cannot control totally their caloric intake.

Dr. Dwivedi: Dr. Smith offered the comment that possibly the answer is low calorie foods. I disagree with that. The answer is to educate the consumer. If the consumer is told that he can have a 2,000 calorie diet in a day, does he understand what those 2,000 calories mean — what kind of foods he can eat within that framework? I think they can do a much better job of eating if they understand calories. If they do they can solve their problems much better than they could by our providing alternatives.

Dr. Schiff: For some ten years the public has been informed again and again that cigarettes are bad for health. Every single package that they pick up informs them that they are going to get some kind of disease. Yet cigarette consumption has increased in the last five years. Education of the public is not sufficient; in this case we have to educate but at the same time we have to do other things.

Dr. Daniels: To be more specific, if you walk into a room of individuals highly educated in nutrition — dieticians and nutritionists — you find just as much malnutrition in the form of obesity as you do in any other group of people in the country. So knowledge is not changing nutritional habits *per se;* other pressures are doing this. Teaching the consumer what is good or bad is not necessarily sufficient, even as regards nutrition.

Dr. White: The important question is: What can we anticipate from the food industry and the confection industry in the way of new carbohydrate sources or syrups and so forth? There has been an incredible change in the kinds of carbohydrates used in the industry in the past few years. That is what we ought to be discussing and recording.

Mr. Khan: I cannot answer the last question that was asked. However, I would like to mention one idea here, that dentistry itself has perhaps in a way contributed to the dilemma we are in today by the fact that it is possible today painlessly to repair, remove, and replace the dentition. This has greatly enhanced the lack of fear. One major motivation for taking care has been removed. We heard that 36% of the people in America claim that they are on a diet. Ask anyone who has had a heart attack or who has suddenly discovered that he suffers severely from diabetes how easy it is to lose 30 pounds. It can be done when you are motivated by fear, and I am afraid that no one today seems to be terribly afraid of dental caries.

Dr. Scala: The point about cigarettes is somewhat misleading in the sense that one of the strongest emerging markets today is the low tar and nicotine cigarette, which in effects says that the public recognizes its frailty and inability to stop smoking, but wants to reduce the risk as much as possible. Indeed, the people at the National Institutes of Health and National Cancer Institute tell us that the low tar and nicotine cigarettes are actually reducing the rate of onset of lung cancer.

I think the consumer is health oriented despite his emotional involvement with food. Statistics show that low calorie alternatives are in tremendous demand. I think most of our market research indicates, however, that it is not always based on the desire to lose weight; the consumer also often wants these low calorie alternatives so that he can eat twice as much. I think it does say, however, that the interest is there. As to dental caries, the people in market research will tell you that the consumer, the housewife, understands dental caries. In other words, she knows and will seek out products that are noncariogenic if she can. If you say, for example, that a new product has no cholesterol and therefore is a substitute for eggs that have a lot of cholesterol, she will buy it. We should think in terms of new components of food. We know certain things especially as related to the phosphates. What new components of foods can we seek which will reduce the cariogenic potential of a given food, especially sweet snacks? I think that is the area in which we are interested, and this is where we must learn to improve on nature. I think things such as the inability to control one's calories represents the same problems that smokers have, and why they lean toward low tar and nicotine cigarettes.

Dr. White: You have provided us with a good summary of the major points made in the first part of this conference — that food is composed of constituents, some of which have beneficial effects, some of which have adverse effects, some of which act in harmony or in opposition to other components of food to provide an effect. We know that we cannot alter drastically the composition of our food supply without its having some effect on the public. The culprit being considered most carefully now, sugars, is a constituent of food that has important food technological functions as well as providing a pleasureable experience when eating the food. It is questionable whether we want or could get to the place where we have a carbohydrate-free food supply.

III. FOOD AND DENTISTRY

John H. Hopper, Ph.D., Chairman

FOOD RELATIONSHIPS TO CARIES

Basil G. Bibby, D.M.D.

Throughout the ages people in many parts of the world have independently reached the conclusion that there was an association between dental decay and the types of foods that were eaten. Thus, Aristotle attributed dental decay to sweet figs sticking to the teeth and in the thirteenth century an Arabian physician wrote that the decay of teeth is caused by "clinging particles of food which decompose, product an acid moisture which eats away and destroys them so that finally, with much pain, they rot away little by little." That is a pretty fair description of what we believe today.

However, there was a period in the 1920's and 1930's when the enthusiasm for nutrition led the medical profession and many dentists to believe that dental caries was the result of deficiencies in the diet. During that period reports were published claiming reductions in dental decay produced by additions of vitamin C or vitamins A and D to the diet or by adjusting the acid-base level of the diet and so forth. These findings still lack confirmation and reasons can be offered to explain the results reported.

As dental research expanded, several types of experiments demonstrated that, apart from fluorine, nutritional adequacy has little to do with the development of caries-resistant teeth. Despite the fact that in conditions of malnutrition the teeth have preference over the bones for the calcium that is available to the body, it does not seem that the body can develop a tooth which will be able to resist the severity of caries attack to which, under today's conditions, it may be exposed.

Several types of research have shown that processes occurring on the tooth surface are essential for the caries attack. These include the demonstration that experimental caries in animals can be prevented by the use of chemicals or anti-bacterial agents which prevent acid formation from carbohydrates in the mouth. Other experiments have shown[1] that there is no dental decay in animals fed by means of stomach tube so no food came in contact with the teeth, but that much caries develops in teeth of corresponding groups of animals fed the same diet in the ordinary way (Table 1). Several modifications of this test, including the feeding of one-half of Siamese twin animals a caries-producing diet, have confirmed that no caries occurs unless food comes in contact with the teeth.

TABLE 1. Effect of stomach tube feeding*

	No. of Animals	Av. Carious Molars	Av. No. Lesions	Av. Extent
Tube-Fed	13	0	0	0
Control	13	5.0	6.7	10.6

*Adapted from Kite *et al.*, [1].

The conclusion that contact between foodstuffs and the tooth surfaces is necessary to produce dental decay leads naturally to the question...whether all foods are equally destructive. While almost all available evidence indicates that carbohydrate fermentation in the mouth is an essential component of caries causation, this does not mean that all foods containing carbohydrate will be equally destructive to teeth. In my opinion, both dentists and researchers oversimplify the relationship between carbohydrate consumption and caries and assume there is direct proportionality between them. I propose to review the evidence we have on this matter, particularly as it relates to the effects of different types of foodstuffs on caries causation. To do this I will first point out the relationships between certain types of foods and their use that have been supported by clinical tests, in other words, tests that relate actual occurrence of dental decay in human subjects to the use of specific foods. Thereafter, I will discuss various properties of foods which probably modify their ability to cause dental decay. Finally, some possible variations in food composition that could modify their cariogenicity will be suggested.

Clinically Established Relations Between Foods and Caries

Carbohydrates: That carbohydrates added to the diet are highly conducive to dental decay was shown in a study of human subjects in Vipeholm, Sweden, in which the inmates of a mental institution were fed a succession of carefully controlled diets of one sort or another over a five-year period.[2] Feeding a carbohydrate diet over a two-year period produced a dramatic increase in caries (Fig. 1),[3] but when this ration of 24 toffees/day was discontinued, caries receded.

Frequency of use: That something other than the total amount of carbohydrate consumed plays a part in determining caries activity is shown in Figure 2.[3] In this test, patients were fed caramels each day during the third year of the experiment which, it will be noted, caused a marked increase in caries. However, in the fourth year of the experiment the same total caramel ration was divided into two parts and eaten at two different times. This change produced a definite increase in caries even though the total amount of sugar eaten each day remained constant. This shows that the frequency of eating sugar is almost as important as the total amount eaten in the causation of dental decay. Further evidence of the importance of the frequency of eating is shown in Figure 3.[4] This gives the results of a study on more than a thousand five-year-old children in Tennessee. The frequency of eating of candies,

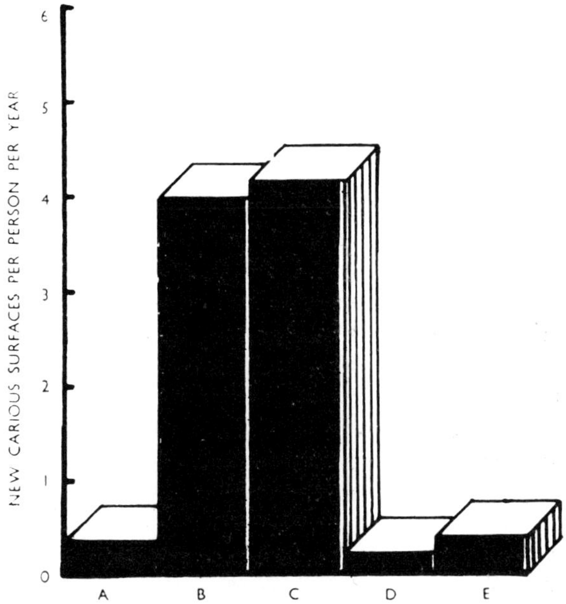

FIGURE 1. Caries in 48 males in Vipeholm Study[2] who used basic diet during years A and D and 24 toffees between meals during years B and C. (Courtesy of G.N. Davies[3])

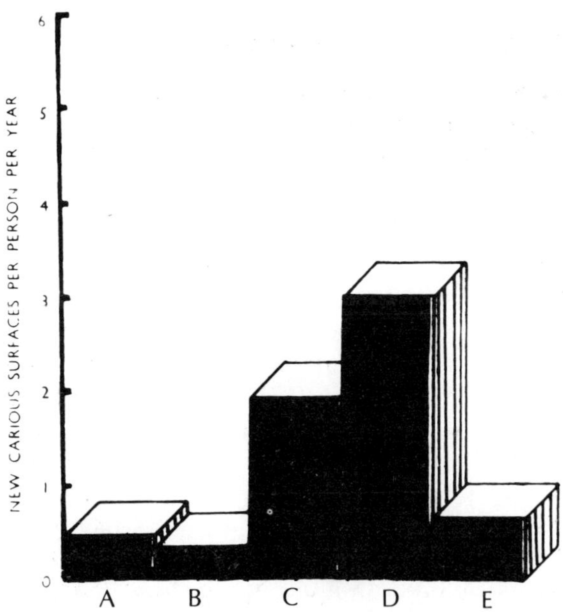

FIGURE 2. Caries in 62 males in Vipeholm Study who ate 22 caramels as two snacks in year C, but as four snacks in year D. (Courtesy of G.N. Davies[3])

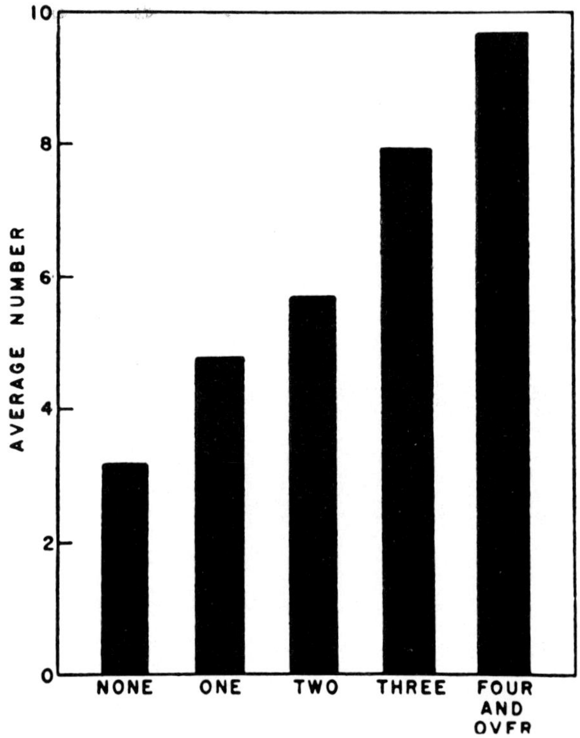

FIGURE 3. Average number of def teeth per child according to between-meal snacks, preschool children West Tennessee, 1956

cookies, chewing gum or carbonated beverages was determinied by child-patient interviews and compared with the numbers of decayed teeth in their mouths. It can be seen that the children who did not eat between meals had the fewest decayed teeth and that the number increased in parallel to the frequency of eating the listed confections. similar results have been reported from studies made in New Zealand and Great Britain.

Food clearance: Another factor that has been shown to have an influence on the carcinogenicity of foods is the length of time they adhere to the teeth after eating. As a part of the Vipeholm Study, Lundquist[5] determined the speed of clearance of foods from the mouth; his findings are given in Figure 4. This shows a relationship between the amount of food that is retained on the teeth after eating and the amount of dental decay occurring in the various groups of patients.

Physical texture: Further evidence that factors related to physical properties of the food are important in caries emerged from the Vipeholm Study.[2] When a comparison was made between the amount of dental decay occurring in the group of patients consuming 75 grams of sucrose a day in liquids, tea and coffee, and in the group consuming much less sucrose in their bread, it was found that almost four times as much decay developed in the latter group

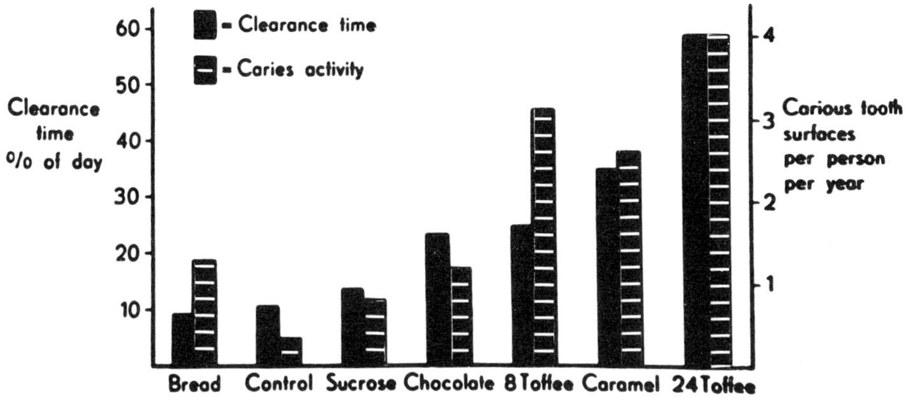

FIGURE 4. Figures giving sugar clearance times and dental caries activitiy for differing forms of foodstuffs. (From Lundquist[5])

(Table 2). The dramatic thing about this finding is that while they ate only at mealtimes, twice as much dental decay occurred in the patients in the bread group despite the fact that they were using much less sugar than those who took the sugar in liquid form. This finding is in keeping with animal tests that show that sugar in liquids is much less conducive to dental decay than when used in dry or solid form. The higher caries occurrence in the bread users could indicate that there was an unrecognized component of the bread that contributed to the caries attack. Adhesiveness of the bread to the teeth might be implicated. How important the factors of oral retantion or food texture are in caries is not known. However, the wide differences that have been shown in the amount of food retained in the mouth after eating (Table 3)[6] make it seem likely that retention must play a part in the ability of individual foods to cause caries.

TABLE 2. Caries from two year addition of sucrose in bread or liquid to basic Vipeholm diet

Diet	Calorie Supplement	Total Sucrose	Meals	Snacks	New Caries Surfaces/Yr
Control	Margarine (45 gm)	0	4	0	0.43
Bread	Bread (345 gm)	50 gm	4	0	2.32
Sucrose	Sucrose Solu.	75 gm	4	0	0.82

(Data from the Vipeholm Dental Caries Study)[12]

Probable Modifiers of Food Cariogenicity

Acid production from foods: The first suggestion that the acid produced by bacterial fermentation of foods would indicate their relative cariogenicity

TABLE 3. Range of food retention in mouth after eating

Food	% CHO	mg Retained
Fig Cookie	70	678
Date	77.5	507
Ice Cream	17	423
Chocolate	50	370
Cookie (shortbread)	59.5	370
Cracker (salted)	70	340
Cracker (oil sprayed)	71	310
Toffee	90	266
Cola Drink	10.5	237
Caramel	56.8	219
White Bread	49	188
Orange Juice	8.5	177
Carrot (cooked)	8.3	2

was made by W.D. MIller[7] who, at the turn of the century, provided the scientific background for our current concepts of dental caries. Although his claim that because potatoes and bread produced more acid on fermentation in saliva than did sucrose is inadequately supported by his experiments, acid production from different foods on fermentation by mouth bacteria has frequently been used as an index of the amount of dental decay they would cause. Recent work has demonstrated that there are tremendous differences between the amount of acid produced from foodstuffs on salivary fermentation when buffers or acid neutralization allow fermentation to proceed to conclusion. Figure 5 shows that even within the same classes of food there are quite wide differences in the amount of fermentation acid which they form.[8]

Enamel demineralization: In polarized light studies of the extent of caries-like change produced in enamel placed in tubes in which salivary bacteria were fermenting foods, the amount of caries-like demineralization did not parallel the amount of acid produced from foods.[9] This can be the result either of the formation of different types of fermentation acids or of the presence in the food of substances which limit enamel demineralization. Both of these have been demonstrated for several foods. Examples of the lack of relationship between acid production and the amount of enamel destroyed by foods are given in Table 4.[10] That the differences in enamel dissolution by breakfast cereals are related to such factors rather than the amount of sugar present for fermentation is shown in Figure 6.[11] The type of dough or mineral or other additives can be seen to determine the amount of enamel dissolved as much as the sugar content. Further evidence along these lines is provided in Figures 7 and 8. In the former[10] it can be seen that a relatively small amount of acid produced by wheat flour demineralizes a large quantity of enamel. The ratio is

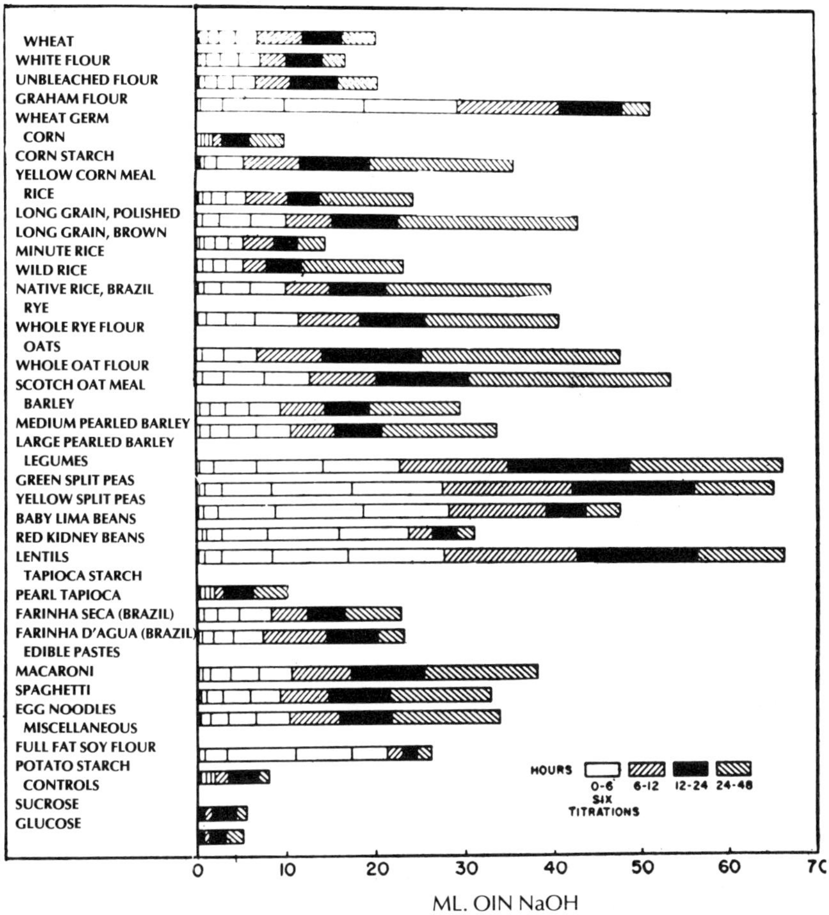

FIGURE 5. Amounts of acid produced during 48 hour fermentation ot starch foods in saliva. Acid was neutralized at 1, 2, 3, 4, 5, 6, 12 and 24 hours to permit continued fermentation. (From Beck & Bibby[8])

TABLE 4. Acid formation and enamel decalcification by certain foods

Food	Acid Formed (ml 0.05M NaOH)	Enamel Dissolved (mg)
Whole Wheat Bread	11.0	0.2
White Bread	8.4	0.4
Corn Flakes Cereal	4.3	0.5
All-Bran Cereal	16.2	0.1
Chocolate Coconut Bar	11.1	1.1
Milk Chocolate	13.2	0.1
White Flour	4.9	1.0
Graham Flour	5.1	0.2

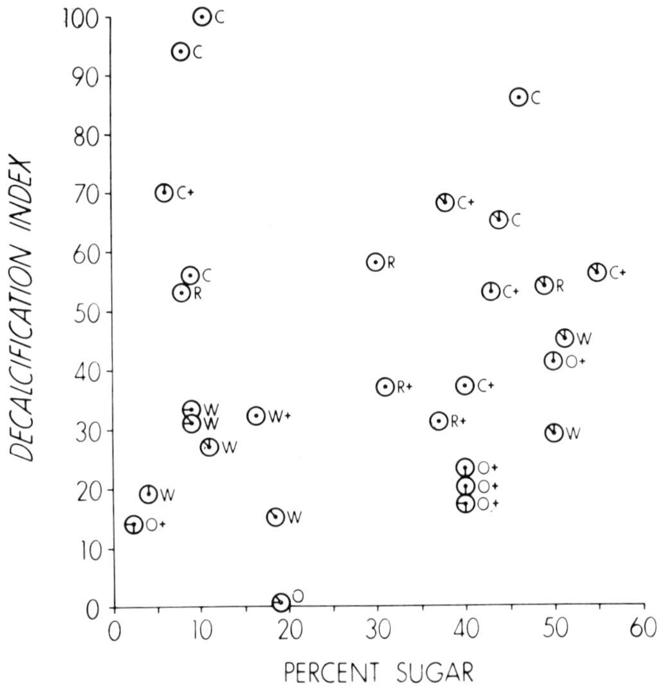

FIGURE 6. Amounts of enamel dissolved on streptococcal fermentation of breakfast cereals with different sugar contents. Key: C, R, O, W indicate dough base of corn, rice, oats or wheat respectively, the + sign addition of another starch, the clock circles the presence of minerals, oils, etc. (From Bibby and Weiss[9])

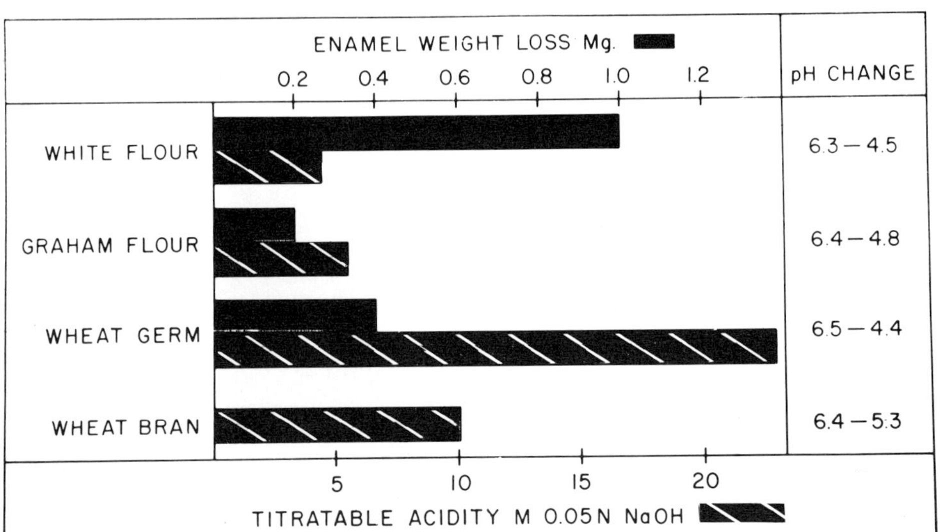

FIGURE 7. Amounts of acid formed and enamel dissolved on incubating enamel blocks in mixtures of cereal products and human saliva. (Courtesy R.J. Andlaw[10])

different with graham flour; even more so with wheat germ. With wheat bran there is a large quantity of acid formed but no enamel demineralization. Figure 8 shows that of the sugar products tested, molasses produces the most acid, but nonetheless it destroys the smallest amount of dental enamel.[12] Table 5 shows that the same lack of parallelism between acid production and enamel dissolution appears when popular candies are tested.[13]

Acid formation in dental plaque: As dental decay attacks teeth from the outside, it seems logical to indicate the cariogenicity of foods by measuring the amount of acid they form in the deposits or plaque on the tooth surface. This is done in several ways. Probe types of pH electrodes can be placed on plaque, plaque samples can be removed and pH measured outside the mouth or electrodes can be fitted into tooth replacements and connected by wires or radio from inside the mouth to pH meters. An example of the various pH

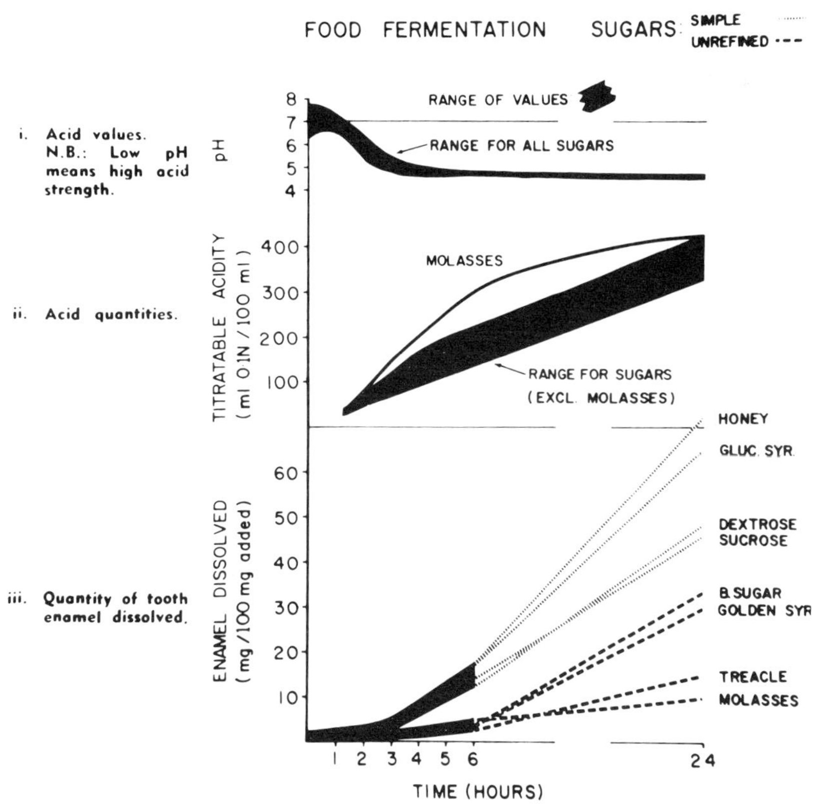

FIGURE 8. Amounts of acid formed and enamel dissolved on incubating sugar products in saliva. (Courtesy B.R. Gillings[12])

TABLE 5. Enamel dissolution — popular candy bars

Candy	Ong pH	Titr. Acid (0.05 *M* NaOH)	Dissolution Index (1)
Butterfinger	6.43	1.95	26
Almond Joy	6.73	1.84	27
Baby Ruth	6.58	2.31	28
Chocolate Caramel	6.45	2.49	28
Milk Chocolate 1	6.55	1.49	29
Caramel	6.45	1.55	33
3 Musketeers	6.85	1.79	34
Milk Chocolate 2	6.35	1.75	35
Milk Chocolate 3	6.35	1.83	44
Mounds	6.92	1.95	48

(1) Sucrose Control = 100

responses given for four foods tested by the first method is shown in Figure 9.[14] A comparison of the results given by the second method for sucrose, caramel, and a caramel made with a sucrose substitute is given in Figure 10.[15] Readings obtained by the third method on different days[16] and for a number of breakfast cereals[16] are shown in Figures 11 and 12. The extent of the pH depressions given by this last, or telemetric method, is accepted under Swiss law as indicating whether a food may be advertised or not as safe for the teeth. While this is a forward step, it is probably premature and lacking in adequate scientific justification. There two main reasons for this opinion. One, as pointed out above, is that acid production from foods does not necessarily indicate the amount of enamel destruction that will occur and the strength of the related caries attack. The second is that tests on caries production in rats by some of the cereals[17] for which pH curves are recorded in Figure 12 gave very different amounts of caries (Table 6) despite the fact that their plaque pH curves were essentially the same.

TABLE 6. Rat caries feeding breakfast cereals

		Caries Scores		Daily Sugar Eaten	
Cereal Type	Sugar Content	Test 1 (100% Cereal)	Test 2 (64% Cereal)	Test 1	Test 2
Plain	8	24.6	16.7	0.27	0.58
Sugar Coated	43	23.6	16.3	1.76	2.90
Enriched	19	9.6	11.7	1.32	1.32
Lab Diet	64		20.2		6.61

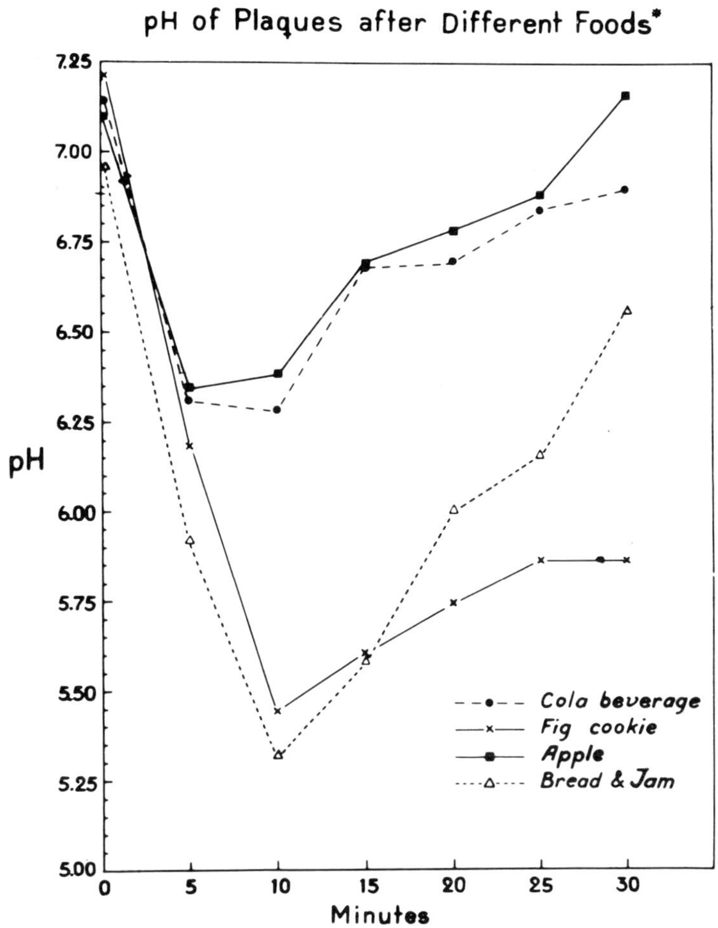

FIGURE 9. Effect of eating several foods in plaque pH. All figures mean of 5 subjects. (From Ludwig & Bibby[14])

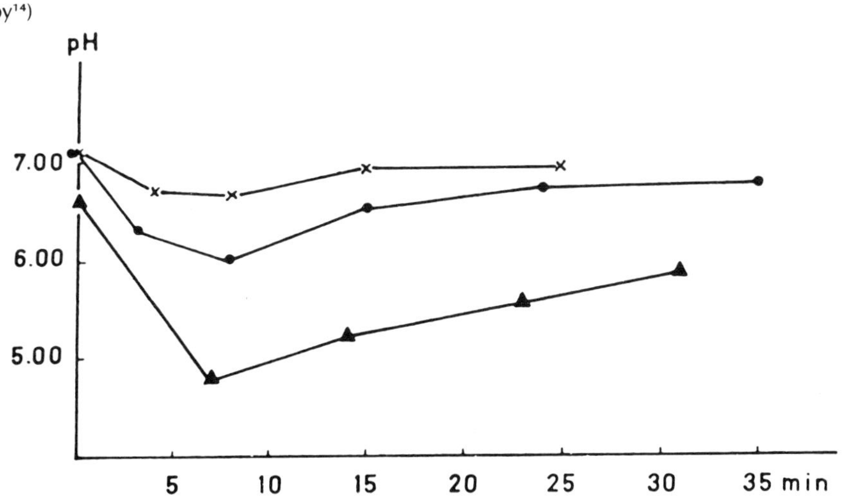

FIGURE 10. Plaque pH after 50% sucrose rinse, Δ; conventional caramel, •; and special caramel, X. (Courtesy G. Frostell[15])

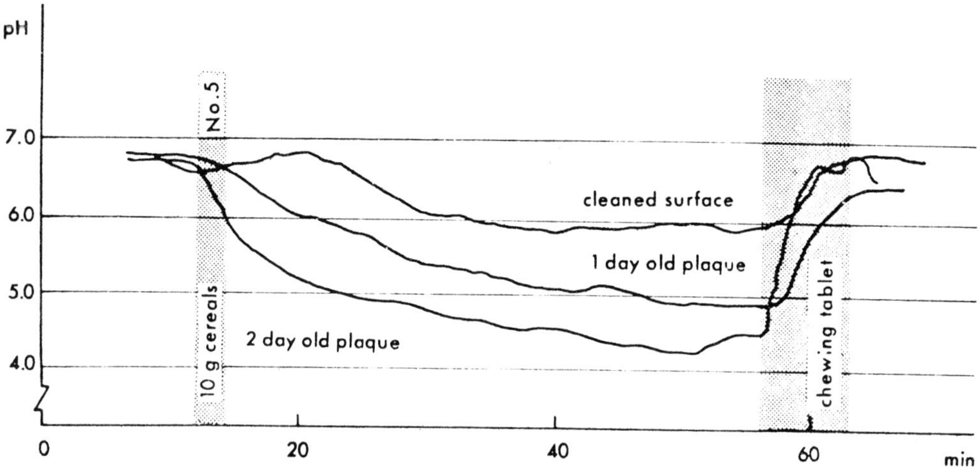

FIGURE 11. pH of interdental plaque after eating breakfast cereal on three subsequent days (telemetric recording). (From De Crousaz, Graf & Bibby[16])

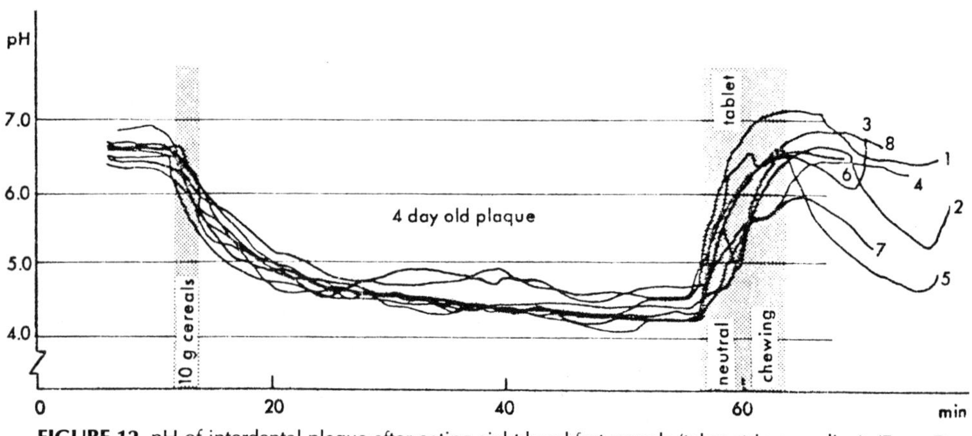

FIGURE 12. pH of interdental plaque after eating eight breakfast cereals (telemetric recording). (From De Crousaz, Graf & Bibby[16])

Animal caries: Experimental caries in animals, although differing in many ways from caries in man, undoubtedly reflect some characteristics of foods that contribute to human caries. It has been much used as a tool for research on some phases of caries, but only occasionally as a tool for indicating the cariogenicity of food. Animal caries without doubt is influenced by a variety of factors. Although the sugar content is certainly one of these, the figures in Table 7 indicate that other factors can be important[18]. Published reports show that the phosphate content[19] or acid buffering capacity[20] of foods exercise a profound influence in caries production in rodents.

The reliability of any of the methods discussed for indicating the cariogenicity of foods in respect to caries causation in the human mouth must await further research. It seems likely that all of them are influenced by factors to be mentioned below.

TABLE 7. 60 day caries on gelatinized and ungelatinized starches

Diet		No. of Animals	Caries Score
Wheat	Regular	24	2.5
	Gelatinized	24	6.42
Potato	Regular	18	16.67
	Gelatinized	23	33.52
Arrowroot	Regular	23	2.87
	Gelatinized	12	24.58
Tapioca	Regular	21	4.14
	Gelatinized	24	32.55

Frostell & Baer[18]

Possible Influences on Cariogenicity of Foods

Protein adsorption on enamel: The action of proteins from the saliva in protecting teeth against caries is generally accepted. The effect appears to be the result of their being adsorbed by the enamel surface. Food proteins also are adsorbed varyingly and are capable of protecting enamel against the action of acid. Of the dozen or so we have tested,[21] casein is the food protein that seems most effective in providing protection against the action of acid (Table 8).

Organic phosphates: A wide range of organic phosphates are adsorbed onto the teeth. Of these, phytic acid of cereals has been most fully studied. It is shown to protect enamel against acid.

Flavors: That flavoring agents can influence enamel solubility has been shown by comparisons of the effects of spices (Table 9).[22] Licorice-flavored candies are less destructive than others of the same type or than corresponding amounts of sucrose. Acid added for flavor effects increases the amount of enamel dissolved and this, in turn, differs according to type of acid used.

TABLE 8. Effect of some proteins on acid solubility of enamel surfaces

Protein	Concn.	Tests	Reduction Mean %
Casein	1%	9	20
Gelatin	1%	9	12.1
Egg Albumin	1%	9	3.2
Gastric mucin	1%	6	25.7

TABLE 9. Effect of water extracts of spices on dissolution of enamel in saliva fermentations of sucrose

Spice Extract	Acid Produced 0.05*M* NaOH	Enamel Dissolved Mg
Sesame	1.61	7.98
Cardamon	1.72	7.79
Clove	1.96	7.44
Cinnamon	1.28	5.18
Ginger	1.40	4.28
Nutmeg	1.29	3.27
Marjoram	1.22	2.47
Garlic	0.52	1.86

Other effects: Of course these are not the only variables to be regarded as factors that could modify cariogenicity. Continuing research undoubtedly will reveal other contributing factors. These could be related to such untested things as trace element content of foods, differences between sugars or the effects of their concentrations or mixtures on biological phenomena such as plaque formation, bacterial metabolism or salivary secretion.

One conclusion that can be drawn with certainty is that a great variety of food characteristics can influence their cariogenicity.

REFERENCES

1. Kite, O.W., Shaw, J.H. and Sognnaes, R.F. The prevention of experimental tooth decay by tube feeding. J. Nutrition 42:89-103, 1950.
2. Gustafessen *et al.* The Vipeholm dental caries study. Acta Odont. Scand. 11:195-388, 1954.
3. Davies, G.H. An appreciation of the Vipeholm dental caries study. New Zealand Dental J. 51:153-157, 1950.
4. Weiss, R.L. and Trithout, A.H. Between-meal eating habits and dental caries experience in pre-school children. Amer. J. Pub. Health 50:1097-1184, 1960.
5. Lundquist, C. Oral sugar clearance. Odont. Revy 3 (Supp. 1):1-121, 1952.
6. Bibby, B.G., Goldberg, H.J.V. and Chen, E. Evaluation of the caries-producing potentialities of various foodstuffs. J. Amer. Dent. Assoc. 42:491-509, 1951.
7. Miller, W.D. The microorganisms of the human mouth. S.S. White, Philadelphia 1890.
8. Beck, D.J. and Bibby, B.G. Acid production during the fermentation of starches by saliva. J. Dent. Res. 40:486-491, 1961.
9. Soni, N.N. and Bibby, B.G. Enamel decalcification in food-saliva mixtures. J. Dent. Res. 40:185-189, 1961.
10. Andlaw, R.J. The relationship between acid production and enamel decalcification in salivary fermentation of carbohydrate foodstuffs. J. Dent. Res. 39:705, 1960.
11. Weiss, M.E. and Bibby, B.G. Enamel dissolution by streptococcal fermentation of breakfast cereals. J. Dent. Res. 49:1481-1486, 1970.
12. Gillings, B.R. A new approach to dental diets. The Dental Outlook (Sydney University) No. 16, 1-4, 1966.
13. Mundorff, S.A. and Bibby, B.G. Unpublished findings, 1976.
14. Ludwig, T.G. and Bibby, B.G. Acid production from different carbohydrate foods in plaque and saliva. J. Dent. REs. 36:56-60, 1957.
15. Frostell, G. Substitution of fermentable sugars in sweets. Nutrition and caries prevention. Stockholm, Almquist and Wiksell, 1965, pp. 60-66.

16. De Crousaz, Ph.A., Graf, H. and Bibby, B.G. Buffering of breakfast cereals and pH of plaque *in vitro* and *in vivo*. Helv. Odont. Acta. 11:157-162, 1967.
17. Chong, U.B., Losee, F.L. and Bibby, B.G. Some effects of breakfast cereals on caries in rats. J. Dent. Res. 52:509-517, 1973
18. Frostell, G. and Baer, P.N. Caries experience of rats fed various starches for study of experimental calculus formation. Acta Odont. Scand. 29:401-413, 1971.
19. Nizel, A. and Harris, R.S. The effects of phosphates on experimental dental caries; A literature review. J. Dent. Res. 43:1123-1136, 1964.
20. Katz, S., Olson, B.L. and McDonald, J.L. Buffering capacity, sugar content and cariogenicity of foods. J. Dent. Res. 53 (Special Issue) Abst. No. 607, 1974.
21. Weiss, M.E. and Bibby, B.G. Some protein effects on enamel solubility. Arch. Oral Biol. 11:59-63, 1966.
22. Clarkson, B.H. and Bibby, B.G. *In vitro* effects of spice extracts on acid formation and enamel solubility. J. Dent. Res. 48:916-919, 1968.

DISCUSSION

Dr. Zoumas: I reviewed the data on the Vipeholm Study and I think that you have to make the point that the levels of chocolate, particularly in caramels and toffees, fed in that study were high. For example, 52 lb. of milk chocolate per year on a per capita basis, and 160 lb. of toffee, and it was a specially prepared toffee, if I remember, that adhered to the teeth. I made a quick calculation of total caloric intake and 640 calories, or about one-third, were coming from toffee. I really don't think that study has too much relevance to the problem here, because the average confectionery consumption in this country is about 16 lb. per year

Dr. Bibby: The manager of the study had a great difficulty in getting the 24 candies into the mouths of the mentally defective people. They were smart enough to realize that it wasn't good. Precautions had to be taken to keep the subjects from putting the candies down the toilet or throwing them over the wall. There are other defects in this study of which I am aware, but the fact remains that it was a heroic effort. If you compare this study with an animal study, you will find the same defects. While admitting it is not perfect, it is the best we have.

Dr. Horowitz: Do you feel that your findings on enamel dissolution can be translated fairly directly to potential for causing dental caries?

Dr. Bibby: I would like someone to supplement my findings and disprove them or support them. I think it is an important measure and one we can't ignore. I think this measure should be combined with pH measurements or something else. I am optimistic that we may be able to find two or three different measures, and perhaps with a mathematical formula transform them into a significant measure of cariogenicity.

HUMAN DIET AND DENTAL CARIES: EFFECT OF DIET IN THE EARLY YEARS

Dominick P. DePaola, D.D.S., Ph.D.

Introduction

Diet and nutrition affect the oral cavity twice: once locally, during the masticatory process and again systemically after nutrients in the food are digested and absorbed. From another perspective, diet also affects teeth during two distinct developmental periods: pre-eruption and post-eruption. Indeed, the classical epidemiologic tetrad used to illustrate the factors involved in the dental caries process indicates that one of the fundamentally important variables is diet (Fig. 1). Althoughthe substrate component accounts for one-fourth of the variables, it is critically involved in each of the other three factors, including: selection and metabolism of microorganisms; the duration of substrate contact during which tooth destruction occurs; and the development and maintenance of the teeth and host defenses. This paper will describe the impact of diet during tooth development on the subsequent resistance of teeth to the caries challenge, and will illustrate the developmental factors that must be considered when one views cariogenicity post-eruptively.

In discussing the relationships between diet, teeth and subsequent resistance to disease, it must be understood that a dual component variable of disease is being addressed. The first variable is microbial (agent) selection, and thus selection of more avirulent strains, modification of the micro-environment manipulated through dietary alterations. The second variable is augmentation of host defense mechanisms, in large part through the influence of appropriate diet intake at key developmental periods. The microbial component is more difficult to assess when observing dietary influences in the developing ecologic niches in the oral cavity, while changes in host resistance are considerably easier to quantitate as a function of diet. Therefore host defenses will be the major variable described here. It must be clear, however, that a particularly virulent or avirulent microbial species and a host with unusually high or low resistance may mask any effects of nutrition on host defense. However, nutritional status may be particularly important in the defense of a host with intermediate resistance from infection by a microbe of intermediate virulence, as illustrated in Fig. 2. It is probable that nutritional factors will influence the great majority of cases of dental caries in humans because human microorganisms have variable virulence and because individuals with highly resistant host defense mechanisms (teeth and fluids) are uncommon. It should be stated, therefore, that for example in terms of dental caries, it would be virtually impossible to produce a tooth developmentally that can withstand an overwhelming challenge in terms of microbial virulence but that given an intermediate challenge it is possible to reduce the resistance to dental caries considerably by producing a tooth that is at an optimal degree of host resistance.

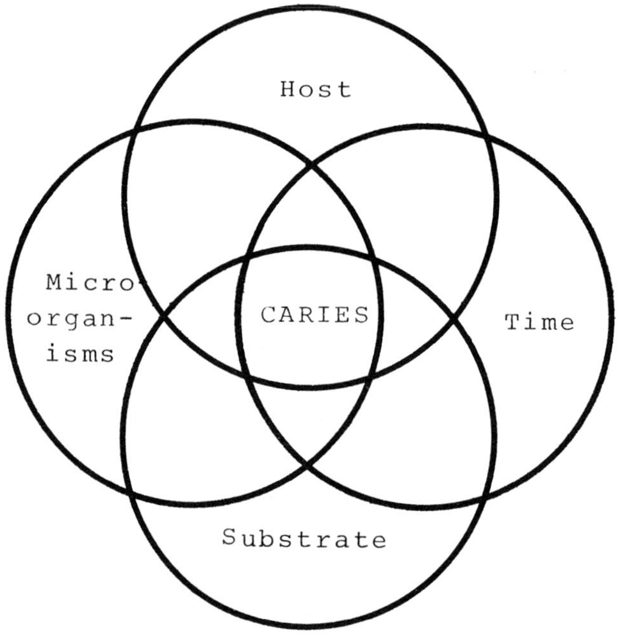

FIGURE 1. Epidemiologic tetrad illustrating the factors involved in the dental caries process.

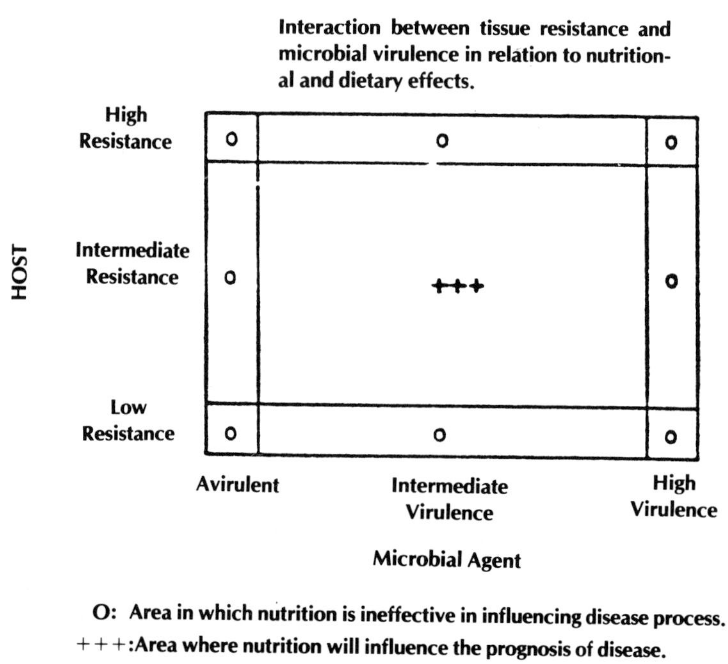

FIGURE 2. Nutritional effects on disease processes will not be seen in extreme cases where the virulence of the microbial agent is high or the resistance of the host is extremely low. However, because of the heterogenous genetic and metabolic background of humans and microorganisms, nutrition will be able to influence the outcome of human disease in a large number of cases. (From Navia[13])

Some fundamental information is presented here about diet and development as a prelude to the work that has been accomplished on diet, tooth development and subsequent resistance to dental caries.

Diet and Development

Organs and organ systems undergo three distinct developmental phases[1]. The first is a hyperplastic growth phase that is manifested by growth via cell division; the second is an intermediate phase in which both hyperplasia and hypertrophy occur simultaneously; the third is a hypertrophic growth phase manifested by growth via cell enlargement. Biochemically, the hyperplastic phase is characterized by obligatory DNA synthesis and thus an increase in DNA, the intermediate phase parallels an increase in RNA and the hypertrophic phase is characterized by an increase in protein synthesis[2] (Fig 3). Each tissue enters into and remains in each of the three phases according to its own unique timetable. For example, any two organs, although ultimately following the same pattern of development, develop in different phases, at different rates and over a variable temporal sequence. Thus, every organ system develops in a sequence by which periods of slow growth are interrupted one or more times by spurts of rapid expansion in cell number and size. The rapid growth spurts, roughly equating with the hyperplastic growth phase, have been termed "critical periods" because they represent those times in development during which environmental stress, such as dietary restriction, may result in irreversible

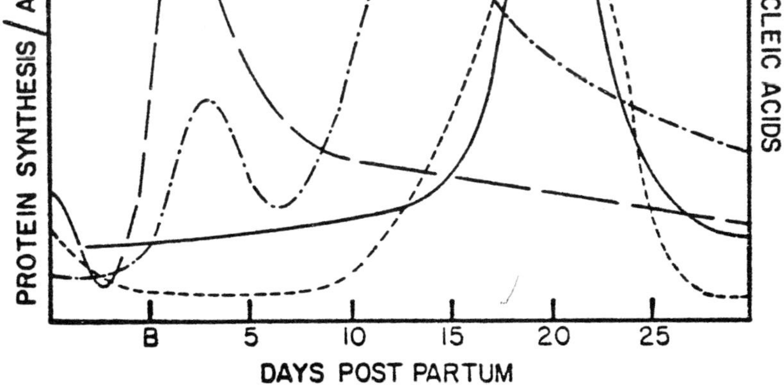

FIGURE 3. An integrated, partially speculative schema of sequential changes in DNA, RNA and protein synthesis in developing organs. (From DePaola, D.P. *et al.*[14])

damage to the developing system.[3] Although each organ system may grow in a differential manner, their development is regulated by both genetic and environmental constraints, thus insuring that haphazard growth does not occur.

Diet and Oral Tissue Development

Because teeth and salivary glands undergo well-defined critical development periods and are therefore particularly sensitive to nutritional stress, their development is associated intimately with the nutrient supply. The dependence of these tissues on available dietary substrate during development has profound implications with regard to oral health maintenance. Much evidence indicates that nutritional imbalance during tooth and salivary gland development alters these structures in such a manner as to profoundly influence the integrity (structure), size, composition, alignment, eruption, and resistive capabilities of teeth to microbial challenge at maturity. Numerous investigators have demonstrated a clear relationship between specific dietary nutrient deficiencies during critical periods of development (either protein-matrix formation or subsequent mineralization) and poorly calcified teeth, which in some cases alter the resistance of the tooth to caries. Shaw and Sweeney[4] and Shaw[5] have reviewed this subject extensively. The nutrient imbalances include: protein, fat, carbohydrate, calories, vitamins A, D, C, calcium, phosphorous, fluoride, and a host of other minerals as well as various amino acids. Rather than describe a wide range of the studies conducted on these nutrients, we will limit this discussion somewhat to protein to exemplify the extent to which diet during development can affect teeth, salivary gland function and subsequent resistance to dental caries.

Navia *et al.*[6] and Menaker and Navia[7] demonstrated that the offspring of female rats fed a low protein diet grew slowly, were smaller in size, had smaller molars, and exhibited delayed eruption of the first and second molars and impaired salivary gland function. The marked reduction in salivary flow exhibited by these offspring may have been responsible for the subsequent increase in caries susceptibility. These studies demonstrated that dental and salivary gland dysfunctions among offspring of protein-deficient rats could be ascribed to protein-deficiency acting at the tissue level (*Nutrition Review*, 1974). Thus, during tooth and salivary gland development, nutritional stress imposed at critical times cannot only induce frank morphological alterations but also influence the functional resistance of oral tissues to bacterial challenge. In developing countries and in pockets of malnutrition in the United States, analogous problems exist in which protein-calorie malnutrition during gestation and the neonatal period may result in a high incidence of enamel hypoplasia and dental caries in the primary dentition. In fact, a relatively common linear hypoplastic defect in the primary dentition of children from developing countries, the "Cauque" lesion, may be related to neonatal infection and low serum levels of vitamin A in this population. Thus, it is not surprising that malnutrition in early life in developing countries may contribute to higher caries experience being seen in the deciduous teeth (*Nutrition Review*, 1974).

It also should be noted that the trace mineral, fluoride, has a well-known, dramatic impact on dental caries, particularly when consumed during tooth development. In the same way, a variety of other minerals may promote or retard the caries process. Navia has classified the relationship between trace minerals and caries[8] (Fig. 4). It is important to note that these minerals play a role in tooth development as well as in post-eruptive remineralization and bacterial colonization of the tooth.

FIGURE 4. Relationship of mineral elements to caries.

Effect	Mineral
Cariostatic	F,P
Mildly cariostatic	Mo, V, Cu, Sr, B, Li, Au
Doubtful	Be, Co, Mn, Sn, Zn, Br, I
Caries inert	Ba, Al, Ni, Fe, Pd, Ti
Caries promoting	Se, Mg, Cd, Pt, Pb, Si

(From Navia, J.M.[8])

Potential Mechanisms Affected by Diet

Knowing that specific dietary nutrients can alter oral tissue development and result in subsequent changes in resistive capability to challenge, the following mechanisms are postulated to be involved in these processes (Fig. 5);

1. Alteration of tooth structure. It is reasonable to assume that a more perfectly formed tooth will be less susceptible to decay. Studies described above on protein and vitamin A implicate this mechanism, as do more definitive studies involving deficiencies of vitamin D, calcium, phosphorus, calcium/phosphorous ratio and fluoride.
2. Tooth alignment. Jaws undergo long critical periods in contrast to teeth, and nutrient deficiencies have been shown substantially to alter jaw morphology and subsequent dental alignment. Tonge and McCance have demonstrated[9] in pigs that severe calorie restriction, when imposed at the appropriate period of development, can produce a delay in formation and eruption of whole dentition with a greater delay in development and growth of jaws, resulting in overcrowding and malocclusion of teeth. In addition, subsequent dietary rehabilitation led to rapid growht of both maxilla and mandible and the dentition, but persistent deformation in the form of malocclusion, small malformed third molars, small molar roots and occasional cessation of tooth formation.

   Poor tooth alignment and crowding result not only in esthetic and masticatory problems but also in increased dental caries. Although dietary imbalances contribute in more dramatic ways to the caries process, this problem does affect human caries and is worthy of further study.
3. Salivary gland development. Menaker and Navia attempted to delineate the mechanism by which neonatal protein deficiency in rats results in increased susceptibility of the teeth to dental caries.[7] They noted that biochemical alterations in salivary gland composition and protein synth-

esis were paralleled by functional changes in the salivary glands. It is probable, therefore, that the increased caries susceptibility caused by neonatal protein deficiency is mediated primarily by salivary dysfunction. Alterations in salivary volume, buffering capacity and protein protective substances are most likely choices for explaining the increased caries susceptibility of the protein-deficient animals. It is interesting to speculate if changes in protein are reflected in altered pellicle forming glycoprotein or in anti-bacterial proteins such as lactoferrin, lacto-peroxidase, lysozyme or secretory immunoglobulin A.[10] Whatever the mechanism, the fact that neonatal dietary deficiency can dramatically alter tooth resistance to the caries challenge in adult life is exciting.

4. Immunocompetence. Malnutrition can affect both cellular and humoral immune mechanisms as well as non-specific immune parameters which may play an important role in conferring resistance to the host when challenged. Cellular immunity is probably not too important in the control of dental caries except as it interacts with the other two systems. However, humoral immunity, especially the secretion of lactoperoxidase, lysozyme and lactoferrin, may be involved intimately in caries protection. Although malnutrition, the most notable protein deficiency, has been shown to decrease the efficacy of each of these systems, the studies usually have been conducted on adult animals and salivary immune effectors have not been assayed.[10]
   Notwithstanding these problems, recent evidence suggests that malnutrition during critical periods of immunodevelopment can alter host resistance at a later time. In humans, for example, it is recognized that intrauterine growth retardation due to maternal malnutrition or placental insufficiency results in profound adverse antibody on post-natal immunocompetence. In addition, significant impairment of antibody formation has been detected not only in the first (F_1) generation of malnourished rats (F_0), but, incredibly, in the second (F_2) generation as well.[11] These facts coupled with the generalized decreased salivary protein synthesis mediated by developmental malnutrition indicate the crucial need for studies on the effects of developmental malnutrition on specific salivary immune effectors.
5. Selection of microflora. Another potential mechanism that needs attention is that dietary patterns during development can create an oral ecological niche that may result in a selection and facilitation of implantation of microflora that may be more or less cariogenic.[12]

FIGURE 5. Mechanisms through which diet during critical oral developmental can alter host resistance.

—Tooth Integrity
—Tooth Alignment
—Salivary Gland Development
—Immunocompetence
—Microflora Selection

Conclusions

Clearly, nutritional imbalances during the development of teeth, jaws, salivary glands and immune system may alter the post-developmental resistive capabilities of the host to dental caries. Thus, the narrow focus that now prevails regarding caries etiology should be expanded to include the very real possibility that nutritional and other environmental stresses during the development of the orofacial and immune systems may predispose the host to dental caries. For example, the concept that a susceptible tooth is required for the initiation of a carious lesion should be expanded to include not only the size, shape and composition of the tooth but also a variety of other host factors such as tooth alignment, salivary function and immunocompetence.

Studies of the effect of developmental malnutrition on susceptibility to dental caries may help to explain the epidemiologic data in which the incidence of caries should not be related to sugar consumption and food consumption patterns, such as seen in studies conducted in Detroit, Columbia and Guatemala. Perhaps the quality of the tooth, saliva and host defense systems, which are never fully addressed, may provide an explanation of those exceptions in conjunction with the fact that a wide variety of food constituents, other than the specific compound being tested, may confer some degree of susceptibility or protection to the tooth.

The present basis of knowledge does not warrant statements that a certain child has more caries than another simply because of neonatal malnutrition. However, the data do suggest that clinicians should be concerned that pregnant women, infants and young children consume nutritionally sound diets. Therefore, it is exceedingly important to begin to translate some of this exciting animal data to the human population. It is evident, however, that in order to counsel the susceptible population adequately regarding dietary intake and dental caries, studies must be completed which indicate clearly that dietary counseling at the clinical level will affect the caries rate. At this point, there is a paucity of human data regarding the clinical effectiveness of dietary counseling as well as data on food cariogenicity. Until studies on food cariogenicity and dietary intervention expand their focus to take into consideration these developmental phenomena and the human clinical situation, one must look upon them with a certain degree of skepticism and continue to counsel vulnerable patients from a rather naive perspective.

REFERENCES

1. Winick, M. and Noble, A. Cellular response with increased feeding in neonatal rats. J. Nutr. 91:179, 1967.
2. Miller, S.A. Protein metabolism during growth and development. In Munroe, H.N., ed. "Mammalian Protein Metabolism," vol. III. New York: Academic Press, 1967, p. 183-233; Protein deficiency and tooth and salivary gland development. Nutr. Rev. 32:24-27, 1974.
3. Winick, M. and Noble, A. Quantitative changes in DNA, RNA and protein during pre-natal and post-natal growth in the rat. Develop. Biol. 12:451-466, 1965.
4. Shaw, J.H. and Sweeney, E.A. Nutrition in relation to dental medicine. In Goodhart, R.S. and Shils, M.E., eds. "Modern Nutrition in Health and Disease." Philadelphia: Lea and Febiger, 1973.
5. Shaw, J.H. Preeruptive effects of nutrition on teeth. J. Dent. Res. 49 (6, suppl): 1238-1250, 1970.

6. Navia, J.M., DiOrio, L.P., Menaker, L. and Miller, S. Effect of undernutrition during the perinatal period on caries development in the rat. J. Dent. Res. 49: 1091-1098, 1970.
7. Menaker, L. and Navia, J.M. Effect of undernutrition during the perinatal period on caries development in the rat: V. Changes in whole saliva volume and protein content. J. Dent. Res. 53:592-597, 1974.
8. Navia, J.M. Prevention of dental caries: Agents which increase tooth resistance to dental caries. Internat. Dent. J. 22:427-440, 1972.
9. Tonge, C. and McCance, R. Normal development of the jaws and teeth in pigs, and the delay and malocclusion produced by calorie deficiencies. J. Anat. 115:1-22, 1973.
10. Alfano, M.C. Nutrition in dental caries in "Biologic Basis of Dental Caries." Menaker, K., Navia, M. and Morhart, R., eds. Harper and Row, 1978.
11. Chandra, R.K. Antibody formation in first and second generation offspring of nutritionally deprived rats, Science 190:289-290, 1975.
12. Navia, J.M. Evaluation of nutritional and dietary factors that modify animal caries, J. Dent. Res. 49 (6, suppl):1213-1227, 1970.
13. Navia, J.M. Nutrition and oral disease. In Caldwell, R.C. and Stallard, R.E., eds, "A Textbook of Preventive Dentistry." Philadelphia: W.B. Saunders Co., 1977.
14. DePaola, D.P., Kuftinec, M.M. Nutrition in growth and development of oral tissues. Dent. Clin. North Amer. 20:441-460, 1976.

HUMAN DIET AND DENTAL CARIES

Steven Kreitzman, Ph.D.

There is probably no dentist in the country who has not advised a patient to cut down on carbohydrates or possibly specified restriction of sucrose. My child's elementary school teacher is absolutely convinced that sucrose is poison and has forbidden all sucrose in the classroom. (Honey is permitted.) I intend to raise two questions: (1) whether sucrose is really this bad and (2) what the dentist or any of us is actually doing when we counsel patients to cut down on carbohydrates.

Taking the second question first, I want you to recognize that we do have accepted dietary standards in this country. The Food and Nutrition Board of the National Research Council has come up with some reasonable nutrient intake guidelines and have made specific recommendations for total caloric intake based on age and sex. The additional recommendation is made in the 1974 RDA publication[1] that people on weight reduction diets should consume the RDA calories in order to insure that they are getting enough micronutrients. There is also a recommendation for protein intake which has been calculated and argued about, and may even possibly be a little low, but we certainly have a recommendation for protein.

The rest of the calories are supposed to come from carbohydrates and fat. Although the NRC does not make a recommendation as to how these calories should be allocated, they do mention that the American Heart Association has fixed a figure of 35% calories from fat as a prudent maximum.

I contend that once you accept that 35% calories from fat you have run out of degrees of freedom. You have fixed a requirement or recommendation for carbohydrate calories. Therefore, when you counsel an individual to cut down on his carbohydrate consumption, the likelihood is that he will increase his consumption of either fat or protein and probably of fat, which I am not sure any of us are prepared to recommend.

I also want to remind people that carbohydrates, fat, and protein in foods do not exist as separate entities. In real foods, they are tied in with important micro-nutrients and by making recommendations for large scale changing of diet patterns we are changing distribution of many nutrients.

Some years ago, we decided to look at what people were actually eating. We tried to find out as best we could what kind of food intake patterns we were able to record in real people. We had large numbers of people keep dietary records, these we fed into the computer. We asked people to record not only what they ate for snacks, but we wanted to know, by brand name where possible, what they actually ate and when they actually ate.

Figure 1 represents the computed calorie intake distribution for 1,200 people. We find that in terms of the percent of the RDA of our "general population," primarily a population of middle class, urban people and not a statistical sample representing the entire population, the mean and median were right about 90% of the RDA for calories.

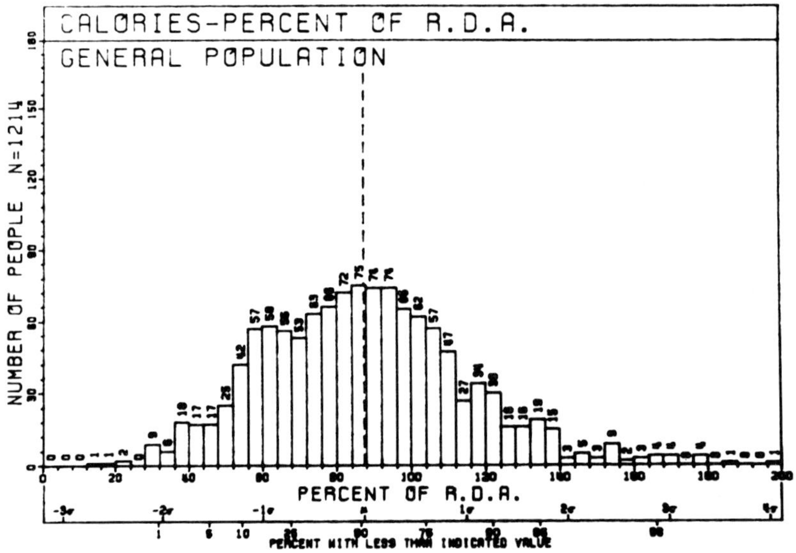

FIGURE 1. Calories-Percent of R.D.A - General Population

Protein, on the other hand, is shown (Fig. 2) to be well above the recommended allowances, with our mean and median about 160% of the RDA. Over half the population were getting two, three and some almost four times the RDA for protein. Clearly there is no room for a suggestion of increasing protein calories.

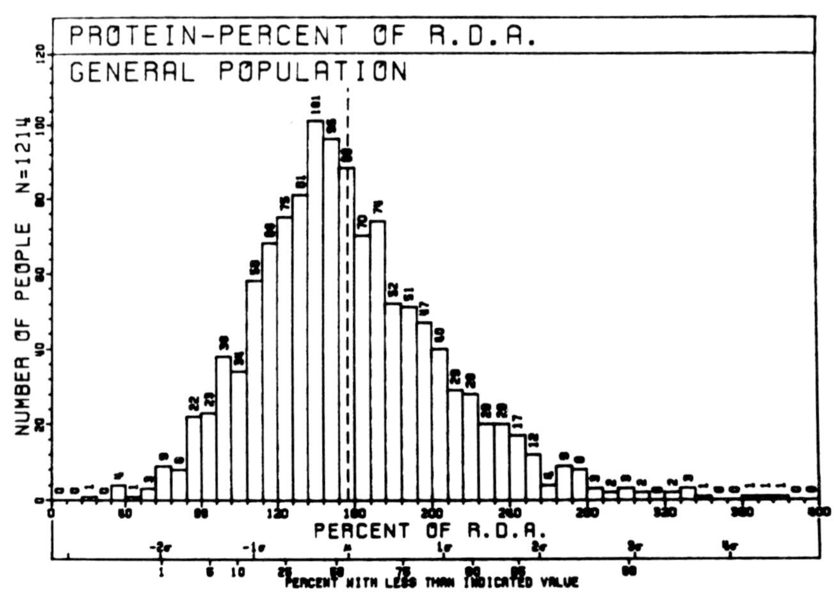

FIGURE 2. Protein-Percent of R.D.A. - General Population

In terms of percent calories of fat (Fig. 3) we find a mean and median of just under 40%. There is no room for a large number of people to increase calories from fat. Some people are consuming enormous amounts of fat.

But when we look at carbohydrate intake (Fig. 4), 100% of the recommended intake or more is consumed by relatively few people, suggesting that at least in the population I have been studying, carbohydrate consumption is too low, not too high. The suggestion to patients that we control caries by drastically changing carbohydrate intake many have some undesired consequences.

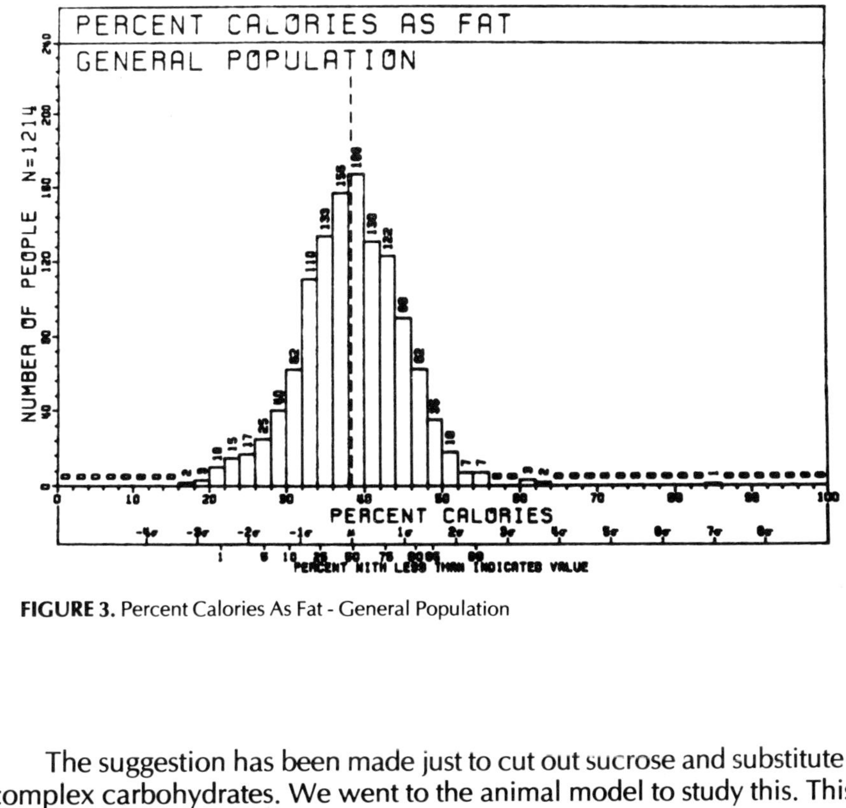

FIGURE 3. Percent Calories As Fat - General Population

The suggestion has been made just to cut out sucrose and substitute more complex carbohydrates. We went to the animal model to study this. This data was presented very timidly a couple of years ago at an IADR meeting.[2] We took our standard 67% sucrose cariogenic diet, and then sequentially reduced sucrose consumption by half. We replaced the carbohydrate by corn starch by halves from 67% down to zero. We found very small reductions in decay, even with no sucrose in the diet. The break point for any observable reduction was somewhere between 8% and 4%.

The Vipeholm Study[3] has been mentioned as evidence for the cariogenicity of sucrose. I do not know how much reliance we should place on a single clinical study from a mental institution. There are many problems with the

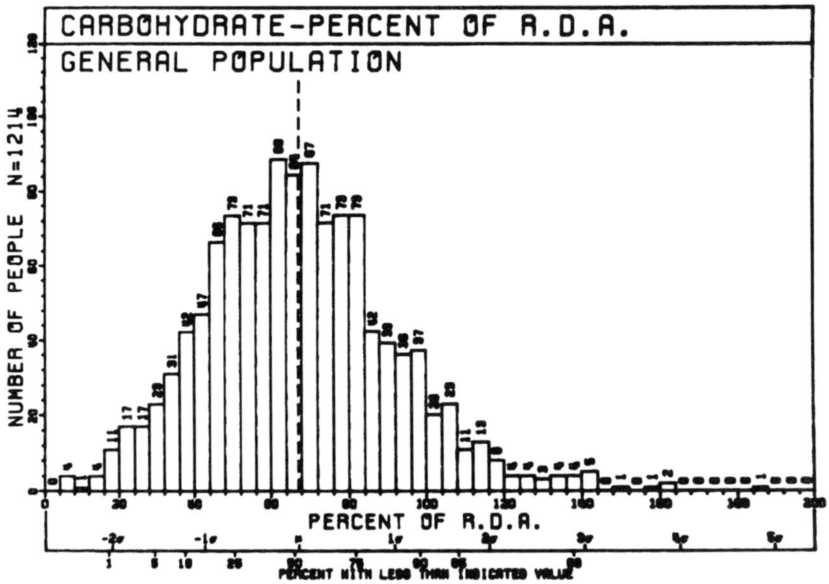

FIGURE 4. Carbohydrate-Percent of R.D.A. - General Population

Vipeholm population. Unfortunately, few people have actually read it. Because of its length, most people only know the study from reviews. There are a number of contradictory studies that have not been very widely recognized. King *et al.*,[4] in English children, for example, found they could substantially increase sugar in the children's diet without increasing caries. These are reputable investigators, and should not be completely ignored.

Following our presentation at IADR, two papers have been published that support our finding that substitution of starch for sugar may not alter caries a great deal. The group in Birmingham[5] has reported reaching a maximal caries challenge at very low levels of sucrose, beyond which caries just levels off. There appears to be a maximum caries challenge at a very low sugar level. Recently, Huxley[6] and his group published a similar type of study. They found slightly different effects in different strains of animals, with a maximum total caries challenge at about 15% sucrose. For smooth surface caries, they found no benefits by reducing sugar intake until they got to extremely low levels of sugar in diet.

This is not to say that we cannot show an effect of diet. From the diet records of our human population—patients of our dental clinic, 500 patients for whom we have a complete dental charting—we have been able to examine a large number of nutrient variables, such as vitamins, minerals, the relationships between vitamins and minerals and between the minerals themselves. Importantly, we also can look at specific foods. We are able to study consumption of soft drinks, tea, coffee, milk, juices, candy, cereals, or supplements. We are utilizing computer generated statistics to find trends in the human population related to dental caries.

We could not predict the level of dental caries in this population simply by measuring the amount of carbohydrate consumed. Our correlation coefficient for carbohydrate with dental caries was .0047. Everybody seems to be eating above the caries threshold for carbohydrates and most of these carbohydrates will support dental caries. We are currently investigating specific patterns of food consumption that associate strongly with caries which are very interesting and which we hope to be able to reproduce.

A discriminate analysis of this population allows the computer to discriminate effectively, between 70 and 80%, as to which patient is going to have high caries and which will not. There are factors in our diet records at least associating with caries repeatedly what the computer is able to recognize. At this stage, I am not ready to say what these are specifically, but there is a relationship with the dietary minerals. I am very reluctant to go any further than that at this time. We need to examine our traditional beliefs carefully before we start changing the dietary patterns of the population with any effectiveness. I am a little concerned about the McGovern recommendation of drastically changing the human diet without thoroughly considering the consequences of those changes.

We now have an effective method of studying what people are eating in terms of specific foods, food types, liquids and retentive foods. It is hoped that we may soon be able to report with confidence the kinds of things that do associate with dental caries in human populations.

REFERENCES

1. Recommended Dietary Allowances, Food and Nutrition Board National Research Council, Washington, D.C. National Academy of Sciences, 1974.
2. Kreitzman, S.N. and Klein, R.M. Non-linear relationship between dietary sucrose and dental caries. J. Dent. Res. *55*:B175, 1976.
3. Gustafsson, B.E., *et al.*,. The effect of different levels of carbohydrate intake on caries activity in 436 individuals observed for five years. Acta Odontol. Scand. *11*:232, no. 3-4, 1952.
4. King, J.D., *et al.*,. The effect of sugar supplements on dental caries in children. Med.Res. Council special report no. 288, 1955.
5. Michalek, S.M., McGhee, J.R., Shiota, T. and Devenyns, D. Low sucrose levels promote extensive Streptococcus mutans-induced dental caries. Infect. Immun. *16*:217, 1977.
6. Huxley, H.G. The cariogenicity of dietary sucrose at various levels in two strains of rat under unrestricted and controlled-frequency feeding conditions. Caries Res. *11*:237, 1977.

DISCUSSION

Mr. Khan: Dr. Kreitzman, I wonder whether we shouldn't take a look at the avalanche that is coming down the mountain. Almost every state legislature seems to be passing regulations about food which contain such numbers as "25% added sugar"; as if 24% is apparently all right, but 25% is not. I think, based on what you just reported, that it is sheer, unadulterated poppycock. I think you and your colleagues ought to let yourselves be heard.

Dr. Madsen: I think, because of the diverse nature of our audience and those in dental research who speak of the Vipeholm Study and rodent study freely, you may have left an impression that you would not want to leave. You say clearly that in the Vipeholm Study, the one striking finding was that the frequency of eating fermentable carbohydrates was the factor associated with the striking increase in dental caries, rather than the total quanity eaten because as much as 300 g a day given at mealtimes did not increase caries. I would also like to comment on the rodent studies. These rodents, unless they are program fed, are eating 20 times a day; therefore, it requires very little sugar, taken 20 times a day, to produce a maximum response. More sugar would not give a greater response. We find in cotton rats that 1 or 2% of sugar in liquid or solid form will produce this response because they are eating 20 times a day. Frequency is a factor of prime importance and one which we must take into consideration. One more comment on an earlier paper by Weiss and Trithout on the correlation made. They did not have to determine the nature of the snack the kids were eating in that western Tennessee community. All they had to do was count how often they ate between meals. When they plotted that versus caries, they got a nice direct response. When you look at what they did eat, most of what was available was about 80% fermentable carbohydrates and mostly sugar-added items.

Dr. Kreitzman: I think the Vipeholm Study now has been discussed sufficiently. I would like to see something else in the literature that either reproduces the findings in that study or comes close to confirming it. It's a wonderful study and we have to go back to it and lean on it, but I think that perhaps something else is needed. The matter of frequency is something that I have always been told is important—and I had no reason to doubt—until I read two papers that call it into question. One study, the 10-state survey, should be reviewed. That survey looked at the frequency of between meal consumption of carbohydrate and attempted to correlate that with the dental condition. If you read the entire paper, you realize that in only one population of the several surveyed was there a correlation. Whoever wrote the summary of the 10-state survey had some preconceptions and repeated the cliche that the frequency was related but did not mention that it was found in only one of the groups studied.

I also refer to a 1973 paper, familiar to many of you, by Bagramian and Russell. They examined epidemiologically the caries: between-meals feeding patterns and found that frequency may not be the factor in all populations. Other things probably much more important than either frequency or total amount of carbohydrate consumed affect the expression of dental caries. According to the literature on minerals, it may be selenium increasing it, or perhaps phosphates, or molybdenum or some other things decreasing it. We all know the tremendous biological change from a trivial amount of fluoride. It changes the occurrence of dental caries, without regard to the level of intake of sugar. No one is suggesting that adding one part of fluoride to the water is in any way going to change the carbohydrate consumption, but it will affect the occurrence of caries dramatically. We need to start looking at other things and not simply concentrate on sugar.

Dr. Newbrun: There have been so many points raised by the three speakers that it is hard to know where to begin. Starting with the Vipeholm

Study which has been discussed by so many people and about which so much has been written, I'm surprised that so many people continue to misinterpret some of the findings. Many people hear what they want to hear. The Vipeholm Study showed a correlation with the frequency of intake of sucrose-containing food items. Bibby talked about that and he also showed the slide of the Weiss and Tritout Study in Tennessee in which they counted the in-between food snacks, all of which contained sucrose. Now people, usually from the food industry, take the Vipeholm Study and say, oh yes, but if you look at the total amount of sugar that was eaten there is no correlation with the amount in quantity, it was only the frequency. But what people should remember is that the Vipeholm Study is an artificial situation, a captive population where the diet was controlled and to that extent was a very good study and will never be reproduced. Dr. Kreitzman, I am surprised that you suggested that it could be reproduced because you know very well it never can be nowadays, because the human experimentation committees would not allow it. The point that I want to make about the Vipeholm Study is that you have a population whose food intake frequency you do not control, then I guarantee that the total amount of sugar eaten, and I am saying sugar, not carbohydrate, is correlated with the frequency. There are abundant studies, funded by the food industry, to document what Dr. Kelly said regarding the fact that we are not eating three meals a day; we are eating — nibbling — continuously.

The whole pattern of feeding has changed from dessert foods to snack foods, and the food industry is well aware of that. I think the first point that I want to make about the Vipeholm Study is that it is an artificial situation, and the fact that you don't find a correlation between sucrose amounts and caries, but only with frequency of intake, does not apply to the general population because in the general population the amount eaten is related directly to the frequency.

Dr. Kreitzman: Let me address that point before you go on. The Vipeholm Study was a very contrived situation. What I am trying to suggest, in the method that I am considering, is that we are going to look at people as they exist in the population, what they are actually doing, and under those circumstances record what things will have an effect and what will not, not what happens in a contrived study. Most people won't conform to what happens in a contrived study. We want to know what happens with free living people, people who don't take food stamps, people who don't participate in all kinds of experimental programs—they go to their private physician, their private dentist. These are the people we are looking at, because these are the people who are interpreting what we are saying and possibly interpreting it incorrectly. I am aware of what you are saying about frequency. Maybe it is so. We have to look at that point more carefully because today there are people who are saying that maybe this is not quite the whole story either.

Dr. Bowen: There is one interesting condition that has not been considered yet. I think the role of sugar in caries among those patients who suffer from fructose intolerance has been shown fairly conclusively. They are virtually caries-free largely because they have abstained from eating sweet-tasting substances. This is a nice example of showing the importance of carbohydrates in dental caries in humans. If Koch had began studying tuberculosis other than in a direct method, would he have ever come up with isolating the tubercle bacillus or would we have come up with the answer of how to prevent the disease or how to cure it? Of course not. As long as we digress from considering the important factors in dental caries, mainly a susceptible tooth, a suitable cariogenic flora and carbohydrate, we are going to go round and round in circles looking for excuses to exonerate either food or microorganisms or some other etiologic agent. One final point: Dr. Kreitzman made the observation that fluoride has a dramatic effect on dental caries and, of course, people don't change their carbohydrate consumption. This is true, and has been used by some irresponsible advisors to the food industry, who say that the fluoridation of water is in fact a license to consume all the sugar you wish because fluoride will protect you from dental decay. That kind of irresponsible statement must be denied as quickly as possible.

Dr. Steinberg: In connection with cariogenicity of foods and the intake on in-between-meal snacks, about seven or eight years ago we did a bottle beverage study in an institutionalized population too, although in a much younger group than the ones in the Vipeholm Study. Even though this was an institutionalized population, we came up with the observation that after three years of consumption of 6 ounces–34 g sucrose–of bottled beverages between meals, added to the 98 that they were already getting in their snacks, the results were seen only on certain surfaces of the tooth structure. When we did an overall comparison of the caries scores, we could not find any differences between the control and the beverage groups. However, when we broke the scores shown to various surfaces of the mouth, we found an effect only in limited areas, for instance on buccolingual surfaces of the posterior mandibular teeth. It appears, at least in this population, that the sugar in a bottled beverage has a limited effect. I feel the one big drawback with the study was that we were dealing with a mentally retarded population that had very poor oral hygiene and a great deal of plaque. This may have biased our study. This is one of the problems of seeking a population in whom you can control all of the variables. An institution is great, in that we do have control over what food the children get. One of the problems when we get diet analysis from non-institution subjects is that their statements are not accurate because many times they do not know what they are receiving.

Dr. DePaola: Unfortunately, caries is a multi-factorial disease. The people who addressed us this morning clearly stated that in so many words. I think to isolate one particular variable, be it the organism, the tooth, or carbohydrate, is doing an injustice to the actual disease. Also, we have a paradox in terms of a clinical situation. I think most of us agree that meal frequency, whatever the meal contains, contributes to the caries process. However, very often in a clinical situation, two things are evident: it is easy to suggest that the patients eat something like potato chips instead of a "Milky Way," which may or may not contribute to the overall health of that individual. I think there is a clear mandate for the food manufacturers to develop nutritious, less caries-producing foods. I am not convinced that we are meal nibblers because there is still a tremendous amount of obesity in the United States. Dr. Newbrun indicated that animal data suggests that perhaps meal nibbling might in fact contribute to a slender population. These things have not been discussed suficiently in relation to our own situtation.

Dr. Kent Stewart: I would like to present a different aspect of this problem; that is, in a study of causality and prevention of disease, there is a role for analytical chemistry, because we need to identify and quantitate the individual components in the diet. Our successes so far with identifying total carbohydrates, total fats, total proteins and minerals, do not, in fact, meet the sophisticated requirements of such diseases as dental caries. If we look at the quantitative data on individual nutrients in our diet, we find that we have little. For example, if we consider sugar—lactose, sucrose, fructose, galactose, etc.—and look at the data we have about the composition of foods and how much of these sugars are there, we find we have very little information.

I think the fact that we have very little data reflects the poor method for determining many of the nutrients. The methodologies that developed in the 40's and were the frontier of the science at that time have been neglected. I think we need new methods of development and new base-line studies on individual components. Let me give an example of sugar analysis. As we look at the current routine methods, they are not very useful because they are not sufficiently selective. In almost all of these studies, total carbohydrate is not, in fact, even measured. It is taken by difference. The individual sugar color reactions do not distinguish between the different reducing sugars and often do not measure cellulose or starch or sucrose or sorbitol. We need new methods which involve a chemical separation and a chemical detection system. I am pleased to report that in my laboratory we have such a method for the common food sugars. I have a chromatogram here for those who are interested that shows how to determine quantities of individual sugars in soft drinks. This method involves chromatography and selective color detection. It also involves sample preparation. In a similar manner, there is an excellent TLC method being used at General Mills for individual carbohydrate determinations. A number of commerical companies are selling liquid chromatographic systems, a third method for doing carbohydrate detection.

I would recommend that as part of this type of study, a subcommittee could be set up by the American Association for Dental Research to develop and provide a compendium of analytical methods for the individual components of the nutrients in the diet. Such a compendium is needed because if you look at the handbook data on, for example, the composition of soft drinks, you find one value. I have in front of me a list of approximately a dozen analyses we did last week on different soft drinks, and the sucrose ranged from 120 mg/ml in creme soda to approximately 60mg/ml in a cola, 14 mg/ml in tonic water, and 0 in club soda; the fructose values varied — 20, 8 and 16 mg/ml where it shows up at all; the phosphate ranged from 0 to 157 mg per liter. All these factors may play a role in the cariogenicity of these foods. I think we need the basic data for it.

Dr. Newbrun: First of all, there is a difference between carbohydrates. Dr. Stewart addressed himself to that to a certain extent. Dr. Kreitzman showed levels of food consumption and he showed carbohydrates. The problem is that the U.S. Department of Agriculture values published in food tables only list fats, carbohydrates and proteins and do not provide data about sucrose. I don't want to imply that glucose and fructose are not cariogenic; we know that they are. However, certainly at the present time, our principle concern undoubtedly should be for human sucrose consumption.

I think all of us, and Dr. Bibby pointed out this problem, we are concerned with how we really measure the cariogenicity of foods. We can study it in humans, but humans are not readily controlled. We can do *in vitro* tests, and Dr. Bibby and many others have worked for years on this. Unfortunately, often in taking salivary sediment and that type of rather primitive experimentation, we really ignore the whole plaque flora. We know that the microflora in plaque is not the same as it is in saliva, but we repeatedly have studies using that type of a model. That is why the model used in Zurich, where you actually have the measure of plaque flora pH drop, is—to the microbiologists at least—a more acceptable model. I recognize, as Dr. Bibby says, that it does not measure caries, it only measures an acid drop. At least it does satisfy the resemblance to plaque. I am sure we all recognize those limitations.

Dr. Steinberg and others of you are also aware that there are many studies in which one particular food has been tested. Dr.Steinberg has tested soft drinks. We have representatives of the food industry here and I recognize your desire to test your particular product—your chewing gum, your breakfast cereal, or your type of candy. The dilemma in doing that is that you ignore the fact that man is omnivirous. He does not eat just one food. Dr. Steinberg saw no dramatic changes in the group that had the soft drinks. Dr. Finn in Alabama did not see dramatic changes in subjects chewing gum. There were differences, but the changes were not as dramatic as you saw in the Vipeholm Study of the 24 chewing gums and the 24 toffees. The breakfast cereal studies done by Nathaniel Rowe in Michigan, the breakfast cereal studies done at Forsyth, and the candy diet studies done by Frostell and his colleagues in Roslagen, Sweden, all required tremendous amounts of work. Anybody who reads them or anybody who has been involved in them recognizes what a tremendous undertaking it is.

Unfortunately, the problem is in the whole experimental design. For example, if you have an individual who, on the average, consumes 100 lb. of sucrose year and if you change it to 110 lb. or to 90 lb. a year, you are not going to see differences. This is the problem, and I am amazed that the food industry will continue to pay for that sort of study because it is money down the drain. You are not going to see any dramatic differences unless you go to the tremendous extreme of the Turku study, where you change 100 food items. Don't try to see a caries change by changing one single solitary food item, because you are not going to see an effect. On the other hand, I am sure that Navia or Shaw or anybody else could do an animal study in which they feed a sweetened breakfast cereal and show you a difference, because there you could control the animal model; in humans you are not going to see any difference because of dietary habits.

Finally, I come to the point that knowledge is the important factor. One gentleman suggested that it was the solution; I am sure that most of you would disagree, because it is not the complete solution. In Scandinavia, where they questioned parents about the dietary habits of the children, it was quite apparent that most of the parents were well aware of the cariogenicity of such food items as soft drinks, and cookies and candies. Yet when they were questioned about whether they wanted to change their children's dietary habits, 60% of the parents said they were not sufficiently concerned to have any desire to change those food habits. So knowledge alone is not the solution and that brings us to the *raison d'etre* for this meeting—that is to get the food industry and the dental profession working together. I recognize the problems in eliminating or reducing sugar content in foods. Yet the food industry can make, as everyone who has ever flown on a plane knows, a coffee cream that does not have cream in it, a chocolate bar that does not have chocolate in it. I think the ingenuity of the food industry is such that there are solutions. We require the cooperation of the food industry. I look forward to the later, more detailed discussion of sugar substitutes.

Dr. Robert Stewart: I want to give a bit of factual information about rampant dental caries or nursing bottle caries. This has been a concern of the baby food industry, particularly since juices are now being marketed in nursing bottles. We did a survey of mothers and their feeding habits, and we found that although only 50% of the mothers were feeding their babies juice, 80% of the mothers fed these from nursing bottles without regard to how they purchased it: whether they purchased the juice as packaged for adults or in a can; 23% of the mothers fed their babies lying down, and 8% of the mothers fed their babies with the bottle propped up. They let the baby go to sleep with the bottle in his mouth. We believe that the real concern here is the method of feeding and not the juice itself. Many juices have a place in infant feeding, but probably not to the extent that they are being used currently. We found, in the 1977 survey, that there is a large increase in the amount of juice being fed to the infants and a decrease in the amount of fruit. The total usage of pureed fruit is still about the same, but there is a decline in the fruit which has pectin and the associated materials that may have some nutrient value. We find that there is an increase in the past five years of the carbohydrates consumption—that is, the total calories as carbohydrates had jumped from 52% to 62%. This is caused primarily by a drop in the consumption of whole milk. The protein levels have gone up, the fat levels have gone down and the carbohydrate levels have gone up.

We can show you the changes that are taking place in the industry, and they are not caused by the removal of sugar alone. One other development point is that there are more strained meats being used, there are more strained vegetables being used, and less of the mixture of the two. Economically, this is costing the mother a little bit more. It may reflect the fact that we have taken all of the salt out of the foods and mothers don't really like their taste. You don't feed foods that the baby rejects for one reason or another. They say, "I don't blame the baby, I wouldn't eat it either" and they never buy it again. That is one of the points that we try to make—that flavor is important in the actual feeding of infants and toddlers. Every mother knows that the baby does not like certain things or completely rejects them; we may try to say that isn't so, but we know that it is.

Dr. Lockhart: In every comment that has been delivered this morning, soft drinks seem to have come out ahead. We know cola does not remain in the mouth very long. The acidity that is created in the mouth is rapidly brought back to normal by the buffering action of the saliva. So far as the sucrose consumption related to soft drinks is concerned, we are nearly at the bottom of the list of purveyors. Even though from 1910 to 1065 the sugar content of the diet has gone up from 15% to 23%, cola is responsible for only a relatively small share of the whole. The balance of the sugar content is pretty well spread around the other 39 food categories that the National Academy has put on its list.

I think what we are talking about, as so often happens, is the lack of information. We have been hearing about the National Nutrition Policy, the national nutrition survey, which has been in the mill for eight years or more, and the Department of Agriculture, which is charged with the gathering of information on what people eat, how much they eat, and when they eat. This is a terrible problem. Fantastic logistics have to be arranged to do this kind of thing.

We don't realize that a great deal of usable information can be gathered from the kind of studies that Dr. Kreitzman is doing. We don't have to have a fancy study. We have to recognize the bits of information that are important, no matter how we get them. How we use them is more important. I think that Dr. Kreitzman is trying to take a step forward. Valuable information will come out of the kind of thing that he is doing and it could be supplemented with information coming from bits of other studies that are being done around the world and in the United States. We must have a system for gathering these bits of information to be put in statistical cells which eventually will have some meaning. We need more information about what people are eating and how they eat it and when they eat it.

Fortunately, the soft drink industry is in a better position to get more information about what people do with soft drinks than some of the other members of the food industry. To some extent we are being forced into this kind of thing because of the way political events related to the food industry are shaping up. Nevertheless, we are getting the information, and when the pressure lets up there will be an opportunity to organize the information. Information must be put into a better framework.

The food industry is one of the most flexible industries we know, despite the great hue and cry regarding changing labels and packing sizes. The formula also can be changed. It has been brought out that a great deal of change has taken place since 1910, not all of which has been bad. Certainly if the food industry is given some hint about the direction in which to proceed, its members will immediately rush to be first in line with competitive products. It is not the arguments that are raised by the nutritionists or government people that will cause us to change; it is the fact that we have a great deal of competition in this country, which is the prime feature in a democracy like ours. The food industry will be anxious and ready to participate in a program that will result in a better life for all the citizens.

Dr. Darby: Looking broadly at dental caries and nutrition, I think it is important for us to get out of the one groove that this subject has been in for so long. We have already heard and discussed the effects of different foods on dental structure or dental dissolution. Now as we are looking in a more sophisticated way at nutrition, we are seeing the same thing in almost every phenomenon that we observe, for example, iron absorption. We can measure the absorption of iron as pure ferrous sulfate, or as various compounds, and we get one answer, but then when we incorporate that into one or another food we get varying effects. I think this emphasis on the foods and the food mixtures that we consume is very important. When we test a single substance, we learn something which we can't necessarily carry over into human experience. We don't eat the same thing every day, as we do under experimental conditions. We are not exposed to the same dietary mix. Further, we have different exposure times to whatever it is we are consuming. By exposure times, I mean, for example, frequency. Finally, in the field of nutrients that do have some relationship to caries, we have fluoride. We do have some cariogenic effect of sugar, depending upon how frequently it is used and how much in contact with the oral flora and what the oral flora is and various other factors, many of which we cannot understand.

There are nutrients, however, which in the past have been experimentally linked to dental caries that have not been investigated in recent years. One of the most striking of these is pyridoxine, which I think would be important to study again. In addition, there are different types of sugars, and other trace nutrients. There are the indirect effects to which Dr. DePaola referred, that also need to be examined; those effects on dental structure that result from fetal nutrition or nutrition in early life during formative stages of the adult tooth. We know that we have many nutrients that affect the soft tissues of the mouth. The indirect effect of these soft tissue changes may or may not be altered by nutrients, and these include vitamin A, vitamin C, niacin, folic acid, vitamin B_6 and iron. The effects of these on the soft structures never have been completely studied, certainly not the effects on the nature, quantity, etc., of salivary secretion. There are many effects that should be defined more clearly for research, such as these indirect effects of nutrition, whether it be from protein or trace elements, on the quality of the tooth structure, occlusion and so on. We should do more research on antimetabolites that decrease plaque formation and are of nutritional or food use, substances that might alter the metabolic activity of the flora.

This complexity is not restricted to the problem of dental caries; we find it in studies of cardiovascular disease, diabetes, and all the chronic diseases in which there is a nutritional risk factor or a potential nutritional risk factor. We must recognize that we have a whole series of diseases that we can minimize by acceptable dietary adjustments — nutritionally minimize that risk, or we can tell people how to do it. We cannot force people to make that adjustment. However, we can help them change; we can make the change easier.

Dr. Hopper: Someone had a question for Dr. Bibby, about plaque formation.

Dr. Bibby: If that is my question to answer, the answer is very simple. I don't know and I don't think anybody else really knows what goes on there. I am aware of the mass of literature on that subject, but a mass of literature doesn't necessarily mean clarification. There is much confusion in a multitude of counsellors.

Mr. Thiessen: One thing that has not been discussed is texture. One of the biggest changes has been in the type of food that is being consumed. Foods are becoming softer and almost gummable. If this trend keeps on, you won't have to worry about caries and worry about teeth, you will be able to gum everything that is submitted to the market — nuts and meats for instance. Instead of having firm hot dogs, we now have mushy ones; the same thing is true in tenderized foods. Is there any relationship between this and plaque formation and caries formation?

Dr. Bibby: This is another area in which there are many ideas but nothing in which you could really put complete trust. The idea that most of us probably have in the back of our minds is that certain foods leave our mouths nice and clean and certain foods leave our mouths feeling junked up, shall we say. The actual attempt to quantitate this or explain it was made by the late Bob Caldwell. He came to the conclusion that too much trust had been put in the texture of foods as a method of preventing accumulation of food on the teeth.

The question of the effect of exercise on the health of gingiva and soft tissues is one of the things that has been talked about a lot. I think everybody will accept the general idea that a thing that has been stimulated is a little better than something that has had no stimulus. It is certainly true if you extract teeth on one side of the mouth, there is no function on that side of the mouth and you get a massive accumulation of debris, of periodontal disease. There definitely is a relationship. But that is on the qualitative rather than the quantitative level, and somewhat indefinite.

Dr. Brin: If the amount of sugar consumed is more critical than the number of exposures — the frequency of exposure, one might expect more dental caries in the obese than in the lean. Is this found to be the case?

Dr. Chilton: The papers presented at the ICOB meeting in Copenhagen by the group from Pennsylvania show that there was no correlation between obesity as measured by skin fold thickness and caries.

Mr. Khan: I am not sure that the facts are correct as mentioned, that foods are getting softer. Over 50% of the snack foods are of the nonsoft, crunchy, peanut type or chip types. I believe the general trend is for more texture and for more toughness as we return to the "more natural" — I think the trend is in the other direction.

IV. APPROACHES TO FOOD MODIFICATION

G. Norris Bollenback, Ph.D., Chairman

PHOSPHATE COMPOUNDS USED IN CARIES RESEARCH

Thomas Schiff, D.D.S.

Our teeth are made of hydroxyapatite—a phosphate. The teeth are constantly washed by saliva, which also contains phosphates as well as calcium and other chemicals. This presents us with an obvious question: Why, in the phosphate-rich environment of the mouth, does the hydroxyapatite dissolve? Why does the body permit this dissolution of phosphates in the saturated chemical factory of the oral cavity?

It follows that if the formation of tooth decay is a simple act of dissolving either calcium or phosphate from hydroxyapatite, why doesn't the presence of saliva—saturated with calcium and phosphate and containing a myriad of other chemicals—act to control tooth decay?

From these obvious questions comes the obvious answer that the mechanism of tooth decay, the role of saliva, and the chemical makeup of the oral cavity are not all that simple or that well understood.

Even as dental science becomes more sophisticated and researchers make serious inroads in the mystery that surrounds cariogenesis, the role of saliva still is not fully comprehended.

Inroads are being made, however, in the fight against decay, and since the days of Stralfors in Sweden, researchers throughout the world have conducted experiment after experiment to this end. Much of the work has been concerned with various chemical compounds and their proposed use as dietary additives to reduce tooth decay. Many of these compounds are phosphates.

Over the years, some of these compounds have been shown to be successful in animal trials, and some have even been successful in human trials. Many of us have been convinced of their validity. None of the compounds, however, has shown sufficient success at reducing tooth decay to convince the greatest skeptic of them all—the Food and Drug Administration. And until FDA is convinced, none of our beliefs makes any real difference.

Phosphate Classification

Six different categories of phosphates have been used by my colleagues in their anticaries research. Although I will mention some of my own speculations about these phosphates and how they work, please do not misunderstand. I do not believe at all that I can explain how different phosphates act on caries, any more than anyone else can do so. My ideas are strictly my own and are presented merely as an attempt to open the way for further discussion of the subject.

The very first trial on a possible anticaries food additive was conducted with dicalcium phosphate dihydrate, an orthophosphate. The trials, which were performed with both animals and humans, were relatively successful.

A white, odorless chemical with very low solubility and extremely high chemical integrity, dicalcium phosphate dihydrate (DCPD) has been used as a polishing agent by the dentifrice industry for at least 30 years. Moreover, it has been proved so safe that it is used regularly as an outside source of calcium and phosphates for pregnant women.

The researchers theorized that when used in combination with refined carbohydrates, dicalcium phosphate dihydrate would be an active buffering agent against plaque and would also work to remineralize saliva.

In its class of orthophosphates, dicalcium phosphate dihydrate was the only compound successful in anticaries additive work. Dr. Hazen Baron of Warner-Lambert Company will discuss in detail the three major human clinical trials he conducted with DCPD. These trials were done with children and used chewing gum as the food medium to which the phosphate compound was added.

Two sodium orthophosphates—monosodium phosphate and disodium phosphate—were used in cereal studies with some degree of success. I hope that my colleagues will discuss these studies in detail, especially the trials in which the two were used in combination.

Logically, I think the sodium salt of the orthophosphate should work much better than the calcium salt because of the solubility difference between the two. The results were exactly opposite, however, in those trials with which I am familiar. One explanation may be that the presence of calcium as well as phosphate is necessary in a local buffering reaction. I believe that orthophosphates have a local, and not systemic, effect on the oral cavity, and that the lack of calcium ion may be the reason for the aforementioned difference.

After orthophosphates, the next group of chemicals considered as possible food additives were cyclic phosphates.

A cyclic phosphate, as the term implies, is a phosphate compound containing a ring or rings of atoms, in this case sodium or calcium or magnesium. These compounds form such well-known anticaries agents as sodium trimetaphosphate, calcium magnesium trimetaphosphate and the like.

Research on trimetaphosphate as a food additive began years ago, under the direction of those great researchers, Drs. Harris and Nizel. Many others have been involved since then, including Drs. Shaw and Navia.

Most of the research on this particular compound has been done with animals, and publication after publication describes successful experiments using hamsters or rats. Animal data suggest repeatedly that sodium trimetaphosphate is a good anticaries agent. Caries reduction of as much as 60 or 70% has been cited in these experiments.

The animal studies have not been verified in human trials, however, a most unfortunate but not unusual situation.

The human animal does not behave like a good experimental animal, as I am sure most of you agree. Because of the irregular eating habits of the animal *Homo sapiens* as well as inconsistent food intakes, data do not reproduce themselves at all well on this most important model.

Even in this troublesome animal, some caries reduction was achieved, however, from using trimetaphosphate additives, although the results of the human studies did not come close to matching the success obtained with animal models. This failure to reproduce animal results in humans left researchers in a quandary about what went wrong, not to mention that it caused them a great deal of embarrassment.

If one could exercise equal control on the human animal's diet for additive intake and uniformity of distribution, I am sure the results would be just as successful. I do hope that the outcome of their human experiments does not cause my colleagues to give up. I encourage them to keep trying.

Other cyclic phosphates—those used in combination as calcium magnesium trimetaphosphates—also showed some degree of success in animal trials.

Phytates, an organic cyclic phosphate category, were also studied for anticaries effects. The phytate experiments were undertaken a number of years ago and, again, animal trials showed some degree of success. To my knowledge, there were no major human clinical trials with this compound. I am sure there were no human trials that showed overwhelming success.

Australia was the source for the next group of experiments. Researchers down under originated the idea of using sugar phosphates with food to prevent tooth decay. Since its inception, that idea has spread around the world and throughout the United States. I recall the time many years ago when a Colonial Sugar representative offered manufacturing rights for the compound to my company. At the time, Monsanto decided we were not interested.

I also recall very clearly what happened when the research literature reported the first clinical successes with sugar phosphates. My supervisor called me into his office and wanted to know why I had not told him originally that this compound was going to be a success.

Well, many years have passed, and the initial successes of sugar phosphates in clinical trials were not reproduced. With all due respect to the compound, I feel that the concept is a good one. Add phosphates to the sugar or refined carbohydrate that a person consumes and that person will have a lower degree of tooth decay. Perhaps this concept is worth thinking about, and may be worth using with some of the other chemicals in trials.

For example, I believe that if all carbohydrates were consumed together with additives such as sodium trimetaphosphate or dicalcium phosphate dihydrate or other limited-success phosphates, the phosphates would be able continuously to counteract the acidic insult on the teeth from the carbohydrates. If we could promote this idea into actuality, we might well conquer the problem of tooth decay.

However, the sugar phosphate concept has met with no better success in the United States than it did in Australia. Dr. Charles Wilson of Bio-Research Associates has conducted some successful clinical trials with sugar phosphates, but his success has not been enough to convince the FDA.

There are other phosphates—the glycerol phosphates—and more specifically the beta glycerol phosphates, which have also shown limited success in clinical trials and more success in subclinical trials.

There are many other partial successes, but rather than list them all, I feel it is best to let the actual investigators share their data with you as they do in reports that follow.

Instead, I would like to tell you the conclusions I have drawn from looking at the overall picture. Remember, my view is colored by the fact that I am a dentist working for a company that is the world's largest producer of food grade phosphates, so I am biased.

However, the picture is clear, without regard to such bias. The research has been diverse, the compounds have been numerous, and all the compounds have been different in their chemical makeup. Yet from all that diversity we still get the same message: A positive relationship exists between phosphates and dental health.

I know that we do not have caries reductions of 100% with any of the aforementioned compounds, but each has had some protective effect. The compounds tested are safe. Dicalcium phosphate dihydrate, for example, is as safe a chemical as one can find.

If all this is true, and it is true that the chemicals are safe and clinical trials have been successful, then what is wrong? What are we missing?

We are missing the cooperation of governmental agencies, especially the Food and Drug Administration, in understanding that tooth decay is not one single disease with one single readily available antidote.

Tooth decay comes in many different forms, from many different sources, and must be fought accordingly, with many different weapons.

Fluoride is one weapon. Phosphates, in all forms, is another.

When we can combine 10% reduction in tooth decay from one source with 10% reduction from another source and another 10% reduction from still another source, when we can combine all the different anticaries agents into safe and effective additives to our daily diet, then and only then will we be triumphant in the fight against the most destructive oral disease of mankind: tooth decay.

MODIFYING THE CARIOGENICITY OF FOODS WITH DICALCIUM PHOSPHATE

Hazen J. Baron, D.D.S., Ph.D.

It comes as no surprise to dental scientists that the level of protection offered by a cariostatic substance under laboratory conditions is considerably greater than is found in a human clinical test environment. When dicalcium phosphate dihydrate is added to the cariogenic diets of caries-susceptible laboratory rodents, a profound anticaries effect is invariably shown. I will review the human clinical trials conducted on dicalcium phosphate (dical) and note the level of caries protection afforded by this compound.

Because dicalcium phosphate has such excellent cariostatic properties under laboratory conditions and is an exceedingly safe compound with no objectionable organoleptic properties, it has been subjected to more human clinical studies than any other phosphate compound. Eight long-term human caries clinical trials have been conducted with dicalcium phosphate dihydrate. In four of these studies, dical was added to such foods as baked goods, taken primarily at regular mealtime; the other four studies incorporated dical into confections taken primarily between meals. As will be shown, the cariostatic properties of dical under conditions of use at regular meals produced results which were not consistently strongly positive. The cariostatic properties of dical added to sugar-containing confections, however, produced unequivocal results in that the dical additive neutralized the cariogenic effect of the sugar-containing confection.

In virtually every article in which various approaches to caries control are discussed, one finds the statement that phosphates offer great promise (based on laboratory experiments), but that clinical results to date have been equivocal. Invariably, the clinical results from the early dical dietary studies are the basis for this statement. Therefore it is important to review these early studies and determine the validity of this observation.

The first three clinical studies on dicalcium phosphate were reported simultaneously in the *Journal of Dental Research* in 1964 (Vol. 43, Supplement to No. 6). The first was by Stralfors, whose study population was over 2,000 nine-year-old school children who attended 13 schools in the Malmo district of Sweden. Seven of these schools were designated as control sites and the remaining six schools were designated as test sites. Two percent dibasic calcium phosphate dihydrate was mixed into four ingredients of the school luncheon food, namely, soft bread, hard bread, and the flour and sugar used for cooking. The test schools received bread, sugar and flour with dical while the control schools got the same foods without the additive. Determination of caries was by radiographs of four proximal surfaces of three maxillary incisors. The caries attack (DFS increment) over the two-year test period was very low on these four surfaces; viz, 0.6 for the control group and 0.3 for the phosphate group, with the difference of approximately 50% being statistically significant. Stralfors cautioned that these caries reduction figures are not to be applied to the dentition as a whole; it would be expected to be lower, with an estimate of perhaps 20%.

Stralfors speculated about the mechanism of action of dicalcium phosphate and made the following cogent observations:

1. In order to be effective, dical must be incorporated into the dental plaque.
2. When acid is produced by plaque bacteria, part of the dical is dissolved. This increases the calcium and phosphate ion concentration and the plaque continues to be saturated with calcium and phosphate despite the fact that the pH has been lowered. As a consequence, the calcium phosphate of the tooth surface is not dissolved.
3. A necessary condition for a good effect against caries should be that the dical is mixed intimately with the plaque-forming ingredients of the diet.

In the study by Averill and Bibby , 548 children, aged 6-15 years, participated in a two-year clinical trial designed to test the effect of 2% dicalcium phosphate additive to the diet. The children were patients in two closed institutions in New York State; one a home for mentally retarded patients and the other an institution for epileptic patients. The dical phosphate was added to the food in the bakery storerooms, mixing it with all of the flour and sugar before they were used for making bread, pastries or desserts or before sugar went to the table. A review of the food consumption showed that 95% of the carbohydrate used in these institutions was phosphate-enriched. Within each institution, the children consumed either the dical enriched diet or the regular, unfortified one. Both clinical and radiographic dental examinations were made. The examination of the children presented technical difficulties: the institutional aides were most helpful in handling patients during the examinations. In some cases mouth props were required to obtain adequate access to the mouth. The level of oral hygiene in these handicapped patients is not defined in the report.

At the conclusion of the two-year study, 277 of the original 548 children remained, and the two study groups had become grossly imbalanced in their age distributions. The authors concluded: "It scarcely needs to be pointed out that the results based on such imbalanced study groups can have little or no significance. However, the results, for what they are worth, are (presented)." The only conclusion that the authors could draw from this study was that under the conditions tested, the phosphate additive in the diet of children failed to influence profoundly the initiation or progression of dental caries. However, they cautioned that although this study seems to show that phosphates have no dramatic effects on human caries, it is not sufficiently defective to justify concluding that phosphates would not, under different conditions, offer demonstrable protection against caries.

The study by Ship and Mickelsen involved 1,672 school-age children distributed among eight boarding schools in North and South Dakota. Four of these schools were designated as experimental sites while the others were designated control sites. In the experimental schools, the children at mealtimes consumed bread which had been baked with flour supplemented with 2% dicalcium phosphate. The control group school children were provided with regular unfortified bread. After the study had started, analysis of the diets showed substantial variation of consumption of the experimental bread, and the dical phosphate was increased in selected schools to bring it to approximately 1 g of phosphate per day. At the end of the three-year study, 732 children of the original study population of 1,672 remained. Annual clinical examinations were conducted on the study participants and some radiographic examinations were made although their number is unclear. At the end of the three-year study period, the authors concluded, there were no differences in caries experience between the experimental and control groups. Their published data, however, refute this conclusion in that the mean DFS three-year increment for the control group was 8.1 while it was 7.4 for the experimental group; the difference, albeit small, was significant at the .02 level of probability.

In 1966, Averill, Freier and Bibby reported a clinical trial they conducted in two rubber plantation towns in Brazil. The study population exhibited an exceedingly high caries activity and a controllable food supply (mandioca) which provides 75% of the caloric intake of this population.

Mandioca contains extremely small quantities of calcium; this population received less than one-fifth of the recommended daily intake of calcium. The experimental subjects were 450 children, aged 7-17 years, in one town in which mandioca had been supplemented with 2% dicalcium phosphate. The 519 control group children, also aged 7-17, in another town consumed an unfortified mandioca diet. Clinical and radiographic examinations were conducted. After 30 months, 216 of the 450 experimental group children remained, and 165 of the 519 control subjects.

The final results showed a modest, undramatic reduction in caries in the experimental group when the DMFS of all teeth was considered. The investigators did note in the experimental group, however, a considerable degree of protection to the molars and premolars that had erupted during the course of the study, with the difference between the experimental and control groups significant at .001 level of probability. In discussing their results, the authors encouraged further investigation of dicalcium phosphate and observed that: "There are sufficient differences between commercially produced dicalcium phosphate dihydrates that solubility or recalcifying effects produced by one might not be given by another."

Thus, by 1966 four clinical studies had been published which showed varying results concerning the degree of cariostatic effectiveness of dicalcium phosphate. Rather than commenting on the design, conduct and control of these studies in light of present-day criteria for conducting clinical trials, suffice it to say that these studies produced results that certainly were not negative but were not consistently strongly positive. By no means did the results from these clinical studies deserve the negative stigma which invariably appeared when one discussed the clinical cariostatic effectiveness of dicalcium phosphate.

Several pertinent observations were made by the original investigators and, in light of subsequent research on this compound, the following comments seem appropriate:

1. Dibasic calcium phosphate dihydrate that has been stabilized during the manufacturing process with tetrasodium pyrophosphate is cariostatically more active than a dical preparation that has been stabilized with trimagnesium phosphate. The former preparation corresponds to Monsanto Grade 210 which none of the four original studies used.
2. Dibasic calcium phosphate dihydrate that has been agglomerated with sucrose is cariostatically more active than dical that has not been coated with sugar.
3. Dibasic calcium phosphate dihydrate must be delivered at the time of cariogenic insult; it will not confer protection against subsequent caries attacks.
4. The most beneficial role of dical would be to supplement highly cariogenic confections with this compound, particularly those confections used between meals. Rather than looking at foods such as bread as vehicles to deliver dical, one should look at specific cariogenic foods or confections which can have their cariogenic potential neutralized with dical.

Taking the foregoing four factors into consideration, clinical trials were initiated to demonstrate that one could neutralize the cariogenicity of a popular between-meal confection consumed by children, particularly American children, through the use of dical. The confection chosen was sugar-based chewing gum which, as will be shown, has a significant cariogenic potential.

Dical chewing gum was formulated by using dibasic calcium phosphate dihydrate that had been stabilized during manufacture with tetrasodium pyrophosphate and agglomerating or spray-drying it with sucrose, thus forming an intimate mixture with a plaque-forming ingredient, as Stralfors had suggested in 1964. Each 3 g stick of chewing gum contained 225 mg of dical that had been treated in this manner. The remaining 1.2 g sugar in the 3 g stick of gum was left untreated.

The first clinical trial designed to test the cariostatic effectiveness of dical chewing gum was conducted by Lisanti, Yacovone and Romenski in Rhode Island between 1957 and 1960. The 349 children who completed this (unpublished) study ranged in age from 8 to 12 years. Their socioeconomic status was similar and they attended three widely separated grade schools in the Cumberland, Rhode Island area. One hundred twenty-four children in school #1 received a regular sugar chewing gum; 131 children in school #2, the sugar agglomerated dical gum, and 94 children in school #3 were not given any gum during the 30-month test period. The children in the gum groups were instructed to chew one stick after each meal and after every snack up to a maximum of five sticks per day. The identity of the gum was not known to the subject, as each stick was packaged in a blank wrapper. The dental caries history of each subject was determined by clinical and radiographic examinations at the beginning of the study and at six-month intervals thereafter. The initial examinations disclosed that the caries level in each group was statistically comparable.

The final 30-month examination (Table 1) showed that the group using regular gum developed significantly more carious lesions per child than either the dical gum group or the no-gum group. The difference in the 30-month mean caries increment between the dical gum group and the no-gum group was not statistically significant.

The second clinical trial designed to test the cariostatic effectiveness of a dical additive to sugar chewing gum was carried out by Finn and Jamison at the Alabama State School for the Deaf and Blind in Talledega, Alabama, from 1963 through 1966 . 606 children were originally selected for study and assigned to three groups according to age, sex, race, infirmity, previous use of a dentifrice

TABLE 1. Dical Chewing Gum Study, Cumberland, Rhode Island

Length of Study: 2.5 years
Treatment Regimens and Population Size

Regular Diet Supplemented With:
Sugar Gum N = 124
No Gum N = 94
Dical Gum, N = 131

	Mean Caries Increment			Group Comparisons		
	Sugar	No Gum	Dical	Sugar vs No Gum	Sugar vs Dical	No Gum vs Dical
DMFS/Subject	13.9	10.6	11.2	3.3 (24.0%[1])	2.7 (19.4%[1])	0.6 (5.7%)
DMFT/Subject	5.6	4.3	4.4	1.3 (24.2%[1])	1.2 (22.4%[1])	0.1 (2.4%)

[1] $p < .05$

and caries experience. The stratified groups were then assigned randomly to one of three treatment regimens: Group 1 chewed a sugar gum, Group 2 a sorbitol/mannitol (sugarless) gum and Group 3 a sugar gum containing 225 mg of sugar-agglomerated dicalcium phosphate per stick. All children were instructed to brush their teeth after meals with a nontherapeutic dentifrice. They were told to chew five sticks of gum daily, with each chewing period to last 20 minutes. Two sticks were chewed before breakfast and lunch, one after school, and two between dinner and bedtime. All gum had the same flavor and was packaged in unmarked wrappers. The gum was distributed daily to each subject by paid supervisors who kept individual records. The clinical and radiographic examinations for caries were made at the start of the study and at consectutive six-month periods. 368 children, ranging in age from 6 to 17 years, completed the entire 36-month study period. Statistical evaluation of the data (Table 2) showed that there was a significantly higher incidence of new caries in the group who chewed the regular sugar gum than in those in the group on dical gum; there was no significant difference in the average caries increment between the groups given the dical gum and the sugarless gum; and the children who chewed the sugar gum had a significantly higher incidence of dental caries than those who chewed the sugarless gum.

The third clinical trial carried out on dical gum was conducted in 11 widely separated grade schools in the Trail-Rossland area of British Columbia,

Canada, from 1968 to 1970 by Richardson, Hole, McCombie and Klothammer. On the basis of age, sex and previous caries experience, the children were separated randomly into three comparable groups: Group 1 chewed three sticks of sorbitol/mannitol (sugarless) gum per school day; Group 2 received no chewing gum, and Group 3 chewed three sticks of dical gum per school day. The sugarless gum and dical gum were identically flavored and packaged. All classrooms within each school contained children on each of the three regimens. The chewing sessions took place under supervision of the classroom teacher just before morning recess, lunch break and school closing. Each stick of gum was chewed for 20 minutes before the children left the

TABLE 2. Dical Chewing Gum Study, Talladega, Alabama

Length of Study - 3 years
Treatment Regimens and Population Size

Regular Diet Supplemented With:
Sugar Gum N + 113
No Gum N + 131
Dical Gum N + 124

	Mean Caries Increment			Group Comparisons		
	Sugar	Sugarless	Dical	Sugar vs Sugarless	Sugar vs Dical	Sugarless vs Dical
DMFS/Subject	7.2	5.1	5.7	2.1 (29.0%[1])	1.5 (21.7%[1])	0.6 (9.4%)
DMFT/Subject	3.8	2.8	2.9	1.0 (24.9%[1])	0.9 (23.0%[1])	0.1 (2.4%)

[1]$p < .05$

classroom. The foregoing procedure was carried out each day that school was in session (200 school days per year). Toothbrushes and a nontherapeutic dentifrice were available to all participants for the duration of the study.

Of the 850 children who started this study, 711 were present for the baseline, interim and final radiographic and clinical dental examinations. Analysis of the data (Table 3) showed there were no statistically significant differences in caries experience whether the children chewed sugarless gum, dical gum, or refrained from chewing any gum.

Recently, the data from the three dical chewing gum clinical trials were subjected to a more stringent statistical analysis which represents the current views of dental biometricians working in the field of clinical caries research. Briefly, the data from each of the trials were subjected to 16 two-way analyses of variance using the net DMFS increment as the response variable (Table 4). The conclusions derived from the original statistical analyses and the more critical analysis of covariance on the three dical gum clinical trials are as follows:

1. Sorbitol/mannitol (sugarless) chewing gum does not promote tooth decay (Trail Study, sugarless vs. no-gum).

2. Sugar chewing gum promotes tooth decay (Cumberland, sugar vs. no chew; and Talledega, sugar vs. sugarless).
3. Sugar agglomerated dibasic calcium phosphate dihydrate added to sugar gum reduces the cariogenicity of the sugar gum (Cumberland, dical vs. sugar; and Talledega, dical vs. sugar).
4. Dical gum does not promote tooth decay (Cumberland, dical vs. no-gum; and Talledega, dical vs. sugarless; and Trail, dical vs. no-gum; and Trail, dical vs. sugarless).

The most recent dicalcium phosphate study to be completed was carried out by Ashley, Naylor and Emslie in 1974. The purpose of this study was to determine the effect of 3% dicalcium phosphate added to boiled candies on

TABLE 3. Dical Chewing Gum Study, Trail, British Columbia

Length of Study - 2 years
Treatment Regimens and Population Size

Regular Diet Supplemented With:
Sugar Gum N + 233
No Gum N + 237
Dical Gum N + 241

	Mean Caries Increment			Group Comparisons		
	Sugarless	No Gum	Dical	Sugarless vs No Gum	Sugarless vs Dical	No Gum vs Dical
DMFS/Subject	5.87	5.89	6.32	0.02 (0.4%)	0.45 (7.2%)	0.43 (6.9%)
DMFT/Subject	3.24	3.15	3.26	0.09 (2.9%)	0.02 (0.5%)	0.11 (3.4%)

TABLE 4. Dical Chewing Gum Studies - Statistical Significance of the Various Pairwise Comparisons Using Different Criteria

	Frequency: 8 Single Comparisons				8 Multiple Comparisons				
					Dunnett		Scheffe		
	.01	.05	.10	Not Sig.	Sig. (.05)	Not Sig.	Sig. (.05)	Not Sig.	Final Verdict
Cumberland, R.I.									
Sugar vs. Dical	0	8	0	0	3	5	3	5	Borderline Sig.
Sugar vs. No Gum	8	0	0	0	8	0	8	0	Sig.
Dical vs. No Gum	0	4	3	1	0	8	0	8	Not Sig.
Talladega, Ala									
Sugar vs. Sugarless	6	2	0	0	8	0	6	2	Sig.
Sugar vs. Dical	3	2	3	0	4	4	4	4	Borderline Sig.
Sugarless vs. Dical	3	2	3	0	0	8	0	8	Not Sig.
Trail, B.C.									
Sugarless vs. No Gum	0	0	0	8	0	8	0	8	Not Sig.
Sugarless vs. Dical	0	0	0	8	0	8	0	8	Not Sig.
No Gum vs. Dical	0	0	0	8	0	8	0	8	Not Sig.

dental caries increments in 11-to 12-year-old London school children. 871 children completed this three-year clinical trial in which the dical fortified sweets or the unfortified sweets were mailed to the children's homes for ad libitum use. Annual clinical radiographic examinations of the study participants were conducted. Although there was some question about the appropriateness of the unfortified boiled sweets as controls, the results demonstrated that the dical additive did reduce the cariogenicity of the boiled candies.

Conclusions

In summary then, the results from the eight clinical trials on dibasic calcium phosphate dihydrate lead one to the following conclusions:

1. It is extremely important that the proper commercial grade of dibasic calcium phosphate dihydrate be used when testing its clinical cariostatic effectiveness.
2. The thorough mixing of dical with sugar, as in spray-drying, contributes to maximum cariostatic effectiveness of this compound.
3. Dical must be delivered at the same time as the cariogenic insult in order to neutralize that attack; it does not appear to confer protection against subsequent caries attacks.
4. Dical is a safe and effective additive for between-meal sugar-containing confections shuch as chewing gum in that it materially reduces the cariogenic properties of those confections.

THE ANTICARIES EFFECTS OF TRIMETAPHOSPHATES

Abraham E. Nizel, D.M.D., M.S.D.

Introduction

As the major chemical constituents of tooth and bone are calcium and phosphorus, it is logical that one would emphasize the ingestion of foods that are rich in these minerals if one wanted to optimize dental health. Lennox in 1931 noted a high dental caries experience in some natives of South Africa who, he claimed, ate foods grown in phosphate deficient soils.[1] To our knowledge this is the first scientific documentation of a possible correlation between phosphates and dental caries. During the early thirties, this postulation of an inverse relationship between the dietary level of phosphate intake and dental caries was experimentally substantiated by a number of different rat feeding experiments conducted independently in several laboratories[2–6]. In fact, to 1964 there had been about 100 different animal experiments run under different sets of laboratory and experimental conditions which pointed conclusively to the fact that a dietary phosphate supplement to an otherwise cariogenic diet could significantly inhibit dental caries development.[7] Since 1964, no doubt there have been at least half again as many similar studies with similar conclusions.

The Discovery and Corroboration of the Significant Anticaries Effects of Trimetaphosphates in the Rodent

In our food and nutrition laboratories at the Massachusetts Institute of Technology, it might be considered serendipitous that phosphate dietary supplements were found to exert significant anticaries effects when added to an otherwise sucrose rich cariogenic diet.

It was the result of a dental caries survey of World War II soldiers that prompted the search for a nutritional etiological factor for the geographic variation of dental caries prevalance in the United States. We found that soldiers from New England had about twice as many carious teeth as did native Texans.[8] Diets containing corn and milk produced in New Englad and fed to one group of Syrian hamsters caused a little more than twice the amount of caries as did identical diets containing corn and milk produced in Texas and fed to another group of hamsters.[9, 10] These experimental findings were the stimulus for collaborative experimental caries research with my teacher and mentor, Robert S. Harris, Professor of Nutritional Biochemistry at M.I.T.

Our next experiment dealt with the caries producing effect of doubling the mineral content of the diet by adding a natural mineral mixture derived from ashing the respective New England and Texas produced foods. The increased mineral content reduced the experimental caries significantly in both diet groupings. A synthetic mineral mix was made to duplicate the natural ash. Different combinations of the components of the synthetic mineral mix were fed as diet supplements and were found ineffective in reducing dental decay until a phosphate, potassium hydrogen phosphate, was added[13] (Fig. 1). When the simplest phosphate compound, metaphosphoric acid (HPO_3) was used as the source of supplementing dietary phosphorus, dental caries was reduced by 70%.[13] We noted that the enamel surface of the rat molars exposed to this phosphate compound had a unique smooth and glossy appearance and the occlusal surfaces were flattened (Fig. 2).

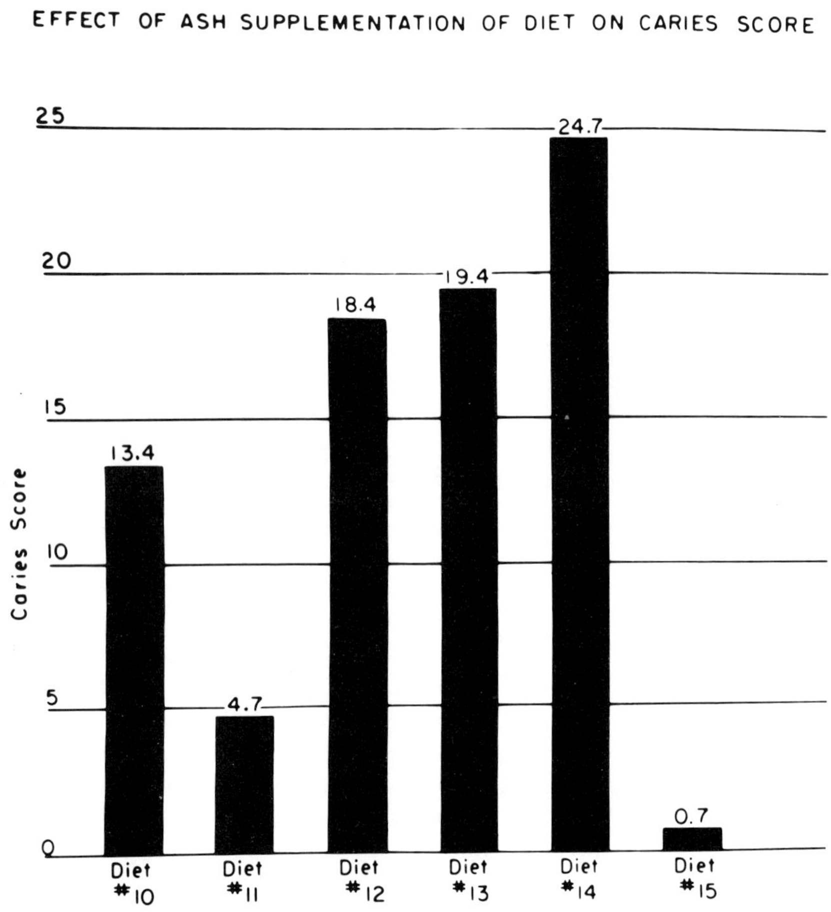

FIGURE 1. Effect of Ash Supplementation of Diet on Caries Score

Our next task was to determine the proper combination of cation and phosphate anion that would exert maximum caries inhibitory effects. To find the best cation, mono- and dibasic salts of sodium, potassium and calcium orthophosphate were fed at various levels. We found that the sodium and potassium phosphates reduced caries much more effectively than calcium phosphate. In comparison to the control group, the caries scores were reduced

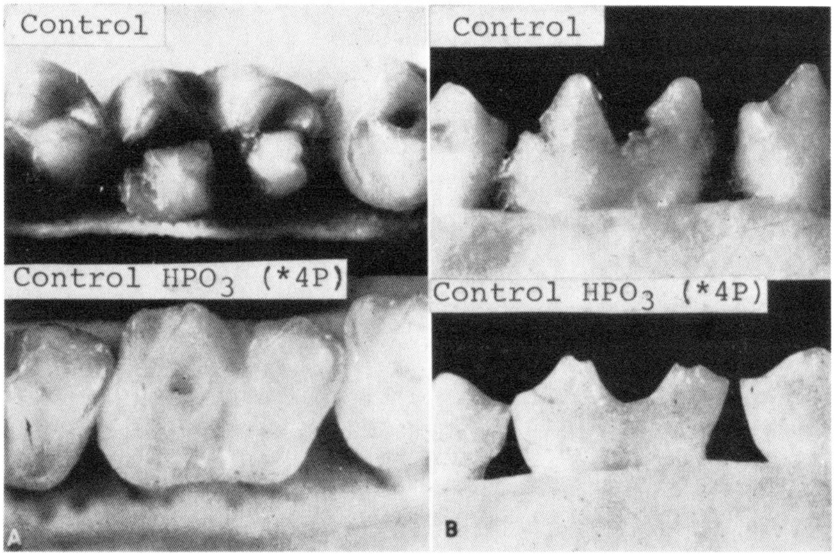

FIGURE 2. A. Occlusal view of hamster molars. Note morphologic as well as caries difference between group on control diet and experimental (control + HPO_3) diet. B. Lateral view of same teeth.

by 81%, 71% and 29% when sodium, potassium or calcium orthophosphate salts, repsectively, supplied the phosphorus supplement[14] (Fig. 3).

To determine the phosphate anion that exerted the greatest anticaries effect, we selected five phosphates representing three different types of phosphate anion: simple (ortho), linear (pyro, tri poly, and hexameta) and cyclic (trimeta-). These five sodium phosphate compounds differed only in their anion structure and were added at equal phosphorus levels to a cariogenic diet. In comparison with the control group, the reductions in caries development were: pyrophosphate, 29%; orthophosphate, 33%; tripolyphosphate, 46%; hexametaphosphate, 51%; and trimetaphosphate, 78% (Fig. 4). Another significant observation was that the group fed the trimetaphosphate supplement had a more lustrous and smoother enamel surface than any other group.[15,16]

Sodium trimetaphosphate, $Na_3(PO)_3$, is a six-membered ring phosphate composed of alternating oxygen and phosphorus atoms. When given orally, appreciable amounts are hydrolyzed in the digestive tract to orthophosphate. Sodium trimetaphosphate is more soluble in water than ortho-, pyro-, tripoly- and hexametaphosphate and has the lowest buffering capacity; it is second lowest in its chelating or complexing abilities (Table 1). On the basis of these comparative physiochemical properties of the five phosphates used as diet supplements, we hypothesized that the ready water solubility of trimetaphosphate may have created a local salivary phosphate concentration that was conducive to remineralizing any demineralized enamel surfaces. Further, the local contact of this cylic phosphate with the enamel surface may have contributed to the improved crystallinity of the enamel surface, which gave it a lustrous appearance.

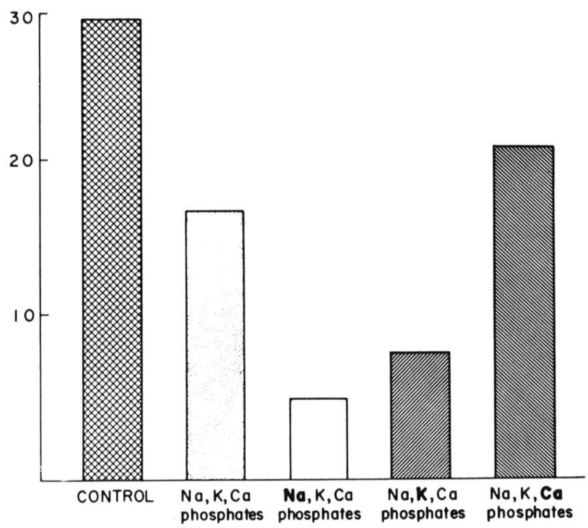

FIGURE 3. Dental caries scores observed in the second molars of rats fed five different diets.[14]

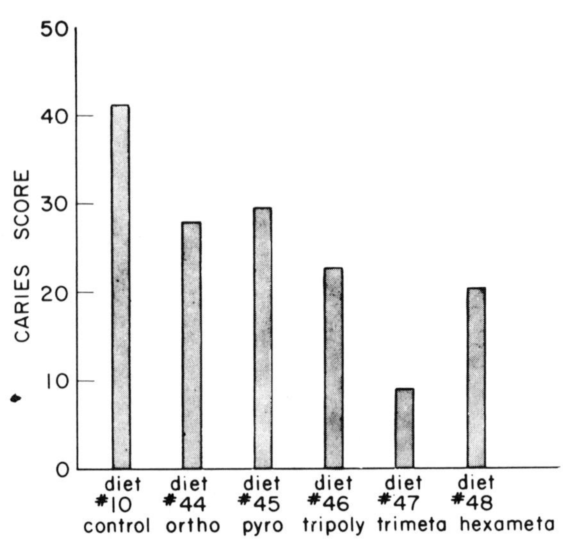

FIGURE 4. Cariostatic effects of several sodium phosphates fed in the diet to rats.[16]

Since our discovery of the significant anticaries properties of sodium trimetaphosphate, there have been at least five other teams of investigators who have confirmed this finding independently.[17–21] Navia and Harris compared the relative anticaries effects of sodium fluoride and sodium trimetaphosphate when fed separately and together as dietary supplements to an otherwise cariogenic diet.[22] At the end of the experimental period, they observed that trimetaphosphate (TMP), fluoride and the combination trimetaphosphate plus

TABLE 1. Ranking of caries reduction, buffer capacity, water solubility and complexing ability of phosphate anions*

	Caries Reduction	Buffer Capacity	Solubility as Na salt in water	Complexing Ability
Pyro-	1	5	4	3
Ortho-	2	4	2	1
Tripoly-	3	3	3	4
Hexameta-	4	2	1	5
Trimeta-	5	1	5	2

*Expressed in terms of degrees of magnitude (l=least; 5=most).

TABLE 2. TMP as chewing gum additive on caries increment[24]

Group	DMFS	% Difference
1. No gum	1.63	0
2. TMP and sucrose gum	1.25	-23.3
3. Sorbitol gum	2.06	+26.4
4. TMP and sorbitol gum	0.85	-47.6

fluoride reduced caries respectively 87%, 65%, and 97% when compared to the control group. These investigators suggested that trimetaphosphate does not prevent enamel solubilization like fluoride. Therefore, they postulated, trimetaphosphate probably does not prevent the initiation of dental caries as effectively as fluoride. But trimetaphosphate probably assists in the remineralization of the tooth and thus prevents the extension of the carious lesion.

One recent animal feeding study is of special interest because it demonstrated that the sugar-frosted, ready-to-eat cereals are significantly more cariogenic than the unsweetened ready-to-eat cereals. When 2% trimetaphosphate was added to the sugar frosted ready-to-eat cereals, the rats had 57% less caries than the control non-phosphated sugar frosted ready-to-eat cereal group.[23]

Effect of Trimetaphosphate in Chewing Gum on Caries Increment in Children

Very recently the final results have been reported of the only clinical study conducted to date in which the anticaries properties of sodium trimetaphosphate have been tested.[24] This study was completed on 349 deaf and blind children, ages 5 to 16, whose diets were under supervision for 24 months while domiciled at school. Three sticks of chewing gum with 1.5% TMP every day was the test material. The children assigned randomly to one of four groups—a non-gum group, a TMP sucrose gum group, a sorbitol gum group and the

TMP sucrose gum group, had respectively 47% and 23% less proximal caries than the non-phosphated sorbitol gum group. Although the groups exposed to TMP had lower DMFT and DMFS increments, the differences were not statistically significant because the occlusal and buccolingual surfaces were not sufficiently protected.

The investigators concluded that the total anticaries action of TMP demonstrated in this clinical trial may have been "marginal" because using a single vehicle may not be the best way for exposing the tooth enamel to the TMP often enough. The fact that the proximal caries increments were decreased significantly prompted them to recommend that future studies focus on 12 -to 14-year-olds who reside in a low fluoride region and who are at the most susceptible age period for rampant interproximal caries.

Mechanisms of Anticaries Action of Trimetaphosphates

From animal and *in vitro* studies, it appears that the major anticaries action of trimetaphosphate is local or topical.

Navia, *et al.*[25] studied the anticaries effect of a 1.31% sodium trimetaphosphate diet supplement when fed to rats during each or in combinations of the four different periods of tooth development, namely pregnancy, lactation, early enamel maturation period and late enamel maturation period. The results indicated that it was the topical action of TMP on the surface of the tooth during the newly erupted early maturation or late maturation period (or both) that was responsible for the low caries scores (Fig. 5). The tooth enamel evidently is permeable enough to take up the phosphate ions, just as it takes fluoride ions from the oral environment. However, the tooth quality, as affected by the systemic intake of phosphates during pregnancy and lactation when the tooth is forming, was not improved enough to resist dental caries. Trimetaphosphate seems to act differently than fluorides on tooth enamel because the latter is effective both systemically and locally whereas phosphates act best locally.

From an *in vitro* standpoint, it has been demonstrated that TMP can modify the enamel surface in such a way as to prevent the adsorption of the protein pellicle which serves as the matrix for bacterial plaque formation.[26,27]

When molar enamel surfaces of rodent fed a TMP supplemented diet were examined by a scanning electron microscope, the surfaces seemed smoother and had less demineralized fissures and less microcavities than in the molar enamel surfaces of rats fed the non-phosphate control diet.[28]

It has been shown as well that TMP dicalcium phosphate can increase enamel hardness, but there is no long-lasting, residual effect as there is with flourides.[29] TMP can remineralize or change the chemical composition of the enamel surface to a more insoluble apatite.[30]

There are some conflicting reports of the effect of TMP in dental plaque bacteria. Handleman and Kreinces reported that with an increase in phosphate concentration derived from TMP, there was an inhibition of both acid production and growth of cariogenic *Streptococcus*.[31] Dennis *et al.* found that TMP resulted in a decrease in total viable organisms and streptococci per mg of plaque.[32] Finn *et al.* found that TMP does not alter the amount of plaque formed

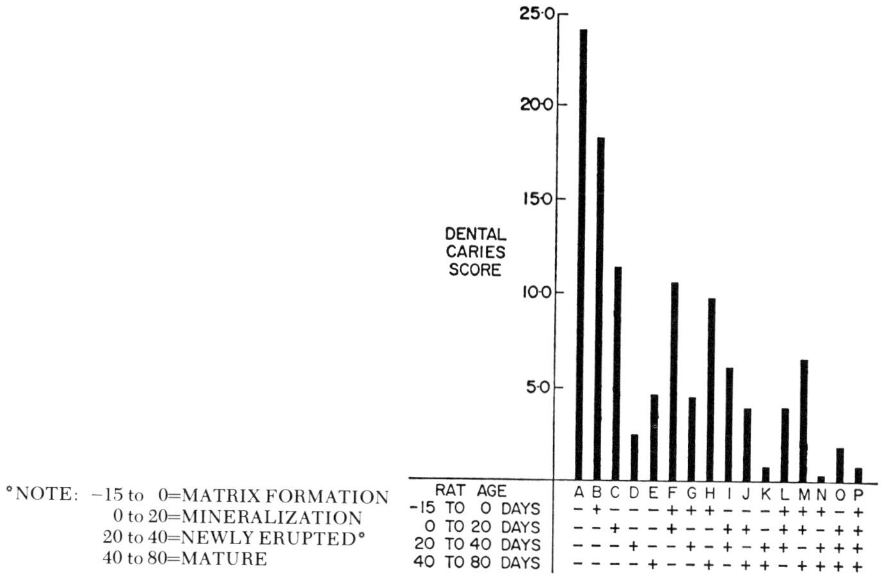

FIGURE 5. Cariostatic effect of sodium trimetaphosphate when fed to rats during different stages of tooth development.[25]

or its microbiologic composition. Neither the ratios of total streptococci to other bacteria nor the ratios of *Streptococcus mutans* to total streptococci seem to be altered.[24]

In summary, the postulated mechanisms for the anticaries effect of TMP are (1) that there is probably a phosphorus ionic uptake by the tooth enamel surface, especially when newly erupted, from salivary TMP, (2) that this phosphorus evidently makes the enamel surface hard and smooth if there is a sustained significant level available, and (3) that this cyclic phosphate can remineralize incipient demineralized enamel.

Conclusions and Opinions

Trimetaphosphate (TMP) has the potential of being an effective food or drink anticaries additive and also may be useful in a dentifrice or oral rinse vehicle. The food carriers for this agent must be a number of different ones such as breads, cereals, flour products and gum so that frequent at meal and between meal contact of the tooth enamel can be made with the phosphate. This is not different from the principles of vitamin and mineral restoration programs used to overcome the nutrient deficiencies created by the food refinement processes. Indeed, 80% of the bran phosphate has been removed during refinement, as is some calcium. Perhaps a sodium calcium trimetaphosphate compound should be used to restore and maintain the desirable Ca:P ratio in the diet.

Because dental caries has a multifactorial etiology, the only rational preventive approach is to use a number of different anticaries agents in a number of different ways (water, foods, drugs). Trimetaphosphate as a sodium or a calcium salt has the potential of being one of these agents. However, its adequate intake can be assured only by incorporating it in a broad spectrum of food and drink carriers. Future clinical trials should incorporate this multi-vehicle approach before one labels phosphate supplementation in humans as "equivocal" from a caries preventive standpoint. Phosphate supplements or additives properly used may be the complementary anticaries agent that dental scientists have been seeking to improve the 40 to 60% caries reduction achieved by currently practiced combined fluoride therapy methods.

REFERENCES

1. Lennox, J. Observation on diet and its relation to dental disease: A further consideration of calcium and phosphorus metabolism in their relation to dental caries.S. Afr. Dent. J. 5:156, 1931.
2. Klein, H. and McCollum, E.V. A preliminary note on the significance of the phosphorus intake in the diet and blood phosphorus concentration in the experimental production of caries immunity and caries susceptibility in rat. Science 84:662, 1931.
3. Klein, H. and Shelling, D.H. The relation of diet to the toxicity of viosterol as a determining factor in the production of experimental caries in rats. J. Dent. Res. 11:458, 1931.
4. Blackberg, S.N. and Berke, J.D. Dental caries experimentally produced in the rat. J.Dent. Res. 12:609, 1932.
5. Agnew, M.C., Agnew, R.S. and Tisdall, F.F. The production and prevention of dental caries. J.Amer. Dent. Assoc. 20:193, 1933.
6. Rosebury, T. and Karshan, M. Susceptibility to detal caries in the rat. V. Influence of calcium, phosporus, vitamin D and corn oil. Arch. Path. 20:697, 1935.
7. Nizel, A.E. and Harris, R.S. The effects of phosphates on experimental dental caries: a literature review. J. Dent. Res. 43:1123, 1964.
8. Nizel, A.E. and Bibby, B.G. Geopgraphic variations in caries prevalence in soliders. J. Amer. Dent. Assoc. 31:1619, 1944.
9. Nizel, A.E. and Harris, R.S. Effect of foods grown in different areas on the prevalence of dental caries in hamsters. Arch. Biochem. 26:155, 1950.
10. Nizel, A.E. and Harris, R.S. The caries producing effect of similar foods grown in different soil areas. New England J.Med. 244:361, 1951.
11. Nizel, A.E. and Harris, R.S. Effects of ashed foodstuffs on dental decay in hamsters. J.Dent. Res. 34:513, 1955.
12. Harrris, R.S. and Nizel, A.E. Effects of food ash, phosphate and trace minerals upon hamsters caries. J.Dent. Res. 38:1142, 1959.
13. Nizel, A.E. and Harris, R.S. Phosphate and dental caries. I. Effect of metaphosphoric acid in the diet of weanling hamsters on dental caries development. J. Amer. Dent. Assoc. 60:193, 1960.
14. Harris, R.S. and Nizel, A.E. Effect of cations on the cariostatic activity of orthophosphates. J. Dent. Res. 44:416, 1965.
15. Nizel, A.E., Baker, N.J. and Harris, R.S. The effect of phosphate structure upon dental caries development in rats. Internat. Asso.Dent. Res. Abstract Number 236, 1962.
16. Harris, R.S., Nizel,A.E. and Walsh, N.B. The effect of phosphate structure in dental caries development in rats. J. Dent. Res. 46:290, 1967.
17. Mühlemann, H.R. and König, K.G. A comparative study of the cariostatic effect of dietary fluorides, orthophosphates, and triphosphates in Osborn-Mendel rats. Helv. Odont. Acta 8:56, 1964.
18. Clay, H. and Navia, J. Sodium trimetasphosphate influence on early development of rat caries and concurrent microbiological changes. Caries Res. 3:326, 1969.
19. Englander, H.R. and Keyes, P. Effect of phosphate supplements on cavitation in hamsters infected with caries conductive streptococci. J. Dent. Res. 49:140, 1970.

20. Larson, R.H. *et al.* Reduction of rat caries by trimetaphosphate on different tooth surfaces: Variations produced by diet and oral flora. Arch. Oral. Biol. 17:883, 1972.
21. Payne, R.W., Kreitzman, S.N. and Simes, I.M. Caries inhibiting ability of trimetaphosphate at low concentrations in solution. Internat. Assoc. Dent. Res. Abstract Number 116, 1973.
22. Navia, J. and Harris, R.S. Longitudinal study of cariostatic effects of sodium trimetaphosphate and sodium fluoride when fed separately and together in diets of rats. J.Dent. Res. 48:183, 1969.
23. Shaw, P. Personal communication.
24. Finn, S.B. *et al.* The effect of sodium trimetaphosphate as a chewing gum additive on caries increment in children. J. Amer. Dent. Assoc. 96:651, 1978.
25. Navia, J.M., Lopez, H. and Harris, R.S. Cariostatic effects of sodium trimetaphosphate when fed to rats during different stages of tooth development. Arch. Oral Biol. 13:779, 1968.
26. Pruitt, K.M., *et al.* Possible basis for cariostatic effect of inorganic phosphates. Nature 225:1249, 1970.
27. Briscoe, J.M. and Pruitt, K.M. Comparison of the effects of linear and cyclic phosphates on the absorption of proteins by human enamel. J. Dent Res. 54:504, 1975.
28. Zuniga, M.A. and Navia, J.M. Effect of phosphates on buccal enamel caries studied by scanning microscopy. Internat. Assoc. Dent. Res. Abstract Number 754, 1972.
29. Koulourides, T. *et al.* Effect of $CaHPO_4$ and trimetaphosphate (TMP) on cariogenicity in humans. Internat. Assoc. Dent. Res. Abstract Number 606, 1974.
30. Gonzalez, M. Effect of trimetaphosphate on the process of mineralization. J. Dent. Res. 50:1056, 1971.
31. Handleman, S.L. and Kreinces, G.H. Effect of phosphate and pH on Streptococcus mutans acid production and growth. J. Dent. Res. 52:651, 1973.
32. Dennis, D.A. *et al.* Effects of sodium trimetaphosphate supplementation of a high sucrose diet on the microbial and biochemical composition of four day plaque and on urine calcium and phosphate levels. J. Dent Res. 55:787, 1976.

DISCUSSION

Dr. Kreitzman: Dr. Nizel, is there any indication given in the clinical study by Dr. Finn about why the sugarless gum group should have had higher caries incidence?

Dr. Baron: Dr. Finn was talking about proximal surfaces of the teeth. In the parameter — all surfaces, all teeth — there was no significant difference between the groups.

Dr. Bowen: We have been looking at the effect of calcium glyceryl phosphate and sodium phytate for a number of years in primates, and we found calcium glyceryl phosphate very effective in reducing caries when added to some of the sugar in the diet of the animals. We were able to correlate this reduction in caries with differences in the composition of plaque. When we attempted to reproduce these results in humans, the results were very mixed. Some people have been able to reproduce the changes in plaque associated with the ingestion of calcium glyceryl phosphate. At the moment, we don't know where we are going to go with calcium glyceryl phosphate. With sodium phytate, we got a fairly big reduction in caries when this was fed to primates. However, Nordbo and Rölla in Scandanavia have observed that they can reduce the amount of plaque in human subjects when the subjects rinse their mouths with weak solutions of either of these substances.

Many people are not aware that calcium glyceryl phosphate is used extensively in the Soviet Union to reduce caries. They claim reduction on the order of 25 to 35% when using this material. It is difficult to get the details of their studies, but I have had first-hand information from Federov that this is a fact.

We have now reached the stage at which approximately 50% of the population in the United States is using fluoridated drinking water. Many people would postulate that the possible action of phosphate is to remineralize the tooth surface which is being attacked by caries. I wonder whether Dr. Baron has considered investigating the effect of combining dical with sodium fluoride. We have some preliminary evidence from work in rats which is not in agreement with Dr. Nizel's observations that sodium phytate in combination with fluoride in the drinking water is synergistic. I think it is something to which we should pay more attention and take cognizance of the fact that more and more people are using fluoridated drinking water. Any agent we examine should be investigated for a possible synergistic effect.

Dr. Baron: I had the idea to put fluoride with dical, for example, in a chewing gum vehicle. As a matter of fact, before the Trail study in British Columbia was initiated, that is exactly what the American Chicle Company was doing. There is a technical problem involved. First, when you are making a 1,500 lb. batch of chewing gum, it is difficult to get a thimble full of sodium fluoride evenly distributed in that batch of gum so that each stick has a comparable amount. Second, many of the constituents in chewing gum contain background amounts of fluoride. When an analysis is made of the chewing gum sticks, the amount of fluoride varies. Third, I would like to consider that sort of product, once the technical difficulties are worked out, as a consumer product. However, a chewing gum with fluoride which is, of course, ingested will probably never be a consumer product. It will be a product promoted to the dental profession to be used on a prescription basis.

Dr. Schiff: Dr. Koulourides has done some studies on enamel slabs which are inserted into partial dentures. He measured the effect of fluoride as well as phosphate and he found some synergism. Some of his data has been published.

Dr. Chilton: Do you feel that the effect on the smooth surfaces in this particular study was from the intrinsic nature of the material which affects smooth surface caries or was it possibly because of the nature of the population? I believe Dr. Backer Dirks presented a chart in one of his papers illustrating how you can show an effect on caries and caries inhibition, depending on the age group which is selected. I wonder whether this was true of the design of the clinical trial.

Dr. Nizel: I did not do the study; it was Dr. Finn's study. One of Finn's conclusions after the study was that the next one should be done with 12- or 14-year-old children, in whom the important effect could take place.

Dr. Navia: I would like to point out something important about the phosphates. The properties of the various phosphates differ tremendously. I think if you look at dicalcium phosphate you think of it as having a certain type of mechanism. When you think about trimetaphosphate you have to consider all of the properties. It is very important in the design of the experiments to realize that these two compounds, though they are included within the generic term phosphates, have very different properties.

In regard to interactions, many years ago Mühlemann and König made tests to find whether there was an interaction between orthophosphate and fluoride, and they found that there was one. When I did my study with TMP and fluoride, there was an additive effect; there was no interaction between the two. We have made extensive studies to discover the mechanism of action of TMP. The more we study the work of Gonzalez, and Fagen and Pruitt, and Caldwell, it seems that the effect of TMP is related primarily to new surfaces and to the capabilities of the particular phosphate to alter the external layers of enamel, perhaps with the dissolution of certain kinds of protein and perhaps with the remineralization effect. The remineralization from trimetaphosphate, if it is present, is a long-term effect. Certainly it is conducive to deposition of very apatitic-like crystals, different from the situation with orthophosphate which leads to a more amorphous type of compound. We must remember, when we talk about phosphates, that there are many different kinds.

Dr. Scala: I think we have identified a point of intervention which can be effective. Dr. Kreitzman and others mentioned the diet surveys which we look at with interest, but which really don't tell us anything until we study them to the point where we conclude that people eat so and so many grams of sugar. That doesn't help us because we don't live as a colony of rats. We eat specific kinds of foods and we have to find those sources of sugar which are, in a sense, hazards to health. I think here we have found a point where intervention can have a definite effect, a positive effect. The findings of the animal studies and the clinical studies seem to confirm one another. Some of the theoretical studies, for example John Gray's work at Procter & Gamble and some of the work at the Forsyth Dental Center by Dr. Moreno, should not be overlooked.

But, again as part of a large food company, I come back to a practical question. What are the points of intervention to which we should address ourselves with regard to phosphates? With the proliferation of sugarless gum on the market, I find it difficult to believe that the only point of intervention will be to neutralize the sugar that is in sugar gum, when we can make perfectly acceptable sugarless gum which does not seem to contribute to the incidence of caries. We have to go beyond that, but the question that I keep asking is, where? My company makes a greater number of beverages and certainly the work of Gray, and some of the *in vivo* work that we have confirmed in our own laboratory, raise the questions: Where should we start adding the phosphate? Should we start adding it? Is it sufficiently accepted? Will we have enough information to start doing some of these things?

Dr. Baron: As for sugarless gum, we have the problem licked. However, only 20% of the chewing gum market is sugarless. If sugarless gum is so great, why aren't all people chewing it? There are organoleptic properties of sugar gum that are desirable and people are going to continue to chew it.

Dr. Scala: My question is: what other sources, or what other points of intervention, should be considered? I think the gum issue seems to be fairly well established. Granted the organoleptic properties are probably very important; also I assume that the FDA is a problem. Someone, somehow, somewhere, some day, must say yes, that a formulation is noncariogenic. Then I think marketing and organoleptic qualities will take over and it will become more widely used. However, gum chewing certainly does not account for much of the tooth decay in the United States. Sugar gum must account for some, according to the studies. I don't know how much, but as Dr. Schiff said, each little step has to count.

Dr. DePaola: The question is difficult — if not impossible — to answer at this time because first you have to establish the cariogenicity of a product. I am not sure whether at this point you can with certainty establish any particular food as being cariogenic. You have to establish which foods are cariogenic before you can make decisions on interventions. I think we are a long way from that right now.

Mr. Khan: One of the questions that we must ask ourselves is how we will reconcile the intervention against dental caries with phosphates and phytate and at the same time answer the criticisms we are already getting from people in pediatrics and geriatrics who are concerned about the intake of phosphates and phytate because of their interference with mineral metabolism

Dr. Kent Stewart: I would like to reinforce that and also insert a note of caution. People are concerned with trace minerals in connection with metabolism. The presence of metaphosphates or phytates interferes with zinc metabolism and iron metabolism, both of which are subjects of considerable concern in the United States nutrition policy. The addition of higher levels of phosphates interferes with calcium metabolism and may cause osteoporosis. Be careful that you don't cure one nutritional disease and initiate two more.

Dr. Vandercook: My research has not been in the area of dental caries, but I gather that there is a great lack of analytical methodology. I think a lot of people in the food industry, food technologists, food scientists and people in government, would like to be able to formulate their products. Not being dentists, there is not much they can do about it until proper analytical methods are available.

Dr. Bibby: As to the point of intervention, it could be answered in two ways. As a dentist, I tend to look at it as the point in the natural history of the caries process in which it is most effective to have the treatment agent. The teeth are most responsive to protective factors when they are young and freshly erupted. So, obviously, if we can get people to use the product at that time, we will have the best result. The other possibility is somewhat remote. I understand, for instance, chewing gum is not used much by the elderly. It is used mainly by adolescents and maybe that would make them the best subjects for some selected placement of the protective agent. If adolescents would use one type of cariogenic food for more than six months, we could probably solve the problem.

Dr. Bollenback: May the difference in results from phosphates be caused in part by trace mineral impurities in the various phosphates?

Dr. Schiff: Most of the phosphates as they are manufactured today have a very controlled trace mineral background. It would be extremely simple today to ask what trace minerals exist in both phosphates and trace it back. I honestly don't believe it.

Dr. Bollenback: Is it possible that the wetting properties of phosphate may have something to do with caries reduction?

Mr. Jorgensen: I don't really believe phosphate salts are considered surface active agents.

XYLITOL

Kauko K. Mäkinen, Ph.D.

The purpose of this article is to review the various products in which xylitol has been substituted for sucrose, and to discuss data that support the reduction in the cariogenicity of that food while maintaining good food characteristics. The term "food" used in this context includes traditional foodstuffs, beverages, candy and chewing gum.

Properties of Xylitol in Relation to Food Manufacture

The properties of xylitol which make it suitable for sucrose substitution include its sweetening power (which equals that of sucrose), nonfermentability in the human dental plaque, regular metabolism in the human body, good solubility in water (179.3 per 100 g water at 25°C), nontoxicity in human use, organoleptic properties, and relatively good suitability for food manufacturing processes.

A particular property of sugar alcohols (xylitol, sorbitol, mannitol, dulcitol, etc.) which is of interest is that they are not subject to the browning reaction (Millard reaction). This reaction occurs when a sugar which carries a reducing carbonyl group, R-CO-R′, is heated together with amino acids or proteins to temperatures of 90 to 120°C. The characteristic caramel taste of brown toffee and the brownish crust of pastry, for example, are results of this heating reaction. Although the lack of xylitol participation in the Maillard reaction may to some extent impair the appearance of certain products, this same property also makes xylitol chemically more stable in food processing and storage of food, and hence may be viewed as a property of major importance.

In addition to the almost absolute inability of human oral microorganisms to metabolize xylitol, those that are often harmful in food manufacture or storage are generally not able to attack xylitol either.

Xylitol is slightly hygroscopic; this sets particular requirements with regard to moisture control during processing and storage of certain xylitol products. Another property of xylitol which is an important difference in relation to sucrose lies in the characteristics of xylitol as a solid substance: xylitol is not known to exist in an amorphous state under usual food technological conditions. Its crystallization properties are different from those of sucrose. The seeding tendency of xylitol differs from that of sucrose and the speed of crystallization of xylitol is higher. In the confectionery industry it is sometimes necessary to boil down sucrose solutions (in the manufacture of jellies, jams, etc.). The evaporation of water takes place differently in the case of xylitol.

Application technology of xylitol is relatively young, but recent progress has been rapid. The literature available already lists a large number of xylitol formulas and recipes for candies, jams, chewing gums, bakery products, other foods, toothpastes, mouth rinses and sweetening tablets. The need for the development of such products for use in diabetic nutrition already has been recognized in certain countries. This use is based on xylitol's minimal effects on insulin secretion and blood sugar fluctuation and on the insulin-independent utilization of xylitol at the first stages of its metabolism in the organism. The use of xylitol as energy substrate in parenteral nutrition is also indicated in certain other clinical situations[1]. The technological application of xylitol in various products has been reviewed by Kracher[2] and other pertinent information was given by Kammerer[3-5]. Table 1 lists some properties of xylitol important in nutrition in food manufacture.

Xylitol Products of the Turku Sugar Study

For the Turku sugar studies[6], the intention was to create as versatile an assortment of food as possible by taking into account the national nutritional habits in Finland and the stage of the technological preparedness existing during the years 1972-1974. Altogether, 12 food and candy factories were involved in the study. In many instances the xylitol and fructose products were made by hand on a small scale, but in the manufacture of soft drinks, ice cream, pastry, chewing gums and many other products normal production lines could be utilized. Table 2 lists all xylitol products used during the feeding study either made by these factories for distribution from the "sugar shop" of the study, or by the subjects themselves at home.

Virtually all xylitol products listed in Table 1 were acceptable for human use with regard to taste, appearance and general properties, and interviews with the subjects revealed no discontent regarding these products. Aversion was not found in any case. Perhaps a suitable proof for this is the rather high xylitol consumption by most subjects throughout the entire two-year study period.[6] The average consumption of xylitol per day and subject was approximately 70 g. Although this dose did not cause any detectable side effects in the majority of subjects, some subjects had transient osmotic diarrhea during the first days or weeks of the study. Exceptionally high doses (200-430 g per day and subject), however, more frequently caused diarrhea or flatulence even at later phases of the study. A number of subjects have continued regular and controlled consumption of xylitol since the termination of the actual feeding study. After five years' consumption, no detectable side effects have been found in these subjects who also include young children.

According to the experience obtained in the feeding study, certain xylitol-sweetened products organoleptically exceeded or equaled the corresponding sucrose-sweetened ones. These included, for example, chewing gum, chocolate, ice cream, pastilles, lozenges, certain canned food and several bakery products. In most cases it was not possible to detect any significant differences between xylitol- or sucrose-sweetened food.

The complex and varied dietary regimen involved in the aforementioned feeding study is naturally unrealistic when considering the needs of normal subjects. The nontoxicity of peroral xylitol in humans and the fact that quite acceptable and appealing food can be prepared from xylitol as the sweetening agent or source of calories may, however, be important when considering the dietary arrangements in special clinical cases.

TABLE 1. Certain properties of xylitol which are important in nutrition and food manufacture.

1. The solubility of xylitol is good (179.3 g/100 g H_2O; 25°C)
2. Xylitol does not participate in the Maillard reaction (browning reaction)
3. The sweetening power equals that of sucrose
4. Xylitol is a natural product
5. Xylitol is normally metabolized in the body
6. The safety of oral xylitol is indisputable
7. Xylitol is not fermented by the human dental plaque
8. Xylitol is easily suited for food manufacturing processes

"Utility Index" of Xylitol Products

Casual consideration may not immediately reveal the utility value of various xylitol-sweetened products for use by normal subjects with regular incidence of dental caries. It may be assumed that while certain products may be of great value in this sense, others do not provide any noticeable benefit, if all possible criteria are used to evaluate such articles. Some products are very suitable, while some are not. Consequently by scrutinizing and evaluating the properties of various xylitol products, one may create, just for illustrative purposes, a particular "Utility Index" for such products. Table 3 describes such criteria which are here used to evaluate the utility and rationality of xylitol-containing articles consumed for the purpose of modifying the cariogenicity of food in normal subjects who have dental caries as a problem. The criteria and the "Index" are thus not directly applicable to diabetics, as these subjects differ to a certain extent from others in metabolism and vulnerability as regards infections. However, xylitol would provide a valuable alternative for diabetics as well. For the sake of simplicity, only articles used in connection with the Turku sugar studies were considered in the evaluation of the xylitol products.

In its simplest form the "Index" would have a maximum of ten points, corresponding to the ten objects of appraisal listed in Table 3. A score of ten would result from ten positive or advantageous properties of the product involved. In a more detailed evaluation, all important properties and aspects would be separately scored, whereby the slightly higher hygroscopicity, and more ready crystallization of xylitol, compared with sucrose, also would be evaluated. For the present purpose, it is sufficient, however, to apply the maximum of ten points and to compare the scores thus obtained with the relative cariogenicity of corresponding sucrose products (Fig. 1). In the determination of the cariogenicity of sucrose-containing food, the experience gathered in several clinical trials was exploited: Vipeholm study[7], Turku sugar studies[6], and the data of Bibby[8]. Naturally, this method suffers from a degree of subjectivity. If food modification is regarded as necessary or desirable in reducing the incidence of dental caries, however, the results shown in Fig. 1 suggest that it would be appropriate to consider substitution of sucrose for

TABLE 2. List of xylitol-containing products made in connection with the Turku feeding studies in 1972-1974.

Product	Content of xylitol (in weight per cent)
I. Industrial products	
A. Pastry	
1. Viennese rolls — of varying appearance and containing varying filling and toppings	8.0
2. Sweet rolls and bone — of varying appearance and containing varying filling and toppings	10.0
3. Sweet loaves — of varying appearance and containing varying filling and toppings	8.0
4. Doughnuts (filled with jam; frosted)	13.0
5. Sweet biscuits (cookies; oat meal or wheat meal)	18.0-21.3
6. Jam-filled shortcakes, pies, etc. (orange, apple, strawberry, Lingonberry, blueberry; with or without glazing, frosting or toppings; 8-10 different types)	10.0-22.0
7. Waffles (wafers) (filled with strawberry, lemon or banana)	33.1
8. Muffins	18.0
9. Chocolate cake	30.0
10. Miscellaneous cakes (layer cakes; 4-5 types)	20.0-24.0
11. Various national dishes (made for special festive days, holidays, memorial days, etc., e.g., Christmas, Easter, Shrove Tuesday, May Day, etc., including Finnish specialties such as "mammi," "tippaleivät," "laskiaispulla," "Runebergin torttu," etc.)	10.0-22.0
The assortment of pastry ranged from 30 to 35 items during the 2-year feeding study	
B. Confections	
1. Chocolate bars and slaps (4-5 different flavors)	30.0-43.0
2. Chocolate-covered candy marmalade	45.0
3. Lozenges (gum pastilles; licorice- and tar-flavored; several types)	33.0-58.5
4. Candies (flavored in various ways; several types including compressed tablets	43.0-100.0
6. Chocolate with jam fillings	43.0
7. Chewing gum (3 different types)	49.0-74.0
C. Jams, marmalades and juices, soft drinks	
1. Orange marmalade	60.0
2. Apple marmalade	60.0
3. Strawberry jam	50.0
4. Lingonberry jam	50.0
5. Concentrated orange juice	50.0
6. Concentrated black currant juice	53.0
7. Soft drinks (including several types containing lemon, orange or grapefruit; Coca Cola and non-carbonated drink)	10.0-11.0

xylitol in certain foods. One may easily arrive at the same result as shown in Fig. 1 by the application of common sense, and this is just as it should be. Table 3 indicates, however, that so many factors determine the rationality or irrationality of a particular xylitol material that the result of intuitive reasoning may not necessarily be correct. If, in addition, some bias is involved, the result is more likely to be erroneous.

TABLE 2. (Continued)

Product	Content of xylitol (in weight per cent)
D. Canned food	
1. Cucumber (sliced or whole; in xylitol syrup)	2.4
2. Red beet (whole; in xylitol syrup)	21.5
3. Pickled pumkin (cut into pieces, in xylitol syrup)	19.8
4. Cucumber relish	5.0
5. Herring (marinated and spice with tomato sauce, wine sauce, ets; five different brands)	48.0
E. Other products	
1. Tomato ketchup	17.5
2. Mustard	21.0
3. Ice Cream (three different flavors)	12.0
4. Cough Mixture	60.0
5. Tonic Containing iron, liver and vitamins	30.0
F. Xylitol in consumer packages	100.0
II. Homemade products	
1. Salad dressing	
2. Various baked dishes	
3. Pastry (in general as in A)	
4. Porridges, puddings	
5. National drinks (including a Finnish specialty "sima," mead)	
6. Alcoholic beverages	
7. Confections (marmalade, candy, etc.)	

A proper example of the latter possibility is a toothpaste containing xylitol. Sugar alcohols, chiefly sorbitol, have been widely used as humectants in toothpastes. It contributes simultaneously to the final texture, sweetness and preservative properties of the product. Some toothpaste brands have contained sorbitol in amounts up to 20 or 30% and even more of the dry matter. When xylitol became commercially available in the present quantities, certain manufacturers started the production of xylitol-containing toothpastes. It is not permissible to present strong dental claims for such toothpastes on the basis of the Turku sugar studies (a sorbitol-containing brand was used as the only toothpaste in that study). Some scientists have, however, upon hearing the Turku xylitol results for the first time, regarded a xylitol-containing toothpaste invaluable from the dental point of view. This idea deserves careful analysis. A toothpaste containing no fermentable carbohydrates may be considered better, from the dental and bacteriophysiological points of view, than one containing a fermentable carbohydrate, *viz,* sorbitol. If a subject brushes his teeth regularly twice a day over a five-year period, the total brushing times add up to 3,650. Even one-minute brushing leaves certain long-lasting chemical effects in the oral cavity. In the case of sorbitol, which is fermented to some extent, it may be assumed that quantitatively much more acid would be formed in

TABLE 3. Criteria for evaluation of the "Utility Index" of various xylitol-containing prducts for the use of normal subjects with regular caries incidence. Comparison of properties of xylitol and sucrose in products used in the Turku feeding studies.

	Object of appraisal	Aspects involved
1.	Physical suitability for techno-chemical processes in food manufacture	Hygroscopicity, easy crystallization, absence of "glass-like" state, etc., may create problems with xylitol.
2.	Organoleptic properties (taste, odor, etc.)	Cooling effect may create pleasant sensations. High sweetness is a positive property.
3.	Compatibility with other diets	Simultaneous consumption of high amounts of xylitol and ethanol, for example, may not be advisable.
4.	Compatibility with other ingredients of the xylitol product concerned	It may be advantageous or disadvantageous if xylitol takes part in chemical reaction such as the Maillard reaction. Generally, inert chemical behavior may be an advantage.
5.	Dental acceptability and rationality (is the dose high enough for positive effects on teeth?)	Nonfermentability by dental plaque indicates a positive property. Additional benefit if it does not irritate oral tissues or if it stimulates salivary flow.
6.	Appearance of side effects (the magnitude of the dose has to be critically considered when evaluating this)	Appearance of osmotic diarrhea may be a negative property.
7.	Storage and shelf life	Nonfermentability by most microorganisms that normally deteriorate food is a positive property.
8.	Price per each lot of xylitol consumed in the form of a product	A bottle of xylitol-sweetened soft drink, for example, is an expensive dose with regard to the proposed effects xylitol has been claimed to exert on teeth. A chicle or pastilles may have more advantages in relation to this appraisal.
9.	Opportunities for unnecessarily frequent use of the xylitol products	For example, it may be expected and normal if ten chicles or 4-5 oz. of chocolate are consumed per day and subject, but it may not be equally assumable that several mustard tubes would be used daily. It would thus be a disadvantageous property of the xylitol product if there are constant chances for the consumption of unnecessarily high amounts of xylitol. Furthermore, in a soft drink sweetened with xylitol only, the daily dose of xylitol may reach undesirably high levels.
10.	Appearance and general properties of the product	It may be generally advantageous if the products can be made to resemble "normal" sucrose-containing ones and if it meets other requirements normally set for a foodstuff in human use.

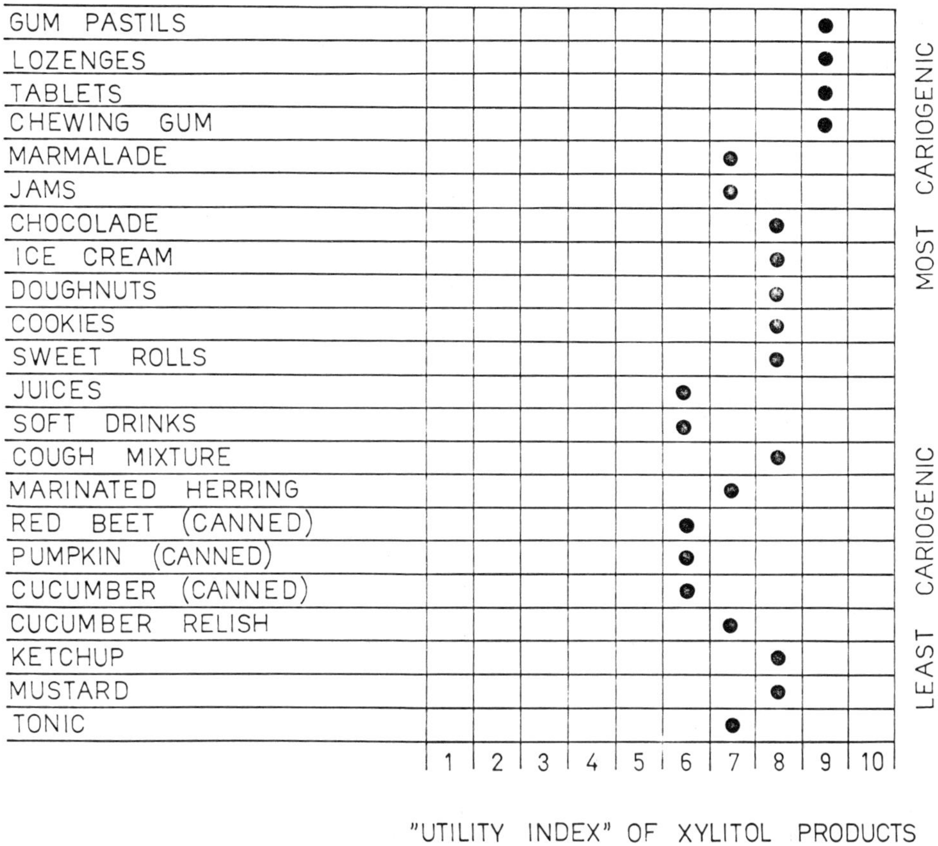

FIGURE 1. Relative cariogenicity of sucrose products used in the Turku feeding studies[6] plotted versus the "Utility Index" of corresponding xylitol-containing products. In the evaluation of the relative cariogenicity, the concentration of sucrose and the frequency of consumption of sucrose-containing food were taken into account. The index was based on criteria described in Table 3 and the text. According to this ranking, the best xylitol products, for the use of normal subjects, would be various pastilles, chewing gum, etc., provided that the other ingredients are not cariogenic.

plaque than would be the case if the paste contained an essentially inert carbohydrate. The coin has its other side too; use of toothpaste, no matter what polyol it contains, initiates salivary flow, with a concomitant increase of all defensive factors of saliva (the flow, itself, is such a factor). Furthermore, sorbitol is not fermented by all oral bacteria, and brushing itself removes part of the plaque. Rinsing removed the largest part of sorbitol from the mouth. What remains after these considerations is: (1) the bacteriophysiological fact: sorbitol is metabolized by plaque bacteria, whereas xylitol is fermented only very rarely; and (2) the clinical fact: xylitol has been shown in clinical trials carried out on both animals and humans to have more advantageous effects than sorbitol. During prolonged and regular use of toothpaste, differences between xylitol and sorbitol may be detectable. The potency of a xylitol toothpaste would be more evident if the mineralization-facilitating qualities of peroral xylitol were to be verified and accepted. A preliminary clinical trial on toothpastes carried out by Dr. Laikko in the Turku Institute suggests that such toothpastes actually do differ from one another with regard to the tooth-cleansing abilities. It is natural that occasional use of xylitol- or sorbitol-containing pastes revealed no differences.

Figure 1 does not include toothpaste or related oral hygiene articles, as they were not tested in the Turku sugar studies. The toothpaste example here merely suggests that before an idea is stifled in its infancy, it should be tested.

Xylitol Products in General

Both the Turku feeding study and other technological experiments have shown clearly that xylitol is suitable for virtually all human food. The addition of xylitol did not impair, and often actually enhanced, the characteristic appeal and acceptability of foodstuffs. The following list describes additional aspects of certain xylitol-containing products.

1. Confections: Xylitol can be used in chewing gums with no difficulty if a few factors such as the relative humidity of air and the grain size of xylitol are controlled. The strongly endothermic reaction when crystalline xylitol dissolves in saliva creates a pleasant cooling effect in the mouth (heat of solution for xylitol is 36.61 cal g^{-1} and for sucrose 4.34 cal g^{-1}). The duration of the sweet taste in chewing gums sweetened either with sucrose or xylitol is approximately the same.

   Chocolate poses no greater problems for the replacement of sucrose with xylitol. A comparison of xylitol chocolate with a product containing sucrose shows only small differences as regards taste and texture. Repeated interviews during the course of the Turku sugar studies showed that xylitol chocolate was considered delicate and "less fatty" than sucrose chocolate. The latter property reflected slight changes in the texture of chocolate sweetened with xylitol.

   Tablets (compressed products) can be made easily from xylitol. The tablet-forming substances have included stearates and deodorized, high-melting point, fat powder.

   Gum products can be made with xylitol with no noticable modifications. The gum-based materials indicated here include gum arabic and certain hydrolysis products of starch.

   Very appealing toffee products can be obtained by the use of xylitol without major difficulties, taking into consideration, of course, the absence of the Maillard reaction and caramelizing when using xylitol. The necessary flavor can be achieved by addition of aromas or a certain minimal amount of sugars (e.g., fructose) which undergo the Maillard reaction.

It is also possible at present to make hard boiled sweets comprised of virtually 100% xylitol. This is possible, despite the absence of the glass-like state of xylitol, by applying the ready crystallization properties of xylitol. The products are quite acceptable and their suckable characteristics compare favorably with corresponding sucrose candies. The cooling effect of such hard-boiled xylitol sweets also is pronounced and may be used to advantage with various flavors and aromas.

2. Products with High Water Content: The similar solubility of xylitol and sucrose is one reason why products such as soft drinks, liqueurs, and concentrated juices are easy to prepare from xylitol. Other similar properties are sweetness and taste. As a matter of fact, xylitol may possess some advantages over sucrose in the manufacture of these products: heating does not cause caramelizing and the product is resistant to microorganisms. The lower molecular weight of xylitol (152) compared with that of sucrose (342) makes xylitol solutions less viscous and gives them a higher osmotic pressure. Unlike sucrose, xylitol does not undergo inversion in an aqueous solution. All these properties are technically important. They would pertain particularly, for example, to milk products containing xylitol, such as sweetened condensed milk or sweetened milk beverages and milk mixture drinks. From the dental point of view, however, there is far less rationale for use of this type of xylitol product by normal consumers than, for example, confections.

3. Bakery products: Sweet yeast dough, biscuit dough and shortbread dough can be made with xylitol with no alterations in the recipe. The degree of browning is less than with corresponding sucrose or fructose products. Xylitol pastry, however, has certain compensating properties: The taste is pleasant and the shelf-life properties are better as a result of increased water-binding capacity. Xylitol also is suitable for butter dough and cakes. Because baker's yeast does not ferment xylitol, sodium bicarbonate can be used to raise the dough.

   Ice cream and other frozen products can in principle be produced by simple replacement of sucrose or glucose with xylitol. The melting properties of xylitol-containing ice cream are altered, however. Xylitol ice cream is softer and smoother than sucrose products, and its melting point is lower. This property should not be regarded as disadvantageous. On the contrary, xylitol ice cream has the advantage that it can be consumed immediately on removal from the deep freeze. Ice cream made for the Turku sugar study was stored for more than one year at temperatures close to −20°C. No significant changes occurred during this storage and there was no crystallization or "graininess" in the ice cream.

4. Other products: Xylitol can be used in yogurt, jelly products, sugar-coated preserves, marinades, sauces and pastes. In some cases the method outlined for sucrose, glucose or invert sugar is not applicable with xylitol, but modified versions have been developed. In general, although all recipes and methods have not yet been refined to give optimum results with xylitol, countless foods and beverages can be produced at present with favorable and often superior results.

Data Supporting Xylitol-associated Reduction of Cariogenicity

Numerous *in vitro* studies have been carried out with plaque and oral microorganisms which indicate the non-cariogenicity of xylitol in humans and experimental animals. These *in vitro* studies naturally indicate the non-cariogenicity only indirectly, but as the number of such studies is very great, the overall information obtained can be regarded as a proof of the advantageous dental properties of xylitol. In addition to the foregoing experiments, long-term *in vivo* clinical trials with human subjects have also been carried out. Virtually all published xylitol studies, with information regarding a few other pertinent unpublished investigations which describe the effects of xylitol in the oral environment, are listed in Table 4. Special reference can be made to the Turku studies[6] which clearly showed that the consumption of a xylitol diet for two years caused little or no caries compared with caries caused when a sucrose diet was consumed. In planning of further human clinical trials with xylitol, the following aspects should be considered:

1. The physiological, microbiological and physicochemical mechanisms of xylitol action are largely known. Accordingly, xylitol should not be considered a "miracle sweetener" or panacea. It is most effective when consumed regularly between meals, preferably several times a day in forms indicated below.
2. Perhaps the preferable administration of xylitol is in the form of products which promote simultaneous mastication or sucking.
3. For dental purposes, xylitol ideally should be used immediately after the exposure of the teeth to sucrose. Xylitol will not have any noticeable effects if it is consumed simultaneously with high amounts of sucrose.
4. Clinical trials should be carried out on subjects who have had dental caries as a regular problem.

TABLE 4. List of important observations in relation to xylitol made in dental studies on animals and humans. The list also notes other pertinent investigations on sugar alcohols.

	Study or result	Reference No.
1.	Sorbitol was attacked by adaptive enzymes and it was slowly fermented by oral microorganisms	9-12
2.	Acid production from sorbitol may increase in time in the oral cavity	13, 14
3.	Sorbitol was considered slightly cariogenic in rats and hamsters	15-20
4.	Marked increase in the capacity of plaque to produce acid from sorbitol was found during 2- or 6-month periods of sucrose consumption	21
5.	*Streptococcus mutans* was able to ferment sorbitol and mannitol. This property has been routinely used to distinguish mutans from other homolactic oral streptococci	22-24
6.	With a manometric technique, human saliva and plaque were shown to degrade sorbitol at a somewhat slower, but constant and continuous rate	25, 26
7.	No critical pH reduction after rinses with 10% xylitol solutions was obtained in man	27
8.	Metabolism of xylitol in certain rat and hamster microorgan isms was lower than that of mannitol or sorbitol	28
9.	Certain enterococcus strains, a micrococcus strain, and a strain *S. mutans* metabolized sorbitol at a clearly detectable rate	29
10.	Of several sugars or sugar mixtures, including sorbitol and xylitol, only xylitol strongly reduced (by 50%) the quantity of human dental plaque during 4- or 5-day periods of neglected oral hygiene	30, 31
11.	Xylitol-containing chewing gum was able in short-term studies to reduce the amount of dental plaque by 30-55%, in spite of neglect of oral hygiene	32-34
12.	In a 2-year feeding study (Turku sugar study) involving almost complete substitution of dietary sucrose with xylitol, the amount of dental plaque in the xylitol group was maintained at a 50% lower level throughout the study when compared to level maintained with sucrose consumption. Xylitol reduced the incidence of caries by 90% and it decreased the acidogenic and aciduric oral flora (fructose reduced the caries incidence by 30%)	6, 35-37
13.	*In vitro* experiments showed that xylitol retarded the growth of the cells of *S. mutans* in a liquid medium more effectively than sorbitol	38, 39
14.	Isotopically labeled xylitol was not bound to human dental plaque to any significant extent, whereas sorbitol and mannitol were bound	40, 41
15.	In an *in vitro* experiment of 10 months, no evidence was obtained of a possible adaptationof *S. mutans* to metabolize xylitol (more recent findings indicate that no such phenomenon was detected even after 18 months)	42
16.	The cells of three oral strains of *Candida* were not shown to use xylitol for growth	43

17.	No evidence has been obtained of the involvement in plaque of microorganisms capable of decomposing xylitol. Such strains have been occasionally described in other reports, however, but they are rare and acid production from xylitol is insignificant	44-46
18.	10 or 20% xylitol in the diet greatly reduced streptococci in microbiological samples of rat molars	47
19.	Human clinical trials demonstrated no great reduction in the incidence of dental caries as a result of the use of a sorbitol-containing chewing gum	48
20.	The use of sorbitol-containing chewing gum did not increase or decrease the normal growth of dental plaque	49
21.	Animal experiments showed the noncariogenicity of xylitol	50, 51
22.	The use of a xylitol-containing chewing gum over a 12-month period reduced the incidence of caries by 90% when compared with that obtained with sucrose-containing chewing gum. No bacterial adaptation to utilize xylitol was observed.	37, 52
23.	Of several sugars, including sorbitol, tested in an artificial mouth system, only xylitol and xylose were considered noncariogenic	53
24.	Radiotelemetric pH recordings of interdental plaque areas revealed a moderate acid formation from sorbitol with a pH value of 6 or higher. In contrast, xylitol caused no drop of the pH at all and can thus be approved as nonacidogenic	54, 55
25.	*Acinomyces viscosus* and *S. mutans* did not ferment or utilize xylitol	56, 68
26.	Xylitol prevented the sucrose-induced acid formation in plaque suspension more effectively than sorbitol even in the simultaneous presence of sucrose when the sugars were tested at a fairly low 0.7% concentration	57
27.	Xylitol most likely interferes with the production of plaque polysaccharides, producing a less acidogenic community of microorganisms on the tooth surface	58
28.	In a feeding study on rats xylitol caused lower caries incidence than sucrose/starch mixtures	59
29.	An experiment with water, xylitol and sucrose rinses showed that xylitol produced the highest pH values in whole saliva immediately after rinse	60
30.	Approximately 200 bacterial strains divided over ten oral species were studied in the presence of various carbohydrates. None of the strains could ferment xylitol	61
31.	30% xylitol diet was shown to be noncariogenic in rats	62
32.	Telemetric recordings of interdental plaque showed that 10% xylitol rinses and xylitol chewing gum were nonacidogenic	63
33.	Sorbitol-chewing gum group showed approximately 10% lower caries incidence compared with control group	64
34.	The noncariogenic nature of xylitol, compared with sorbitol, fructose and sucrose, was demonstrated in a rat feeding study	65
35.	The lower cariogenicity of xylitol, compared with sucrose and sorbose, was shown in a rat experiment.	6
36.	Continuous consumption of xylitol over a period of 3.2-4.5 years showed no microbial adaptation concerning its use by bacteria for acid production in dental plaque	67

REFERENCES

1. Mäkinen, K.K. Experientia, Suppl. 30, 1978. In press.
2. Kracher, F. Kakao + Zuker, 27:68-75, 1975
3. Kammerer, F.X. Dtxch. Zahärztl. Z. 26:1056-1062, 1971
4. Kammerer, F.X. Kakao + Zucker, 24:184, 1972.
5. Kammerer, F.X. Süsswaren 16:22, 1972.
6. Scheinin, A. and Mäkinen, K.K. Acta Odont. Scand. 33:Suppl. 70, 1975.
7. Gustafsson, B.E., Quensel, C.-E., Swenander Lanke, L., Lundquist, C., Grahnén, H., Bonow, B. and Krasse, B. Acta Odont. Scand. 11:232, 1953.
8. Bibby, B.G. J. Amer. Dent. Assoc. 90:121-132, 1975.
9. Grub, I.C. J. Dent. Res. 24:31-44, 1945.
10. Shay, D.E. J. Dent. Res. 33:717, 1954.
11. Shockley, T.E., Randels, C.I. and Dodd, M.C. J. Dent. Res. 35:233-240, 1956.
12. Crowley, M.C., Harner, V., Bennet, A.S. and Jay, P.J. Amer. Dent. Assoc. 52:148-154, 1956.
13. Frostell, G. Acta Odont. Scand. 22:457-475, 1964.
14. Gulzov, H.-J. Vergleichende biochemische Untersuchungen über den Abbau des Sorbit durch Mikroorganismen der Mundhöhle. Munich, Hancer Verlag, 1968.
15. Klapper, C.E. and Voler, J.F. J. Dent. Res. 33:666, 1954.
16. Shaw, J.H. and Griffiths, D.J. Dent. Res. 39:377-384, 1960.
17. Frostell, G. *in* Nutrition and Caries Prevention, p. 60. Stockholm, Almquist and Wiksell, 1965.
18. Mühlemann, H.R., Regolati, B. and Marthaler, T.M. Helv. Odont. Acta 14:48-50, 1970.
19. Larje, O. and Larson, R.H. Arch. Oral Biol. 15:805-816, 1970.
20. Böhmer, U., Kater, H.J., Schneider, P. -Th., Welzbacher, H. and Buttner, W. J. Dent. Res. 50:752-753, 1971.
21. Frostell, G. *in* Nutrition and Caries Prevention, p. 60, Stockholm, Almquist and Wiksell, 1965.
22. Fitzgerald, R.J. and Keyes, P.H. J. Amer. Dent. Assoc. 61:9-19, 1960.
23. Edwardsson, S. Arch. Oral Biol. 13:637-646, 1968.
24. Guggenheim, B. Caries Res. 2:147-163, 1968.
25. Gülzov, H.-J. Dtsch. Zahnärtzl. Z. 26:1121-1128, 1971.
26. Gülzov, H.-J. Internat. J. Vit. Nutr. Res. (Suppl.) 15:348-357, 1976.
27. Hassel, Th. M. Dtsch. Zahnärtzl. Z. 26:1145-1154, 1971.
28. Gehring, F. Dtsch. Zahnärtzl. Z. 28:769, 1974.
29. Gehring, F. and Patz, J. Dtsch. Zahnärtzl. 29:1026-1029, 1974.
30. Scheinin, A. and Mäkinen, K.K. Int. Dent. J. 21:302-321, 1971.
31. Scheinin, A. and Mäkinen, K.K. Acta Odont. Scand. 30:235-257, 1972.
32. Mouton, C., Scheinin, A. and Mäkinen, K.K. Acta Odont. Scand. 33:27-31, 1975.
33. Mouton C., Scheinin, A. and Mäkinen, K.K. Acta Odont. Scand. 33:33-40, 1975.
34. Mouton C., Scheinin, A. and Mäkinen, K.K. Acta Odont. Scand. 33:251-257, 1975.
35. Mäkinen, K.K. and Scheinin, A. Acta Odont. Scand. 32:413-421, 1974.
36. Larmas, M., Mäkinen, K.K. and Scheinin, A. Acta Odont. (Suppl. 70):173-216, 1975.
37. Larmas, M., Scheinin, A., Gehring, F. and Mäkinen, K.K. Acta Odont. Scand. 33 (Suppl. 70):321-336, 1975.
38. Mäkinen, K.K. J. Dent. Res. 51:403-408, 1972.
39. Mäkinen, K.K. and Scheinin, A. Acta Odont. Scand. 30:259-275, 1972.
40. Mäkinen, K.K. and Rekola, M. J. Dent. Res. 55:900-904, 1976.
41. Mäkinen, K.K. Proceedings "Microbial Aspects of Dental Caries." Stiles, H.M., Loesche, W.J. and O'Brien, T.C.O. eds. Sp. Suppl. Microbiology Abstracts, Vol II:521-538, 1976.
42. Knuuttila, M.L.E. and Mäkinen, K.K. Caries Res. 9:177-189, 1975.
43. Mäkinen, K.K., Ojanotko, A. and Vidgren, H. J. Dent. Res. 54:1239, 1975.
44. Karle, E. and Gehring, F. 11th Session of Internat. Assoc. of Dental Res. (Central Eur. Div.) Abstract No. 2, 1974.
45. Karle, E. and Gehring, F. Dtsch. Zahnärtzl. Z. 30:356-363, 1975.
46. Gehring, F. Dtsch. Zahnärtzl. Z. 26:1162-1171, 1971.
47. Narkates, A.J., Navia, J.M. and Bates, D. 54th Session of Internat. Assoc. of Dental Res. Abstract No. 455, 1976.
48. Møller, I.J. and Poulsen, S. Community Dent. Oral Epidemiol. 1:58-67, 1973.

49. Ainamo, J., Sjöblom, M., Talari, A. and Tiainen, L.J. Clin. Periodont. In press.
50. Karle, E. and Büttner, W. Dtsch. Zahnärztl. Z. 26:1097-1108, 1971.
51. Grunberg, E., Beskid, G. and Brin, M. Intemat. J. Vit. Nutr. Res. 43:227-232, 1973.
52. Scheinin, A., Makinen, K.K., Tammisalo, E. and Rekola, M. Acta Odont. Scand. 33:269-278, 1975.
53. Koulourides, T., Bodden, R., Keller, S., Manson-Hing, L., Lastra, J. and Housch, T. Caries Res. 10:427-441, 1976.
54. Hassel, Th. M. Dtsch. Zahnärtzl. Z. 26:1145, 1971.
55. Schneider, P. and Mühlemann, H. Schweiz. Mschr. Zahnheilk. 86:150, 1976.
56. Noguchi, T. and Mühlemann, H. Helv. Odont. Acta 20:45, 1976.
57. Plüss, E.M. J. Clin. Periodont. In press.
58. Wood, J.M. Unpublished results, 1976.
59. Green, R.M. and Leach, S.A. 55th Session of Internat. Assoc. Dental Res. Abstract No. 207, 1977.
60. Mäkinen, K.K. and Mäkinen, P.-L. 24th ORCA Congress Abstracts, p. 83, 1977.
61. Havenaar, R., Huis in 't Veld, J.H.J., Backer Dirks, O. and de Stoppelaar, J.D. 24th ORCA Congress Abstracts, 84, 1977.
62. Moll, R. and Büttner, W. 24th ORCA Congress Abstracts, 86, 1977.
63. Mühlemann, H.R., Schmidt, R., Noguchi, T., Infeld, Th. and Hirsch, R.S. 24th ORCA Congress Abstracts, 87, 1977.
64. Møller, I.J. Dtsch. Zahnärztl. Z. 32:66-70, 1977.
65. Karle, E.J. Dtsch. Zahnärztl. Z. 32:89-95, 1977.
66. Battelle-Institut report, Battelle-Institut e. V., Frankfurt am Main, 1977.
67. Mäkinen, K.K. and Virtanen, K. To be published.
68. Mühlemann, H.R., Schmidt, R., Noguchi, T., Infeld, Th. and Hirsch, R.S. Caries Res. 11:263-276, 1977.

OTHER SUGAR ALCOHOLS AS SUCROSE SUBSTITUTES

Albert T. Brown, Ph.D.

Of central importance in the etiology of dental caries is the metabolism of dietary carbohydrates by the plaque microflora. Microbial accumulation on oral hard surfaces leads to the production of bacterial products, particularly organic acids, which collectively demineralize oral hard tissue.

Sucrose has been implicated as a causative agent of dental caries more than any other dietary carbohydrate. The reason for this may be that sucrose contributes directly to the three biological determinants of plaque formation—adherence, aggregation, and growth. For example, sucrose contributes to the processes of adherence and aggregation by serving as a precursor of glucan synthesis via the action of glucosyltransferase enzymes. It contributes to growth by serving as a substrate for energy yielding glycolytic metabolism which serves to sustain life functions of oral bacteria and results in the production of the organic acids generally thought, at least in part, to be responsible for the demineralization of oral hard tissues during the caries process.

In recent years, attempts have been made to decrease the frequency and incidence of dental caries by providing dietary substitutes for sucrose which have a sweet, pleasing taste without harmful side effects, yet produce a significant decrease in the level of dental caries because they are more metabolically inert than sucrose in regard to their interaction with the plaque microflora. It should be stressed that it is the collective metabolism of a given carbohydrate by dental plaque which dictates its effectiveness as a cariogenic agent.

A class of compounds which have been explored in recent years as dietary sucrose substitutes are polyhydric alcohols or polyols. Two of these polyols, in addition to xylitol, are mannitol and sorbitol.

As the metabolic interaction of carbohydrates with dental plaque is of primary importance in the etiology of dental caries, the remainder of this presentation will deal with the metabolism of mannitol and sorbitol by selected components of the plaque microflora.

In contrast to xylitol, which is a five-carbon polyol, mannitol and sorbitol are six-carbon polyols, both of which can be produced by reduction of the six-carbon keto sugar, d-fructose. The importance of the structural relationship of sorbitol and mannitol to fructose will become apparent as the metabolism of these polyols by the plaque microflora is discussed in more detail. It should also be noted here that mannitol and sorbitol *per se* are not the form in which these polyols undergo metabolic transformation by the plaque microflora, but rather, the polyols are metabolized after prior conversion to their phosphorylated derivatives, mannitol-1-phosphate and sorbitol-6-phosphate, respectively. The comparative structures of these polyol phosphates are shown in Fig. 1.

Generally speaking, when one refers to mannitol and sorbitol metabolism by dental plaque, one is talking about polyol metabolism by streptococcal components of the plaque microflora. For example, all *Streptococcus mutans* serotypes utilize both mannitol and sorbitol as a primary energy source, as will oral isolates of *S. faecalis* and *S. faecium*. In addition, a few isolates of *S. sanguis*

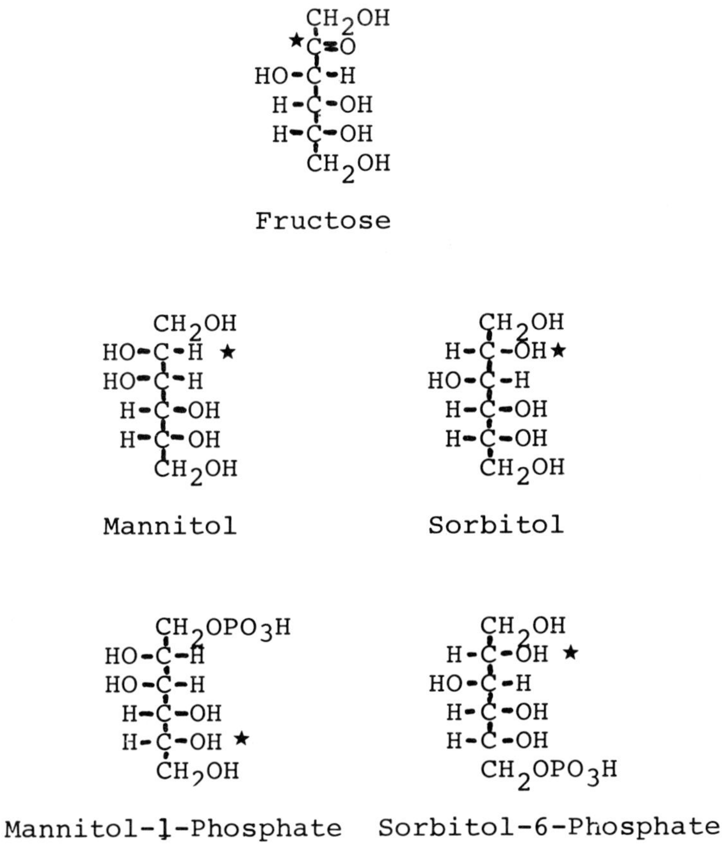

FIGURE 1.

and *S. salivarius* will grow on mannitol. Although some isolates of the genera *Actinomyces* and *Lactobacillus* grow in mannitol, most other components of the plaque microflora are metabolically inert in regard to these two polyols. However, because streptococcal species are usually the predominant cultivable organisms in supragingival plaque, the metabolism of mannitol and sorbitol by members of this genus is worth discussing.

Mannitol and sorbitol are metabolized in the following manner by all oral streptococcal species studied. Extracellular mannitol and sorbitol are actively transported into the cell in the presence of a phosphoenolypyruvate (PEP) phosphotransferase system and appear inside the cell as mannitol-1-phosphate and sorbitol-6-phosphate respectively. The metabolic fate of mannitol-1-phosphate and sorbitol-6-phosphate is as follows: the polyol phosphates are oxidized by separate and distinct NAD-dependent polyol phosphate dehydrogenases and in the process are converted in this single oxidative step to the glycolytic intermediate, fructose-6-phosphate. The enzyme responsible for the NAD-dependent oxidation of mannitol-1-phosphate is mannitol-1-phosphate dehydrogenase, that for sorbitol is sorbitol-6-phosphate dehydrogenase. It should be stressed that mannitol-1-phosphate dehydrogenase and sorbitol-6-phosphate dehydrogenase are completely reversible, each readily catalyzing the NADH-dependent reduction of fructose-6-phosphate to mannitol-1-phosphate and sorbitol-6-phosphate respectively. The importance of the reverse ability these reactions will become apparent when the role of mannitol metabolism in modulating sucrose-dependent glucan synthesis is discussed.

Once mannitol and sorbitol are converted to the glycolytic intermediate fructose-6-phosphate through the sequential action of PEP phosphotransferase and the NAD-dependent polyolphosphate dehydrogenases, they are metabolized via the remainder of the glycolytic sequence and are converted to equimolar quantities of the fermentation products ethanol, formate, and lactate. It should be noted here that the heterolactic fermentation observed when oral streptococcal species are grown on mannitol or sorbitol is in direct contrast to the homolactic fermentation usually observed when these organisms are grown on other carbohydrates such as sucrose or glucose. The organic acids, formic and lactic, which are products of the glycolytic metabolism of polyols by the streptococcal components of the oral microflora, have at least the potential to participate in the destruction of the hard tissue of the host under the appropriate environmental conditions. These metabolic reactions are indicated in Fig. 2.

Although mannitol does not contribute directly to the biochemical process of adherence, current evidence supports the idea that mannitol metabolic pathways may indeed have a role in modulating sucrose-dependent adhesive glucan synthesis by oral streptococci. It is well established that glucans are the primary determinants for the adherence of *S. mutans* to the tooth surface and thus play an important role in the formation of dental plaque. It is also known that free fructose is an inhibitor of sucrose-dependent glucan synthesis by *S. mutans* and is also a product produced by the action of glucosyltransferase on sucrose. Recent observations by Kornman and Loesche have shown that high concentrations of free mannitol are found in the culture supernatant after cell suspensions of *S. mutans* have been exposed to levels of sucrose sufficient to result in glucan synthesis. The reverse reaction catalyzed by the mannitol-1-phosphate dehydrogenase from *S. mutans* may provide them with one step in a metabolic sequence in addition to glycolysis which serves to remove the glucosyltransferase inhibitor fructose from the extracellular environment. This sequence, shown in Fig. 3, would serve to convert extracellular fructose to extracellular mannitol, which exerts no inhibitory effect on glucosyltransferase, the enzyme responsible for sucrose-dependent glucan synthesis. In consequence, a role for mannitol utilizing metabolic pathways in modulating glucan synthesis by oral streptococcal species is a distinct possibility.

Important metabolic pathways in microorganisms are generally under stringent cellular control and important regulatory enzymes are generally conserved during the process of microbial evolution. The fact that mannitol metabolism is under stringent cellular control in oral streptococcal species may indicate that the ability of these organisms to metabolize mannitol is of some importance for their survival and proliferation in the oral environment. Both

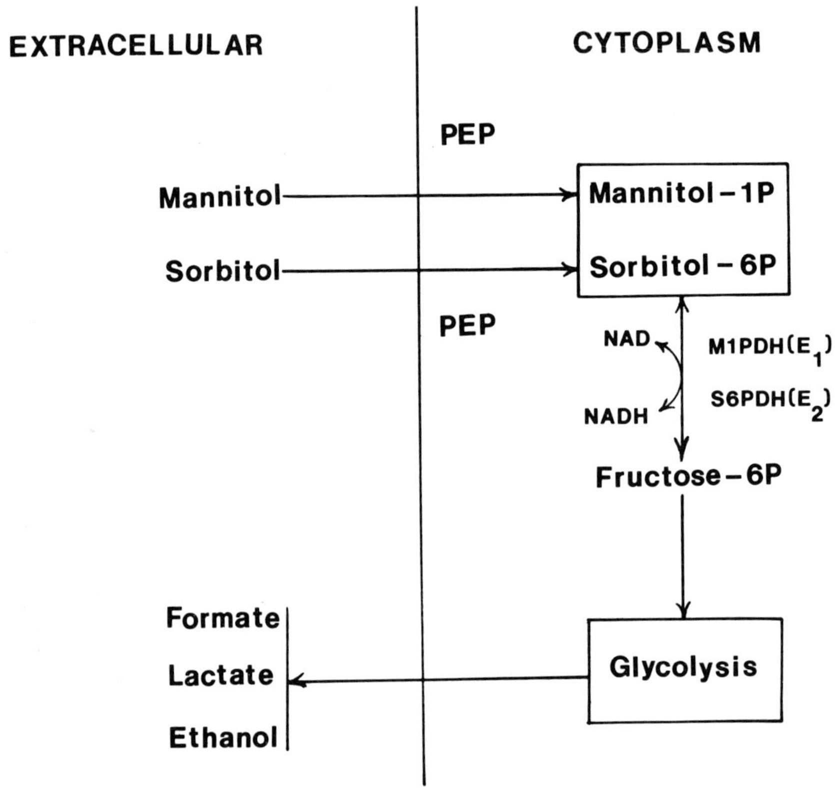

FIGURE 2.

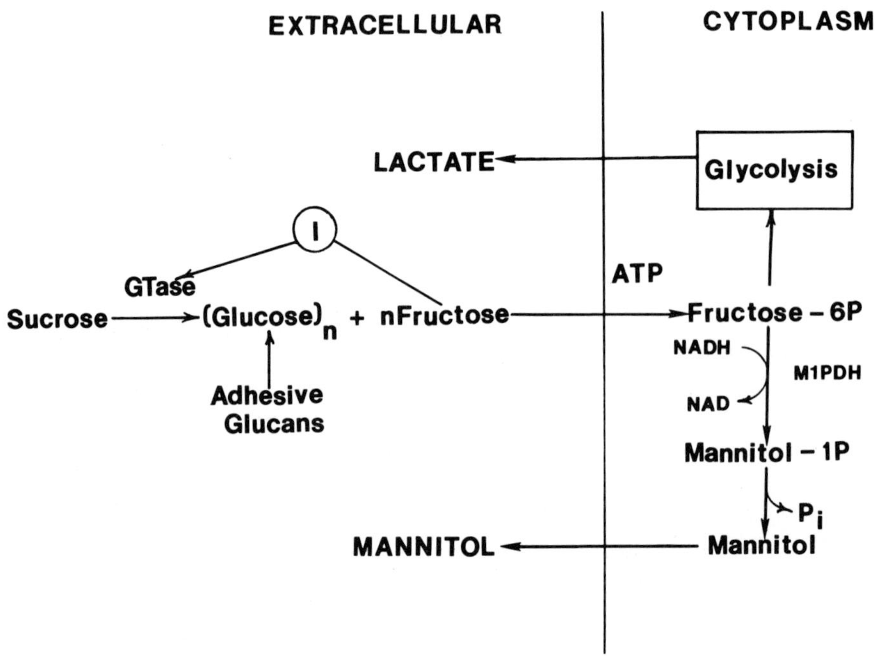

FIGURE 3.

mannitol synthesis and mannitol degradation in oral streptococcal species are under cellular control; these controls are exerted on the forward and reverse reactions catalyzed by the mannitol-1-phosphate dehydrogenase.

The entry of mannitol carbon into the glycolytic sequence is conserved, as shown in Fig. 4, when the extracellular pool levels of ATP and fructose-6-phosphate are high through inhibition of the forward mannitol-1-phosphate dehydrogenase reaction by these two biologically active compounds. In contrast, fructose-6-phosphate is preferentially metabolized via the glycolytic sequence rather than being converted to mannitol when cellular ATP levels are low through an ADP-mediated inhibition of the reverse reaction which catalyzes the conversion of fructose-6-phosphate to mannitol-1-phosphate.

In summary, mannitol and sorbitol interact directly with streptococcal components of the oral microflora by serving as primary energy sources. Acidic fermentation products produced during the catabolism of these polyols by oral bacteria have at least the potential for hard tissue demineralization. In addition to serving as a primary energy source and supporting the growth and acid production of oral streptococcal species, the ability to metabolize mannitol may contribute to plaque accumulation—and hence—caries incidence—in a more indirect way by positively modulating sucrose-dependent adhesive glucan synthesis.

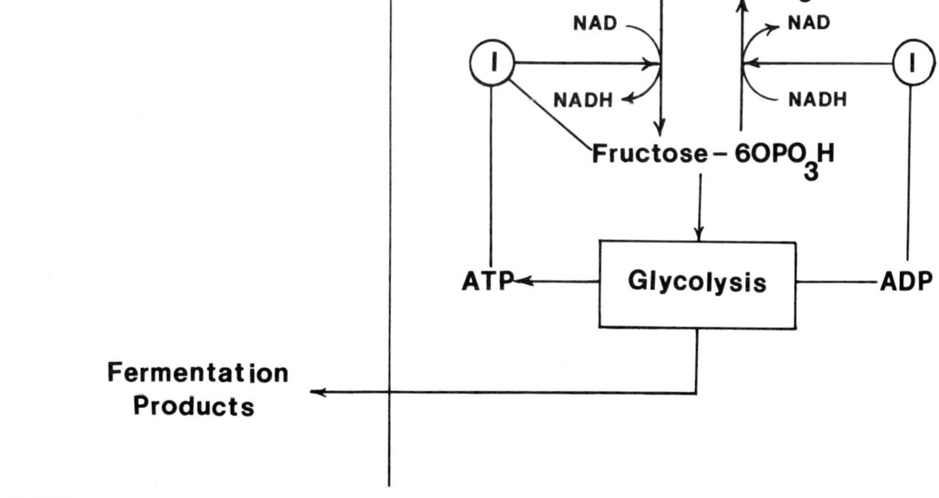

FIGURE 4.

In addition, mannitol and sorbitol may be important ecological determinants in plaque. The widespread use of mannitol and sorbitol as sucrose substitutes may provide certain streptococcal species which can utilize these polyols to a competitive advantage in the oral environment. The production of mannitol from sucrose by oral streptococci may well be a source of this polyol in plaque. The very fact that oral streptococcal species are capable of utilizing mannitol as a primary energy source could mean that the mannitol produced from exogenous sucrose may be selectively utilized by these organisms when their extracellular sucrose levels are depleted. Although they are metabolically active with the oral microflora, it is important to stress that current data support the observation that both mannitol and sorbitol are probably less cariogenic in humans than sucrose.

DISCUSSION

Dr. Brin: The achievement of Professors Scheinin and Mäkinen in introducing xylitol into the caries field is certainly to be commended, not only because of the professional achievement, but because they carried out a two-year feeding trial which is rather unprecedented; the logistical management of such a trial is an engineering and administrative accomplishment.

In the Russian literature a study is described in which xylitol was given in large doses for constipation. It worked for short periods, but was not considered a useful laxative as the people soon adapted to it. However, whatever laxation does occur, even though the incidence and severity are not important at normal intake levels, is the result of the osmotic action of the unabsorbed residue in the GI tract. This may have inadvertent but profound health benefits. Our studies, for instance, demonstrate that xylitol completely spared deficiencies in thiamin (vitamin B_1), riboflavin (vitamin B_2), and partially for pyridoxine (vitamin B_6) in rats. In a completely adequate vitamin diet, body weight change was between 138 g without xylitol and 149 with xylitol. The liver weight was 10.2-10.4 g.

In a thiamin-deficient diet the weight gain was 20 g without xylitol, but 140 g with xylitol, putting the body into the normal weight range. Liver thiamin was raised from 4.2 to 10.3 units, which is in the normal range for liver thiamin. This could not be the result of dehydration because we know that erythrocyte transketolase was also normal in these animals.

In a riboflavin deficient diet, the weight gain was 60 g without xylitol, but when xylitol was added at a 20% level to the riboflavin deficient diet, body weight was increased to 138 g, again in the normal range. Liver riboflavin increased from 7.6 without xylitol in the riboflavin deficient diet to 10.3 units with xylitol.

With vitamin B_6 there was a partial restoration of normalcy; body weight went from 72 without xylitol on a pyridoxine deficient diet to 114, which is about halfway back to normal body weight, and liver pyridoxine was increased from 8 to 10 units. Accordingly, there may be some inadvertent health and nutritional benefits from the presence of xylitol in the diet.

Dr. Fisher: I feel qualified to speak only on the much discussed subject of chewing gum. It is only natural that chewing gum is an easy target because of the highly competitive advertising and the commonplace nature of the product itself. I would like to comment on several previously cited studies and reviews of clinical studies which we had done by an outside consulting laboratory and subjected to professional dental criticism. The answer keeps coming back to us in much the same fashion—that really there is not a significant, or at least not a highly significant, difference between the effects after chewing regular sugar-containing gum and sugarless gum. We have considered this observation philosophically and technically for quite a number of years. We felt that if it were ever clearly demonstrated in a practical sense that the differences with which we were dealing were not significantly small, but large enough for us to consider as of practical significance in the real world, we would take the plunge. We have done that, but with a question remaining in our minds about the real effect of sugar-containing gum versus sugarless gum.

The last clinical study in which we were involved to the extent that at least we contributed the gum for the study and made a financial contribution to assist in the work and had no control in the design of the study or the conclusions that were drawn from it, was the three-year study by Professor Slack in Crete. During that period, he studied children who were consuming regular sugar-containing gum at the rate of five sticks per day. Although his hypothesis in the beginning was that this was going to prove that sugar in the form of chewing gum was harmful to the teeth, his conclusion was that chewing gum is neither helpful nor harmful to the teeth. He wrestled with his statistics, as many others have done.

We regard consuming five sticks of chewing gum a day as exceptional, certainly not representative of the real world; this is an extremely high consumption rate. The question boils down to whether sugar in the form of chewing gum consumed at a one-stick or two-stick level a day really is contributing anything. Obviously, we have a great deal of interest in and hope for xylitol. If one can say anything at all at this point, xylitol is noncariogenic. That has been confirmed by Dr. Koulourides and Dr. Mühlemann and a number of other investigators. We make no claims for xylitol in the present *Orbit* formulation, other than it does a great deal for its flavor in terms of coolness and sweetness and therefore it is of value.

We are conducting our own clinical studies and trying to confirm the findings that Professor Mäkinen has reported. We are optimistic that there is more to xylitol than sweetness and flavor and coolness.

Dr. Rao: I would just like to mention that recently some British chemists have synthesized a new derivative of sucrose—this is a tetrachloro derivative and it is reported to be about 500 to 600 times as sweet as sucrose. There is no aftertaste, it is nonfermentable and has stability. Everything seems to be very good. However, no clinical, toxicity and anticaries studies have yet been performed. It may be of some interest to you.

Dr. Schiff: In your studies, Dr. Mäkinen, in which the xylitol groups were compared with the sucrose groups, you showed that the sucrose groups started with a zero DMF rate. I want to know how do you do that. All groups at the start had zero DMF and then went upwards. I am not sure if I understood what you were showing with that.

Dr. Mäkinen: It was the change in the DMF rate.

Dr. Roussos: I would like to ask Dr. Brin: Is it correct that xylitol has alleviated vitamin deficiencies?

Dr. Brin: Yes.

Dr. Roussos: How do you explain that biochemically? How could you replace a vitamin, which is an essential nutrient, with xylitol?

Dr. Brin: You can't do it biochemically. There are other explanations. During the early 1960's penicillin was used to promote growth in animals; sorbitol as used on occasion to increase absorption of vitamin B_{12}. We used it in our thiamin deficiency system and found that both of these increased thiamin excretion in urine. In the studies that I just showed, I did not show the data because of the time factor. Xylitol is much more effective than sorbitol in correcting thiamin deficiency. The only explanation is that the residue in the GI tract must modify the bacterial flora to produce more thiamin or increase the absorption of thiamin or riboflavin, or both. We are currently doing studies in which we hope to determine whether this is the case. The fact that the thiamin and riboflavin deficiencies are relieved is clear, as shown by correction in the body weight, by the levels of the vitamin in the liver, and by enzyme activities which require the coenzymes of those vitamins in the tissue.

Dr. Roussos: So you are saying that salvaging of the preexisting vitamins might occur.

Dr. Brin: No, they can't be doing that. In the case of thiamin, it is generally accepted that the thiamin-deficient animals actually excretes it. In man this was shown by Najaar at Duke University 25 years ago. Thiamin-deficient men, as well as animals, excrete thiamin in their feces. Thiamin is synthesized microbiologically in the GI tract below the point of absorption, or where the GI tract may be able to absorb it at a lower level.

Dr. Baron: Professor Mäkinen, in the clinical data that I have seen from the Turku studies, I have noticed that the radiographic and clinical diagnosis of caries was not done in a way consistent with the method recommended by the American Dental Association; for example, in the testing of cariostatic agents. It is my understanding, and correct me if I am wrong, that a large number of so-called lesions in the Turku studies were in fact white spots, demineralized areas in the teeth, that you called early caries, and many of these white spots reversed; they disappeared in due course and were diagnosed as caries reversals. Under the diagnostic criteria that we in the United States use for conducting clinical caries trials, can you tell us what actual caries reductions or net DMF increments were seen in the sucrose or the xylitol studies? I am interested in the chewing gum study primarily but also in the full feeding study. Is there a way of converting your data to eliminate the white spots, so to speak, and evaluate solely the large initial lesions?

Dr. Mäkinen: First of all, I understand the clinical radiographic methods which were used in the Turku study were the conventional ones. I am not a clinician; my colleague performed the clinical examinations using the probe and mirror technique and normal radiographs as usually used elsewhere. The statements which claimed that we had used special microscopic methods and some strange type of dyes to determine caries are absolutely false. We never have done this type of examination. We tested the microscopic method of Theilade and Theilade but found at an early stage of the trial that this was not a suitable method to detect caries. As far as I know, we used normal conventional radiographic methods; that much for the first. I think most of you have read the *Acta Odontologica Scandinavica* Supplement which describes the methods we used in the study. From those data, you also can determine what we did.

In the results there were differences in the index, therefore they started from zero. The present reduction in caries in the xylitol group normally, if it was full substitution or partial substitution, approximated some 85 to 95% when compared to sucrose. We have compared xylitol consumption and sucrose consumption. So that is the first value. The fructose consumption reduced incidence some 30 to 35%. As far as the white spots are concerned, I am not the clinician. I only can repeat what I saw from the radiographs and from the photographs which were taken. There were cases in which the white spots disappeared; the consumption of xylitol was associated with the disappearance of these white spots.

CURRENT OVERVIEW - SYNTHETIC SWEETENERS

Edgar W. Mitchell, Ph.D.

A variety of organic chemicals have been examined for use as sweeteners. These chemicals vary widely in chemical class and physical characteristics. Many occur naturally, some are synthetic. They are ranked in Table 1 according to their relative sweetness when compared to a sucrose standard with a sweetness of 1. A number of factors such as concentration, temperature, pH, type of medium used in the taste test, and sensitivity of the taster influence sweetness, and even the sweetness of sucrose, the usual standard, changes with age because of hydrolysis. Three synthetic sweeteners in the table are currently of interest because they are at present on the market and are being reviewed for toxicity, or because of their pending approval for marketing. These three are sodium cyclohexylsulfamate, more commonly known as cyclamate, sodium saccharin, and aspartylphenylalanine methyl ester, or aspartame. The difference in the chemical structures of these chemicals is shown in Fig. 1. Note that cyclamate is a sulfamate, saccharin is a sulfonimide and aspartame is a dipeptide containing aspartic acid and the methyl ester of phenylalanine.

Because of regulatory activity of the Food and Drug Administration, only one of these is available on the United States market at the present time. However, this single agent, saccharin, has again come under scrutiny by the Food and Drug Administration because of studies which have linked saccharin to bladder cancer in male mice. In addition, there are some epidemiologic studies which some believe link it to an increase in bladder cancer in human males.

On April 15, 1977 the Commissioner of the Food and Drug Administration proposed to revoke the interim food additive regulation permitting the use of saccharin in certain human foods; to prohibit the use of saccharin in animal foods; to eliminate saccharin from all cosmetics and most human drugs and all animal drugs; and to permit the marketing of saccharin as a single ingredient drug sold over-the-counter pending submission and final action on new drug applications for such products. The period for comment on the ban has been extended to October 3, 1977. In Canada, saccharin will be banned in all soft drinks and beverages October 1, 1977, in foods December 31, 1977, and in all drugs as of December 31, 1978. Legislative efforts have been made in the United States to put a moratorium on the ban, but as yet no legislation has been enacted.

Regulatory action in 1969 banned cyclamates from use in food, drugs and cosmetics in the United States. The ban was based primarily on chronic toxicity studies in rats using a cyclamate-saccharin combination and with cyclohexylamine, a breakdown product of saccharin. Two studies demonstrated that bladder tumors develop in rats when they are fed high doses of the combination. Since that time a number of studies have been conducted both by manufacturers of cyclamates and by independent investigators. The Food and Drug Administration is now conducting hearings and receiving testimony

TABLE 1. Relative sweetness of various organic chemicals

sucrose	1
lactose	0.4
maltose	0.5
galactose	0.6
D-glucose	0.7
D-fructose	1.1
invert sugar	0.7-0.9
D-xylose	0.7
sorbitol	0.5
mannitol	0.7
dulcitol	0.4
glycerol	0.8
glycine	0.7
Na 3-methylcylopentyl sulfamate	15
p-anisylurea	18
Na cyclohexylsulfamate (cyclamate)	30-80
chloroform	40
glycyrrhizin	50
aspartyl-phenylaline methyl ester	100-200
5-nitro-2-methoxyaniline	167
5-methylsaccharin	200
p-ethoxyphenylurea (dulcin)	70-350
6-chlorosaccharin	100-350
n-hexylchloromalonamide	300
sodium saccharin	200-700
stevioside	300
2-amino-40nitrotoluene	300
narigen dihydrochalcone	300
p-nitrosuccinanilide	350
1-bromo-5-nitroaniline	700
5-nitro-2-ethoxyaniline	950
perillaldehyde anti-aldoxime	2000
neohesperidine dihydrochalcone	2000
5-nitro-2-propoxyaniline (p-4000)	4000

regarding the original tests and tests conducted since 1969. Abbot Laboratories contends that cyclamates are not carcinogenic and that there is sufficient evidence of their safety that they should be placed back on the United States market. Cyclamates are presently available in Canada and a number of other countries as a non-prescription drug. The future status of cyclamates in the United States is not clear at present.

The third synthetic sweetener currently receiving attention is aspartame. It was approved for use in foods in July of 1974, but a stay order for its marketing was issued in December 1975. Aspartame was approved for use as a sugar substitute in dry free-flowing form or as tablets for sweetening hot beverages. It

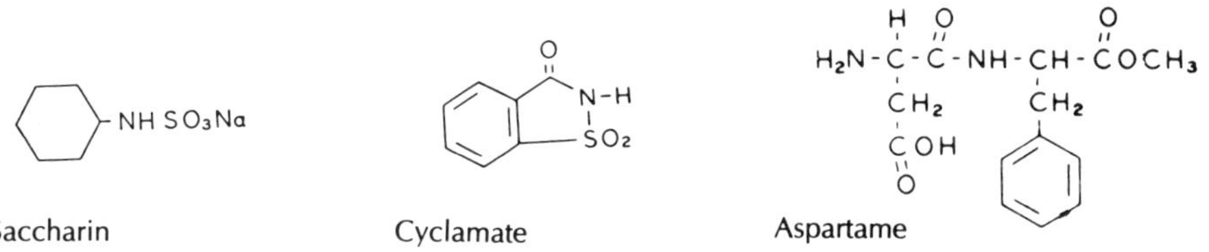

Saccharin Cyclamate Aspartame

FIGURE 1. Chemical Structures

could also be used in the manufacture of cold breakfast cereals, chewing gums or in dry bases for "instant" foods and drinks. It was not approved for uses requiring cooking because prolonged high temperatures can cause significant breakdown to diketopiperazine, which is significantly less sweet than aspartame. The stay of marketing order is in effect until questions about discrepancies in the raw laboratory safety data and final reported data have been reviewed and evaluated thoroughly. This review is in progress.

A combination of saccharin and cyclamate was used widely in foods, drugs and cosmetics prior to the removal of cyclamate from the market. When cyclamates were removed in 1969, it was estimated that approximately 17 million pounds of cyclamates were consumed in the United States yearly. This amounted to an average per capita ingestion of 100 mg per person per day, which, at the time was 1/50th of the generally accepted safe daily intake of 5 g per day. Manufacturers of cyclamates believe that recent studies have demonstrated that 2.5 g per day can be consumed safely.

The estimated consumption of saccharin per year is approximately 5 million pounds. This is an average of approximately 30 to 50 mg per person per day, and represents approximately 1/30th of the once generally accepted safe daily intake of 1 g per day. It is estimated that approximately 70% of saccharin which is consumed is in the form of soft drinks. Estimates are based on total consumption of dietary foods, drinks, confections and drug preparations.

The manufacturer of aspartame has estimated that if aspartame could completely replace sugar in the diet (which it cannot), the daily intake would be approximately 0.03 oz. or 0.8 to 1 g per day. Aspartame does provide some calories in the diet because it is metabolized as a protein. Saccharin is not metabolized in the body and neither are the cyclamates, but the latter can be metabolized to cyclohexylamine by intestinal bacteria.

When synthetic sweetners are used as flavoring agents in toothpastes, mouthwashes and certain other drug products that are not actually swallowed, they are used in low concentrations and their consumption is small compared to that in foods or beverages. The advantage of using synthetic sweeteners is obvious, particularly in fluoride toothpastes and mouthwashes used in maintaining oral health. Many people would not brush their teeth regularly if they did not have a toothpaste which had a pleasing flavor. In fact, some studies suggest that people will not maintain a regular pattern of brushing their teeth unless they can use a toothpaste. A number of topical fluoride preparations used in the dental office for periodic treatment of children's teeth employ artificial sweeteners because the taste of some of the fluorides is very bitter. The loss of the use of artificial sweeteners in these products would likely contribute to noncompliance with regular good oral hygiene practices by patients. At the present time it is difficult to formulate an acceptable toothpaste without the use of an artificial sweetener. The available alternative sweetening agents are not compatible with current toothpaste formulations.

The American Dental Association has recommended that saccharin be retained for use in fluoride toothpastes, mouthrinses and dietary supplements at least until a suitable alternative can be developed. The Association has pointed out that consumption of saccharin from dental drug products is low. When a person brushes the teeth twice daily with 1 g of a fluoride toothpaste, it is estimated that 0.1 g may be ingested per brushing. With the concentration of 0.2% saccharin used in most toothpastes, a person might ingest 0.4 mg of saccharin daily from the product. A similar amount would be ingested with daily use of a fluoride mouthrinse. Chewable fluoride tablets would provide up to 2-3 mg of saccharin per day.

When cyclamates were banned, saccharin was still available and continued to be used. Aspartame has been incorporated into toothpastes in some foreign countries with varying degrees of success, but at the present time saccharin is the only synthetic sweetener available in the United States.

DISCUSSION

Dr. Finley: In the discussion, Dr. Mitchell has pointed out that the soft drink industry, of course, is a very significant user of artificial sweeteners, saccharin in particular. I think too, that we are all quite aware of the problems faced; we are currently facing the demise of saccharin in Canada. I think that is where most eyes are going to be focused in the next few months to see how the industry moves. I can tell you now that some diet formulations in Canada are using so-called high fructose sweeteners. Whether we will continue to see these types of formulations, we don't know. Their success remains to be seen. The other artificial sweeteners that have been mentioned, such as cyclamates, we know we can use effectively. We have done so in the past. With aspartame sweetener we have some difficulties because it is not stable in acid systems such as in soft drinks; the sweetness characteristic tends to be lost after perhaps two to three months, depending upon the formulation. The usefulness of aspartame for soft drinks appears to be limited.

Probably the greatest confusion that developed in Canada was in relation to fructose. It was compared to saccharin because of the loss of saccharin. It is not a substitute for saccharin. It is a slightly sweeter sugar than sucrose and thus has the ability to reduce the level of sugar and enhance the amount of calories in a product. It is unfortunate to have had the confusion which occurred in Canada. There appear to be no problems at the moment related to considering fructose as a saccharin replacement. In this particular case, diabetics would have to consider fructose as they would sugar and handle it in their dietary exchange lists exactly as they would sucrose. That was the issue in Canada.

Dr. Michaleis: I think it is important to consider all the metabolic effects of sweeteners. There is a great need to determine realistic levels amd the effects that they have on human subjects. At Beltsville today we are attempting to start human studies in which we are looking at lower levels of carbohydrate in the diet. I feel that any time you consider the effects of sweeteners in connection with dental problems, you cannot avoid considering other metabolic consequences.

Dr. Dwivedi: I do not agree with the Food and Drug Administration's general attitude that saccharin is carcinogenic. It might be carcinogenic or harmful at the concentrations that were tested, but possibly there is a threshold level below which it is not. However, the FDA is the regulatory agency and we had to go along with it. At this time there is a great need to look into some additional intense sweeteners. I prefer to call them intense sweeteners rather than synthetics, because some of the natural sweeteners are intense sweeteners that can be used in place of saccharin. In the past few years, it became clear that so-called synthetic sweeteners are nonmetabolizable sweeteners. They really will not be looked upon very favorably by the regulating agency. We should concentrate more on the intense natural sweeteners or semi-natural ones such as aspartame. I would urge industry to do what it can in this respect.

Dr. Roussos: I am disturbed with the approach of the workshop. I have heard twice thus far the comment that this is strictly a caries workship. We have to realize that there are several other diseases as well as nutritional problems which have been variously linked with the problem of sweeteners. The Department of Agriculture, I am sure, is concerned with diabetes and cardiovascular disease. We have the caries program and we have the problem of obesity and we have the problem of nutritional inadequacy. We also have another major problem, the problem of money. If an industrial concern is planning to develop a sweetener, obviously it must develop one that will be satisfactory as much as possible in all areas, not just caries. You cannot separate these problems.

Regarding the comment that it would be better to stick with the natural sweeteners, I would like to indicate, first of all, that the USDA has carried out all tests necessary for the FDA clearance for the hydrochalcones, neohesperidine principally. It is safe. Now this is particularly suited to two areas that have been repeatedly mentioned today, toothpaste and chewing gum. It has a lingering cooling effect which will make it particularly applicable here. It also will be applicable to pharmaceuticals. Of course it won't be applicable to other products in which the lingering effect is unwanted. There are other sweeteners, e.g., monellin. This is a sweetener that the National Caries Program has supported. It is the sweetest natural substance that we know in the world at present. It is 3,000 times as sweet as sucrose on a weight basis and 90,000 times on a molar basis. It is a protein. In its natural form it is being used in Africa, and has been used for years. In view of the limitation that the FDA has put on cyclamate, aspartame and probably saccharin, these are other areas one ought to consider. There are other potential sweeteners.

The point to remember is that when you consider a sweetener, you don't consider dental caries alone, you consider obesity, which means you have a sweetener which is noncaloric and several times sweeter than sucrose. Xylitol, sorbitol and other of the natural sweeteners like fructose or glucose do not meet these criteria, apart from other problems that they might have such as the osmotic diarrhea or flatulence. These are problems that must be considered seriously in making any recommendations.

Dr. Dwevide: Industry has not taken the initiative in considering some of the intense sweeteners which are probably safe, if you refer to neohesperdine, dihydrochalone and monellin. A few smaller companies have filed petitions. Even in those instances, I don't know if they are considered high priority products. I think that major food companies should take the initiative, work together, and get some of these sweeteners approved.

Dr. Newbrun: I don't think this conference in unaware of the fact that we have to look at other than dental effects. At the National Academy of Sciences symposium, several speakers pointed out the problem that exists with the high intake of glutamate and the similar effects of the high intake of aspartic acid and the possible neurological effects. Dr. Mäkinen spoke about flatulence, the effects of the polyalcohols, so I think we are all aware that one has to look at the total effect. In looking for suitable sugar substitutes, there is no magic bullet. There is no single sugar substitute which is going to be a substitute for sugar or sucrose in our food products.

I think the way the food industry and the dental profession should look at sugar substitutes is, first of all, to consider those foods which are taken in large portions — that includes soft drinks, and those which are taken in intermediate quantities, and those that are taken in small quantities. There are certain sugar substitutes which will be a substitute at one level but cannot be used at another, quite apart from availability and cost factors. I think if we look at the potential sweetening agents in each of these categories — the large, intermediate and small intake — a great variety of sugar substitutes potentially are available. I don't think that they have been developed adequately by the food industry.

Dr. Michaleis: I agree that the individual has to be considered too. A certain percent of the population is potentially carbohydrate sensitive. It may be of some benefit to use natural sweeteners in the sense that the body handles them better, but those individuals may have to use other forms of sweetening agents.

Dr. Glass: We have enough problems with existing carbohydrates. I think it is a waste of time to discuss carbohydrates or other sweeteners which are not yet approved by the FDA.

Dr. Dwevedi: If the sweeteners are not approved by the FDA, it does not mean that we should not look into them. It is very important that these intense sweeteners be made available to certain groups of people who want to regulate the caloric content or their carbohydrate or sugar content.

Dr. Rao: I would like to mention some new developments regarding the carcinogenic testing of saccharin. There seems to be some indication that the saccharin that has been tested was contaminated with a minor amount of trace impurities, as many as about 12 minor trace impurities in the commercial saccharin, for example. A couple of groups have tested saccharin in the Ames bacterial mutagenic tests. The saccharin produces negative results. However, if you extract commercial saccharin with chloroform, the chloroform extract gives a positive Ames test. A number of people are looking at trace contaminants. These are primarily the starting material *o*-toluidine sulfonamide, and the breakdown products during the synthesis, benzoyl sulfonic acid and a number of related aldehydes and acid derivatives. So it could very well be that in the next five to ten years saccharin could be cleared. There is some hope for it.

Dr. Warnecke: Dr. Mäkinen, you mentioned the fact that the consumption of xylitol was 70 g per person per day. Can you give some idea what the consumption of fructose and sucrose was in the diet in that study?

Dr. Mäkinen: The average daily consumption of sucrose per subject was slightly higher than that of xylitol. That was true of fructose as well. If xylitol was consumed 70 g per day per subject, the approximate dose was some 90 g per day subject for both sucrose and fructose. That was in the full substitution studies. In the chewing gum study, it was 6.75 g xylitol per day per subject.

Dr. Horowitz: I would like to return to the question raised by Dr. Baron. I don't think he was implying necessarily that unorthodox methods were used to record dental caries in the Finnish study, but that they were not the conventional methods used in American studies to record decay. Certainly, as stated in the report, decalcification was recorded at a stage that would not be called carious by most investigators in the United States. Going through the Finnish data carefully, a lot of the treatment effect was caused by changes in this category of decay as it was called in Finland — the very small lesions with no cavitation that had disappeared after one or two years of investigation, depending on the study. We spent a fair amount of time trying to reconstruct the data to determine what we would have gotten if we had been doing the study according to the criteria recommended at the ADA conference on clinical testing in 1968, which are almost identical, if not identical, to the criteria we have used. Because of the many permutations in the Finnish studies, in which recurrent decay was used, we were not able to reconstruct those data according to our criteria with any certainty at all.

Dr. Shaw: I would like to ask Dr. Mäkinen, in connection with the xylitol products, how many of those are now on the market in Finland and to what extent are they accepted and used? Is there any sense in which they really are accepted by your people and purchased eagerly?

Dr. Mäkinen: I think that the first commercial xylitol product, chewing gum, was launched in Spring 1975. Since then the number of these products has been increasing rapidly. Let me say that in three months, xylitol gum became the number one gum in Finland because of its taste. Finland is a small country and therefore it is possible to inform both dentists and the public about a new product without presenting therapeutic claims, just saying that this is better than the normal chewing gum containing sucrose. Since then, these products have been increasing, perhaps too rapidly in the sense that we have not been able to test all of them. We have only tested those in which there was full substitution of sucrose by xylitol, and a particular type of chewing gum.

In spite of this, we do have toothpaste, mouthrinses, wafers and all kinds of products containing xylitol. In many of them it is not necessary to have xylitol at all because the concentration is so low. The product we can really consider is chewing gum. The gum with the full substitution is working but we know nothing about the beneficial or detrimental effects of say, xylitol toothpaste. The public has accepted all the xylitol products eagerly, because of their quality. Xylitol seems to be suitable to the various commercial products that I have listed — certainly based on the organoleptic properties of xylitol and the solubility, and on the fact that it is suitable in bakery products as well. We have had some five-year experience in using xylitol in various products, both industrial and home-made. From a dental point of view, only a limited number of products are rational.

Returning to the methods which we use to assess caries, no matter what kind of methods we used, we can still point to the difference in comparing sucrose and xylitol. One criticism has been that we used dental students, and that we should have used children. That was impossible because the cooperation of children is very poor in the instance of full substitution in the two-year-long trial. I remember very well when we used dental students they tried their best to get rid of dental caries and plaque. They brushed their teeth, used toothpaste, dental floss and everything possible, but still the difference was revealed between fructose and sucrose on one hand, between xylitol and sucrose on the other.

Dr. Smith: When these products are sold, are they sold at a premium price?

Dr. Mäkinen: The price is higher than for sucrose products. It is still accepted because of the information given to the public. The price is almost twice that of sucrose products.

Dr. Madsen: If I understand correctly, all the products in the Turku studies used xylitol exclusively, or at least did not contain any fermentable sugars. Recently, Mühlemann has published in *Caries Research* an article that dealt with rat caries, plaque and *in vivo* telemetry that showed even the very smallest amount of fermentable sugar — sucrose, in the presence of a large amount of xylitol still renders the product cariogenic. So it would appear from the data that the product must contain xylitol exclusively, or at least be free of fermentable sugars.

Dr. Mäkinen: In our products, we replace sucrose with xylitol usually up to the same amount in which sucrose occurs in a product so that there was a 1:1 substitution. That was true in the full substitution study. You must remember, however, that in the chewing gum trial which lasted for only one year, we gave the subjects chewing gum containing xylitol or sucrose only, otherwise the dietary habits and oral hygiene were normal.

Dr. Navia: Some years ago we did several small studies using xylitol in what was essentially a starch diet. In our studies we could not detect any beneficial or therapeutic effects for xylitol. We have tried in several other ways. We realize that if we take isolates of *S. mutans* from the rat and try to grow them in xylitol, they do not grow. However, other organisms that are present, *S. sanguis* and lactobacillus, seem to at least be responsible for the caries. We have not done an extensive study of which organisms are capable of fermenting xylitol. But when we had only partial substitution, we did not see any therapeutic effect. I wonder with human subjects if we must have a complete substitution to find a significant effect. At least in our studies when we only substituted 5%, we saw no great improvement.

Dr. Kreitzman: We have just completed the first part of an animal study using xylitol, and xylitol mixed with sucrose. Both were substituted at the level of 17%. The first time through we did not find any statistical difference. We do get a caries reduction, but we do not find a statistical difference between results in the xylitol plus sucrose study and that using xylitol by itself. We have not done the replication study yet. We hope to have that completed soon.

Dr. Madsen: Your rats had no problems at the 17% level in the diet?

Dr. Kreitzman: The rats did have some problems, although not to the extent that we could not complete the experiment. We have the saliva data, and we have the linking data with these animals. We did not lose a sufficient number of animals to prevent us from completing the study. We have plenty of animals.

Dr. Michaleis: We did a series of experiments with rats with different sugar alcohols, with carbohydrate as 50% of the diet, and then the sugar alcohol replaced that much of the glucose. We had to get somewhere below the 5% level before the liver enzyme responses were normal. They may not have had diarrhea, but they had other metabolic parameters that were definitely inhibited by this sugar.

Dr. Schiff: I want to ask a question of Professor Mäkinen about the chewing gum study. The gentleman from the Wrigley Company said that using five sticks of chewing gum a day in a study is an enormous number. I have just found out that 4.5 sticks a day were used in the Turku study. I think that we ought to know that in both studies the amount of chewing gum used was five sticks day.

Dr. Briner: I have had similar experiences with xylitol in rats, using a 5% level in the diet. We reported and got an LD_{40} for the rats. They had diarrhea and died at levels up to 10%; topically used we have seen no effect.

Dr. Brin: We have just completed a two-year toxicology life-time study in rats and mice at levels up to 20% of xylitol in the diet with no difficulties so long as the animals were adapted to increments of xylitol over time. Now, this is well known for all of the polyols and there is no reason why xylitol should be any different from sorbitol or mannitol. You feed it at 5% of the diet for a week and then increase it to 10% and then to 20% and you will have no problem. The data that we showed in the vitamin deficiency studies resulted from feeding it at 8% level of the diet for two weeks, and then to 20% for two weeks and we had no problems at all.

Dr. Michaleis: What parameters were you measuring?

Dr. Brin: We were using body weight as a parameter.

Dr. Briner: We were looking at enzyme responses in various tissues.

Dr. Dwivedi: Actually there is a limit in human subjects to the adaptability to different polyols. Based on our understanding of the metabolism of polyols, you cannot use 10% level of any polyol, whether sorbitol, mannitol, or xylitol, in the human diet. It will cause diarrhea. Humans cannot adapt to that extent.

Dr. Brin: Our experience has been that they do adapt. In Dr. Kreitzman's study, which was initiated at the 17% level, he did have some laxation. But Dubach adapted people to 220 g per day.

Dr. Mäkinen: Concerning polyols in general, the metabolism differs greatly from one to the other. The metabolism of xylitol occurs mostly in the liver cell. Some 80% of the xylitol metabolism takes place there, and German studies have shown that the metabolic capacity of humans to xylitol, oral xylitol and parenteral as well, is 0.6 kg/per day, meaning that the metabolic capacity is rather high; it is much higher than for sorbitol and mannitol. The second point I wish to repeat is that the 70 g of xylitol which we used in Turku sugar studies produced no osmotic diarrhea. The third point is that we did not start the two-year dietary feeding study without the previous knowledge that xylitol was absolutely safe. We knew from the studies carried out in West Germany, Japan and other countries that oral xylitol in the doses which we planned to use was absolutely safe. The two-year study, which has now continued with a smaller number of the same subjects for a five-year period, has shown that the oral xylitol is absolutely safe.

Dr. Navia: I want to make it clear that the results which I got were with 5% xylitol in a diet that contained 62% corn starch. I have been able to adapt the animals as Dr. Brin indicated. I have fed the animals a small amount of xylitol during a ten-day period before weaning, and then started to raise the level, and I have gone as high as 20%.

Dr. Roussos: I would like to ask Dr. Brin a question with regard to adaptation of the rats to xylitol. I can't recall the concentration of xylitol you used in the previous study in which you reported that it had cariostatic properties. Your survival rate, I believe, was about 35% even though you had adapted the rats. Your paper claims that you had three different stages of adaptation.The only thing I can't recall is what concentrations you used.

Dr. Brin: The final concentration was 10% of the diet. The adaptation was not proper and, as it turned out, the diet was crushed rice without any vitamin or mineral supplement or protein supplement. It really was a very poor diet.

Dr. Roussos: So you would say that even the cariostatic properties that you claimed are not reliable.

Dr. Brin: I wouldn't say that. If they had been of the order of what was observed with sorbitol or mannitol, we would not have bothered to publish the paper. We recognized its limitations when we published it. We are sorry a better diet was not used. Of course, this study was actually done 10 to 12 years ago. However, having a 90% reduction in caries was so dramatic that it was worthwhile to publish the findings simply to encourage other people to work in this area.

Dr. Roussos: I agree with what you say. However, you agree that you had a 35% survival rate and, also, according to those studies, even fructose was cariostatic. In other words, if you compare it with sucrose it lowered the caries incidence. How would you interpret such a study which is contrary to what is known?

Dr. Brin: Fructose was cariostatic also in the Turku feeding trial to a degree. There was 30% less caries if I recall.

Dr. Roussos: That does not mean that it is cariostatic, it is less cariogenic.

Mr. Khan: I think those of us in the food industry would very much like to hear what those who are here from the dental field would like to see us do. We talked about possible food modification. The only things we talked about were phosphates and similar substances. I think there was an allusion to the question of texture.

Dr. Newbrun: I am glad you raised this point, especially as a representative of the baking industry. The people in the baking industry always say if you take sucrose out you don't have the right crumbling qualities and consistency. We have to go on testing. We have to go on doing research, even with products that have not been approved, because how else are we going to get them approved. But let us say, for argument's sake, that the dihydrochalcones are approved. I think right now the food industry should be testing them, because when you put in dihydrochalcones and they are so sweet, you have to find other bulking agents. Fiber bulk has been discussed already. This is a very open field and research is very much needed to find out if you take sugar out and put in something like dihydrochalcones, whether cellulose or carboxycellulose can be substituted as bulking agents. These are areas that should be investigated.

Dr. Daniels: Are you saying in essence that there is nothing that we can do now? Because that is what we are after. We are asking you what can we do now. We agree with you that as they come closer to becoming legitimate entities which can be used, we are foolish if we don't start product development work on them. But at least a certain percentage of us are asking: What about now? If you are telling us that we have to wait for a legal artificial sweetener and the legalization of bulking agents in order to do anything about dental caries, I think it might be a little counterproductive.

Mr. Khan: You are implying that: (1) one way or another a reduction or an elimination of sucrose in bakery products would be useful. It is contrary, however, to what has been said about the concentration or the amount related to the frequency of intake; (2) you imply that the other components in bakery products are not something we need to worry about; (3) there is an absolute prohibition by the FDA on the inclusion of noncaloric sweeteners in an otherwise caloric food. The limitations of the uses of the noncaloric sweeteners are narrowly defined.

Dr. Newbrun: I can't tell you which products or what you can add to foods or use in foods specifically, that you don't know already in terms of caries reduction. We have been talking about phosphates and the limitations in the sugar substitutes, which are as apparent to you as they are to me. I was talking about future development and not waiting until a food is approved, because it will only be approved if, first of all, the food industry will support that type of research and secondly, it has to be tested. But now coming to Mr. Khan's question, I was thinking in terms of frequency of consumption, because bakery products, particularly cookies, biscuits and sweet rolls are the sort of foods which are eaten between meals. It was in that sense I was talking in terms of frequency, because bakery products are high frequency items. I don't see that this is contrary to anything I have said earlier.

Mr. Khan: The other point is that you wish that we would use a noncaloric sweetener in the presence of the otherwise carbohydrate source. This is really whistling in the dark as far as FDA is concerned. Until somebody at the National Institute of Dental Research provides some very strong evidence that the inclusion of a noncaloric sweetener is instrumental at least in solving the dental caries problem, I think that the FDA would not consider the mixing of starchy foods with noncaloric sweeteners.

Dr. Newbrun: We have to separate two things: one is a therapeutic effect and the other one is a nonpathologic effect. The fact that something is safe does not say it prevents anything. It just is not therapeutic, it is not cariogenic or odontopathic. Here, I think, one gets into trouble. The scientific literature claims that xylitol is not cariogenic. When it is translated into lay literature, claims are made that it protects against caries. I think that these two effects must be distinguished. I don't think, if you come up with a product, that you can say it is going to protect against caries if you remove sucrose. Removal of sucrose will not protect against caries, it just won't cause caries. Somebody earlier referred to a Swiss government's recognition of food or candies or gum as "tooth safe." That means it is is not caries producing. It does not mean that it has a therapeutic effect. You will not get the FDA to recognize any of these foods as protective, but I think that the claim can be made that it is potentially safe.

Dr. Roussos: I think two points were brought up with regard to the reluctance of the food industry to use something that has not been approved by FDA and I can appreciate that. Monellin, for instance, has been used in a pilot trial as a sweetener in a chocolate candy. It can withstand the processing conditions. Of course, the product won't be as palatable as one with sucrose because of the lack of bulking effect. As Dr. Newbrun has indicated, this can be overcome by other normal metabolizable bulking agents such as xanthin, for instance, or many others that exist or can be synthesized. I recognize that it is a matter of cost. Industry will not undertake something unless it can see a profit. However, the National Caries Program has a mission to eliminate or reduce caries. One of the major approaches is to modify the diet. One way of modifying the diet is to eliminate cariogenic substances such as sucrose, fructose, and glucose. I don't care what has been said, foods that contain these substances as well as cooked starch are cariogenic. You can't get away from that fact. Moral support must be mobilized from the industry and the public as well as the scientific community, including the dental community, to look for sugar substitutes.

Dr. DePaola: The immediate need is the need for funding; it is for funding for mission-related rather than target-related research. I think some examples were shown today. It is clear that diet is involved in dental caries. I have not heard anyone discuss other aspects of disease which also affect the diet. Dr. Darby suggested that we need to have some research on pyridoxine which may not give short-term corporate benefits. A study to help general oral health might be in keeping with corporate responsibility. The same kind of analogies could be made with candies and chocolate. Right now, because the industrial support is mostly for third-party clinical trials, and a very low level of support for nutrition studies by the National Institute of Dental Research, I think that the most immediate need is for support for nutrition research. Then some of the questions related to cariogenicity of specific foods will be answered.

Dr. Bowen: I am not speaking on behalf of the National Institute of Dental

Research, other than to make the observation that it can fund only the applications concerned with nutritional research that come in. If such applications don't come in, they can't be funded. Reference has been made twice today to pyridoxine, suggesting more work should be done. I want to tell you that we carried out a study for four years in which we added pyridoxine hydrochloride up to substantial amounts in the diet of monkeys. We got absolutely no reduction in caries. We found no metabolic changes in the dental plaque. We looked at all the organic acids. If people would consult the literature, they might find a few things there which, if reexamined with new thoughts and new emphasis, might product benefits; we would not continue to chase shadows until we find a few shadows that are worth chasing.

Dr. Schiff: I have heard what we in the industry can do today. We have heard and read hundreds and thousands of pieces of literature regarding *in vitro* and *in vivo* studies that say that certain compounds are safe and effective. The FDA has not approved them, but they are safe and effective. Why don't you put them into the products?

Dr. Daniels: Are they safe and effective?

Dr. Schiff: They are safe products which reduce caries a certain percentage. You may not claim them today, because they have not been accepted by the Food and Drug Administration yet.

Dr. Daniels: Are they approved for use?

Dr. Schiff: Yes, they are approved for use.

Dr. Daniels: Isn't xylitol being used?

Dr. Schiff: Xylitol is being used. How about using calcium phosphates? How about using other phosphates?

Dr. Daniels: I think calcium phosphates are being used. I would like to discuss metaphosphate. One very important issue was brought out today. I heard that 50% of the diet is decimated with starch, sucrose, fructose, lactose, and so on. A comment was made that you can't treat dental caries without treating general health at the same time. We live in a meat-eating society which a natural sweetener (monellin) for which to the best of my knowledge the tion in the medical community that believes that osteoporosis would be reduced in the aged if this were not the case. All of our animal nutrition data seem to tell us that 1.5 or 1:1 calcium to phosphorus is desirable. I heard a recommendation to use a high phosphate compound that is unbalanced; dicalcium phosphate makes some sense in the human diet. Among the other compounds mentioned, just one of them is legal, dicalcium phosphate, which might actually ameliorate some medical problem. But you are recommending a natural sweetener (monellin) for which to the best of my knowledge, the toxicology studies do not satisfy the U.S. Food and Drug Administration. That's why it is not legal and that is why industry won't use it. But the data do not exist. It has not been accepted by the U.S. government, nor has aspartame been accepted. You can't expect industry to use these things. The question is, can I alter the products so long as the alteration is within the bounds that exist as legal and proper and will improve the condition?

Dr. Newbrun: Let's take the example of dihydrochalcones. I have known about them for at least seven years, and part of the problem is that the safety testing of the dihydrochalcones as far as I know, has been done only by the Department of Agriculture. Why hasn't the food industry been testing them? It doesn't take seven years to run animal experiments. The food industry has not been involved in the development of the hydrochalcones at all to my knowledge, at least as regards safety testing. The drug industry does do its own testing. They don't leave it to the Department of Agriculture or to the universities to do it. Why hasn't the food industry been involved? Why have I seen no work coming from the food industry on the dihydrochalcones?

Dr. Daniels: I'm sorry, but you do see literally millions of industrial dollars spent on research on other products such as aspartame, cyclamates and monellin. You are picking a particular compound in which the agricultural community has a vested interest. Why don't they do their own research? Industry is being indicted for not doing research on additives, and industry is criticized first for the use of additives and then can't get them approved in a relatively legitimate process. I don't think the indictment is quite fair.

Dr. Kent Stewart: There are some new avenues opening up for funding. The current agricultural bill that was passed and due for signature has 5 million dollars in it this year for agricultural research on nutrition additives. This will be available for anyone who has good research projects. I understand that a peace treaty has been signed between HEW and USDA regarding nutrition research. The USDA will handle the nutrition research directed toward free living individuals and HEW will hand nutrition research related to clinical situations. I think things are a little bit better for funding along these lines.

Mr. Jorgensen: I was surprised that the food industry did not answer the question of dihydrochalcones. I think the reason why the work was supported on aspartame and not on dihydrochalcone was that one was a good sweetener and the other was not.

Mr. Khan: Let me assure you that there are very few substances that are permitted to be used that are not being used. Let me also assure that the people who are licensed by the USDA at this time to manufacture dihydrochalcone are fully aware of the fact that hundreds of companies are doing experimental and developmental work. It is not customary for the food industry to publish ahead of time what it is going to do; it is a competitive industry.

The last question you asked was why don't we do the testing, why is the Agriculture Department left to do it? First of all, as somebody has already indicated, it is a substance with limited usefulness. Secondly, to do a complete testing job today costs at least $750,000. That is not the kind of money anybody throws away lightly, especially when one vocal misanthrope can knock the whole thing into a cocked hat by making up a cock and bull story about how it does this or it does that.

Dr. Bowen: I would like to add to my response to Dr. DePaola's concern about the lack of support in nutrition research in NIDR. The National Caries Program, in fact, is the largest supporter of research dealing with sugar substitutes in the entire National Institutes of Health. It supports far, far more even than the people concerned with diabetes.

Dr. Shaw: In my way of thinking, the use of 23.5% of sugars in diets in the United States is intolerably high, not just because of dental caries. Here are substances which, by and large, are very pure. They make no contribution to the diet in the manner of protein, minerals or vitamins. Here you have a major portion of the diet that is contributing nothing but energy—now energy is important, I'm not denying that—however, you are automatically saying that everything else in the diet has to provide on the average 50% more in order to end up with a well balanced diet.

Industry asks what can we do right now? In my way of thinking, there are a number of products on the market advertised as foods which should be removed. I say this with absolute sincerity and earnestness. When industry is putting out products that have, as in the case of the cereals in particular, around 50% or even 35 or 40% sugar, it ought to be ashamed and take them off the market. I think that you can go down the line on a lot of things like that and come to the point at which you are not enticing the public to maintain its sugar level of intake at an average of 23.5%. Because, if the average is 23.5%, you know very well that for some people it is going to be 35 or 40 or 45%.

Now somebody is going to say that it is not really proved that sugar(s) cause dental caries. It's true that dental caries has been with mankind for all the years of recorded history and that you can go back and exhume skulls for many, many decades, even centuries, and there is always a little bit of tooth decay in any population. There will be a lesion in every five or ten skulls, or something like that. However, you find nothing like the problem that exists in the modern population. Indeed, if you look back carefully in the records, caries did not become a problem until around the medieval period. The increase since that time has been terrific. I know of no instance recorded in the animal literature in which you get caries without either sugar or highly cooked starch. This, of course, automatically means that there are going to be some sugars in that cooked starch, or at least some relatively low weight polysaccharide which in all probability is as cariogenic in the animal situation.

I give you a case in point. Four years ago, I was asked by one of the food manufacturers to go to their headquarters and sit down with a number of their people and talk about the cause of dental caries. I did this on an innocent sort of basis. I gave what I thought was a very fair evaluation of a host's susceptibility and resistance, of the role of bacteria and of the role of foods. Afterward, various people were sitting around, some from advertising, some from food formulation, dso forth. I was asked about some of the things that we have on the market today. I said O.K., how much of the sugar, for example, in your syrups really has to be there to qualify as a syrup. The answer was that they could cut it down to a third of what it is and keep the viscosity of the syrup with other things, and it will be perfectly palatable and perfectly salable. I know very well that company has not touched that product and yet here is something that could very well be done tomorrow; cut down the amount of sugar in a product that is used in a situation which is very likely a highly cariogenic one. So it's really begging the issue to say, first, that sugars are not involved or may not be involved, or perhaps they are not involved in dental caries, because it is very clear that in some fashion or another, whether directly or indirectly, they are.

Secondly, I think that there are many products on the market today through which, if you genuinely want to help, you can do so.

Dr. Navia: About seven years ago, there was a conference set up by Dr. Bibby in Rochester on the role of foodstuffs in dental caries. A lot of things that we are talking about here were also discussed at that time. Several things came out of the conference. Personally, it stimulated me to work on the sugar substitutes and to develop animal models for the study of the cariogenicity of foodstuffs. I think that what Dr. Bibby said pertaining to the concept we have about the cariogenicity of foods is important—that sugar is a factor and that this cannot be denied. It is also true that there are many other factors within food that modify and alter the cariogenicity of foods. Therefore, thinking of the kinds of things that could be done with the knowledge that we have today, the understanding that we have of caries, sugar and fats, textures and hardeners, we can try to develop a program through which we look at a food and then modify certain aspects of the food which probably would decrease its cariogenicity without the need for special things. The paradox is that we have developed *in vitro* methods and we have developed animal model methods, we have developed very different kinds of indirect methods to test the caries promoting properties of a food. However, what we lack at this time is a single study in humans to tell us whether a certain food is cariogenic or not and how cariogenic it is. This is important at this point, because if we had that, it would be the reference point for all of us to continue to do a lot of short term animal *in vitro* experiments that would guide us in the design of better foods. I think that they can be done. But we need research and we need funding. Somebody has to put up the money and to have the interest in the study.

Dr. Clydesdale: I heard that we should stop eating sugars and cooked starch. That is 50% of our diet and that bothers me. Another comment that I hear is about the monodimensional thing that disturbs me a little bit. I will not argue about the 23% sugar question. I don't think anyone in this room is going to question the fact that sugar is involved in dental caries, but I think to say such things as you should take a 30 to 40 to 50% sugared cereal off the market is another matter. Let's just think about where that fits in terms of food composition. That is a weight by volume which most people don't think about—that's equivalent to about 2½ to 3 teaspoonsful per serving because it is weight by volume. That is what a child would put on his cereal anyway. This is not in defense of it, this is just how much it is—a 40-50% sugared cereal is equivalent to that. Now, as concerns weight by weight sugar—are we going to outlaw dried fruit too? It is over 50% sugar by weight and not by volume. So if we make a recommendation to take a cereal off the market that has some added nutrients plus some calories in it and it is taken with milk, are we also—unfortunately to be consistent—going to make the recommendation to take dry fruit, jams, dry milk and a few other products off the market?

V. METHODOLOGY TO ASSESS CARIOGENICITY

Anthony R. Volpe, D.D.S., Chairman

CARIOGENICITY AND CLINICAL TRIALS

Robert L. Glass, D.M.D., Dr. P.H.

In recent years one has heard a lot of discussion about dental caries in general and the cariogenicity of foods in particular. This suggests that foods are either non-cariogenic or cariogenic. These, like many other discussions of dental caries, are gross oversimplifications. Existing knowledge suggests that while some foods may be noncariogenic, other foods may be placed within a hierarchy of cariogenicity. The situation concerning cariogenicity is further complicated by the fact that the cariogenicity of a given food substance may be altered according to the conditions and frequency under which the particular food is ingested.

At the outset it must be made clear that the association between refined carbohydrates and dental caries is well established. We have known this for a long time, since the days of Hippocrates and certainly since the days of W.D. Miller. However, the situation is complicated; there is not a one to one correspondence between the incidence or prevalence of dental caries and the ingestion of refined carbohydrates. Several studies failed to demonstrate the expected association between caries and snacking, and between caries and snacking with foods containing highly refined carbohydrates. Time does not permit a detailed discussion of the design of clinical trials. Suffice it to say that certain types of clinical trials of the cariogenicity of foods may be carried out.

It is important to point out that there are two all-pervasive problems underlying such studies in human subjects. The first involves the reluctance or even unwillingness on the part of some committees on human studies to consider clinical trials involving certain refined carbohydrate control groups. This is an acknowledgement of fact and for the moment not a criticism. However, in 1974 the American public spent something on the order of 7 or 8 billion dollars on dental care. Much of it was dental caries-related and this large sum of money, plus the suffering involved, seems to deserve some studies of the amelioration of cariogenicity of foods. Some believe that clinical studies of the cariogenicity of foods may and should be carried out. However, such studies must be designed well to increase the probability of benefit to society. Perhaps they should be limited to efforts to reduce the cariogenicity of those foods at the top of the hierarchy of cariogenicity.

The second conerns the actual design of the trials and may involve certain intractable problems. The desired purpose of the study may be to determine the cariogenicity of a selected food; however, the human diet consists of about 12% protein, 42% fat, 46% carbohydrates, plus other nutrients. Under the circumstances it is clearly impossible, for example, to feed a human being something like bread alone for two years if this is the food under consideration. On the other hand, human studies are necessary and certain compromises in design and a little common sense may be required in their interpretation.

Another important issue concerns the sensitivity of clinical trials. Somebody commented that they were a waste of time because one could not detect changes. However, others believe that the existing clinical techniques are sufficiently discriminating to detect differences in the cariogenicity of foods. There have been a number of different designs; Dr. Steinberg referred to his beverage study, Dr. Schiff addressed the general subject of trials of phosphate, and Dr. Baron focused on the trials principally made by Dr. Sidney Finn and his group to evaluate the cariogenicity of chewing gum and the neutralizing effect of phospate.

In discussing clinical trials, one would be extremely remiss if one did not mention the Vipeholm dental caries study. This is a classic study in spite of its deficiencies. It will never be repeated; in fact, it need not be repeated. Without going into much detail (Fig. 1), they had a control group, a so-called sucrose group which was fed sucrose in a solution; a bread group; a chocolate group; a caramel group; an 8 toffee group. These toffees, as pointed out yesterday, were unusual. There were extemely large and were a mixture of complex and simple carbohydrates. There were designed to be large so that the patients participating in the study would not swallow them. This study is complicated, but a classic.

The data shown in Fig. 2 and 3 are derived from the Vipeholm study. Figure 2 sums up the effect of taking refined carbohydrate, in this instance sugars, at mealtime. The vertical axis shows relative caries activity and the horizontal axis grams of sugar per person taken at mealtime. The relative risk and the attributable risk of reasonably large amounts of sugars at mealtime is minimal. The data in Fig. 3 provide the basis for our concern with respect to the frequency of eating or the frequency of snacking. In the first series of dots under unity on the vertical axis in Fig. 3 is shown the relative caries activity of sugar in a sticky form between meals. Some of the subjects in this group were taking up to 300 g of sugar per day, but at mealtime. However, other subjects were eating something less than 150 g maximum between meals, but in a sticky form. This illustrates the tremendous relative risk, or increase in risk, of caries in relation to extended frequency of eating. The frequency of eating was extended to the point at which "eating" was virtually continuous between meals. These data are shown in a different format in Fig. 4.

Some years ago, we carried out a study that has been the subject of considerable comment; it concerned ready-to-eat breakfast cereals. In Fig. 5 are shown the analyses carried out for presweetened cereals, regular cereals, and all types of cereals. This type of analysis was done for each year of the study and the entire study period. Note that the study included 979 subjects. From a design standpoint, we were in a position to keep this group together for two years. In order to do this, free dental care was provided. Some of the people

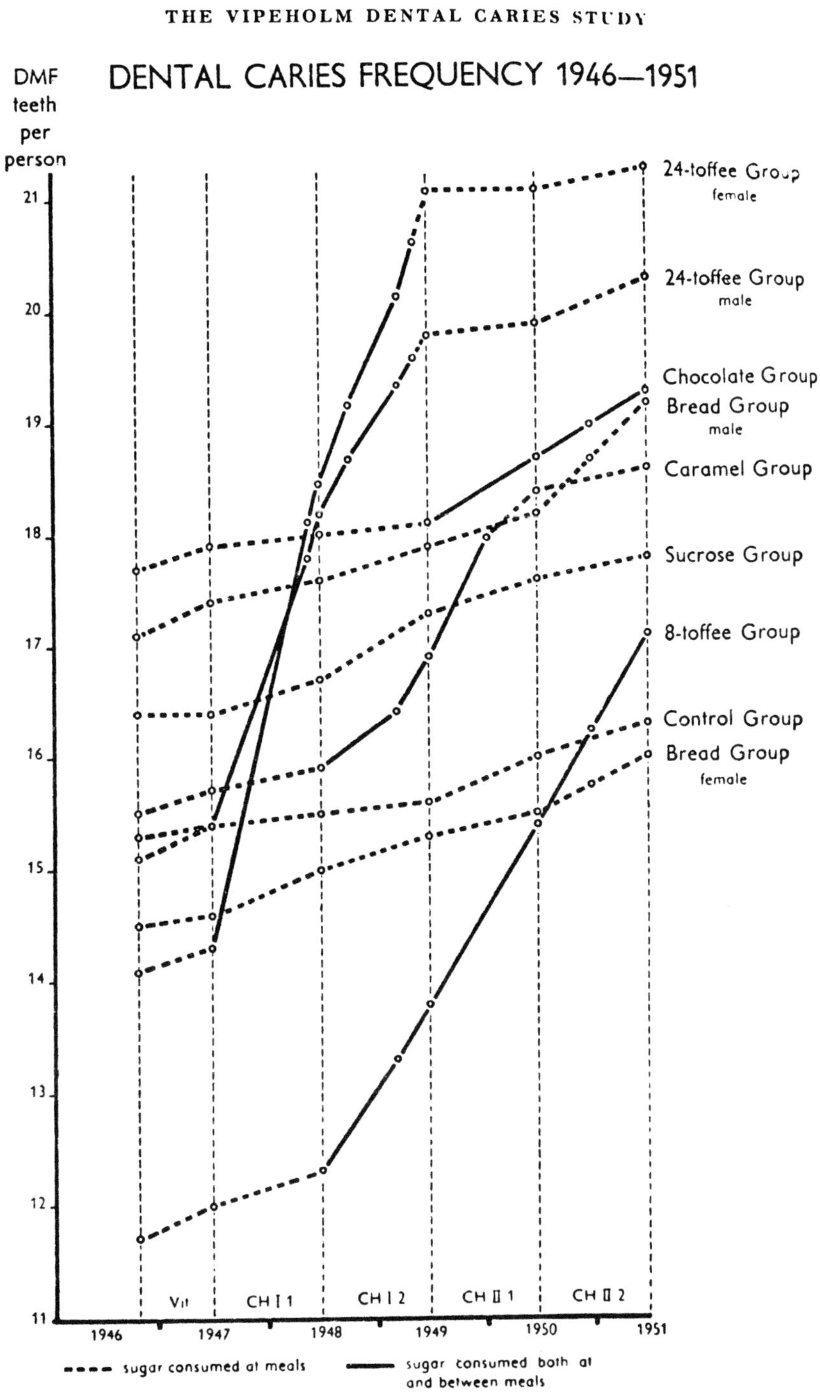
THE VIPEHOLM DENTAL CARIES STUDY
DENTAL CARIES FREQUENCY 1946—1951
DMF teeth per person
21
20
19
18
17
16
15
14
13
12
11
24-toffee Group female
24-toffee Group male
Chocolate Group
Bread Group male
Caramel Group
Sucrose Group
8-toffee Group
Control Group
Bread Group female
CH I 1
CH I 2
CH II 1
CH II 2
1946
1947
1948
1949
1950
1951
sugar consumed at meals
sugar consumed both at and between meals

FIGURE 1.

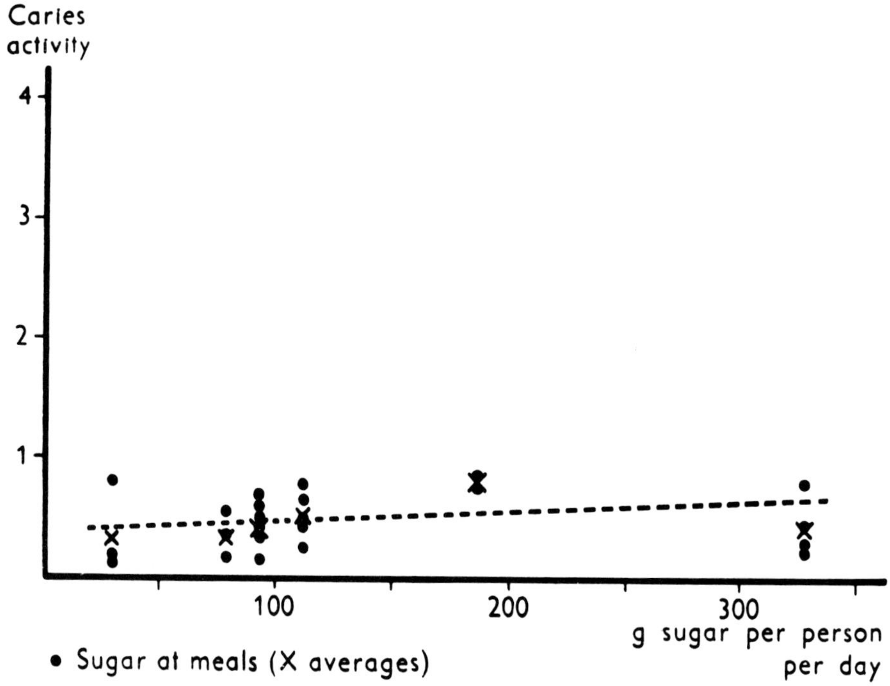

FIGURE 2.

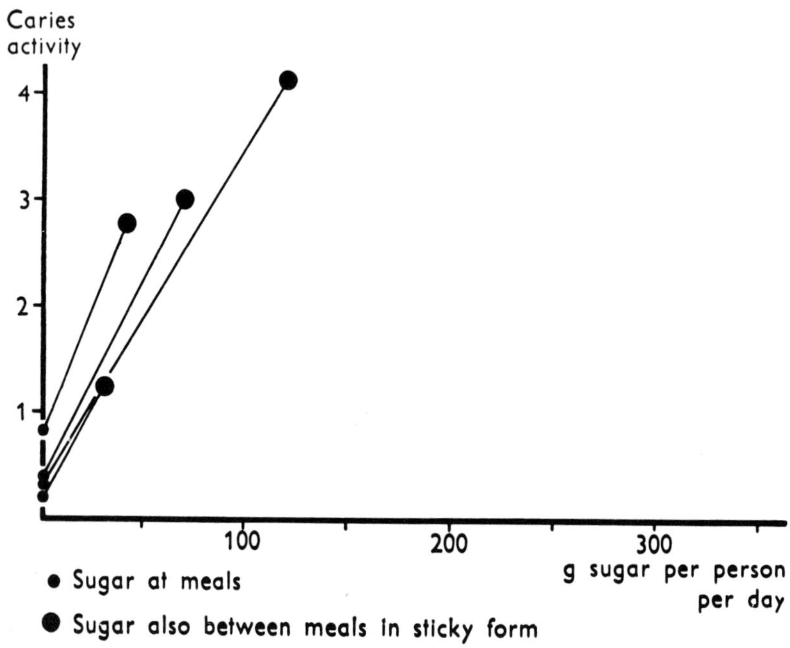

FIGURE 3.

FIGURE 4. Influence of sugar supplement on caries

Group	Number of subjects	Tooth surfaces becoming carious per person per year
Control diet	60	0.30
Control diet plus sugar in liquid form[1]	57	0.67
Control diet plus sugar as sticky toffee[1]	48	4.02

Source: Vipeholm Dental Caries Study as adapted by Volker.

[1]These groups consumed comparable amounts of sugar, over 100 pounds per person per year.

joined the study just to get the free dental care, because they did not eat much cereal. Cereal distribution was carefully recorded. Nutritionists from the Harvard School of Public Health recorded 487 dietary histories of a random sample of the whole group. Consumption of ready-to-eat breakfast cereals ranged from near zero to one serving daily. Cereal was taken with milk 94.7% of the time. Milk, of course, changes the consistency of the cereal, reduces its retentiveness and increases the buffering capacity. Whether they were low consumers, medium consumers, or high consumers of cereal, the figures are substantiated by the dietary histories. This technique of dividing the group into low and high consumers is one developed by Kelley. We found no significant differences in caries increments, without regard to the variable examined. The amount of dental care that subjects needed on their permanent teeth as well as their deciduous teeth during the course of this two-year study also was analyzed. The range of cereal consumption was extensive and it is quite clear that some youngsters just do not like cereal.

The results of this study have been corroborated by two other studies, one by Rowe and his group at the University of Michigan, another by Finn and Jamison at the University of Alabama. Examination of the correlation coefficients between cereal consumption and a number of variables that may be indicative of caries activity showed near-zero correlations for the first year as well as the second.

Analyses were carried out of the dietary histories of 487 subjects who were interviewed by nutritionists, using food models to help the mother being interviewed to get some idea of the amount of foods ingested. Figure 6 shows the correlation coefficients. The most interesting measure is that of the new decayed and filled surfaces. It made no difference whether you looked at calories, proteins, fats, carbohydrates, calories from snacks, or carbohydrates from snacks, the correlation coefficient was extremely low. This finding is consistent with findings from other dietary studies.

The reason for the apparent lack of association is that it is not sufficient to look at carbohydrates alone or calories from carbohydrates. One must consider a number of variables, including the retentiveness of the food, the frequency of eating and the amount of the refined carbohydrate present.

Analyses of age, caries increments, and dental restorative treatment needs according to cereal consumption: first year.

	Low consumers		Medium consumers		High consumers		
	Mean	SD	Mean	SD	Mean	SD	F
Regular cereals							
Age	9.94	1.30	9.93	1.27	9.94	1.25	0.02
Net increment*	1.96	3.27	2.23	3.18	2.25	2.90	0.79
Caries incidence rate†	2.35	4.09	2.74	3.79	2.80	3.64	1.16
Permanent treatment	1.88	2.75	2.34	3.28	2.19	2.74	2.04
Total treatment	2.75	3.46	3.55	4.28	3.25	3.64	3.53
No. children	264		451		264		...
Range of consumption in boxes per year	1-9.2		9.3-19.1		19.2-115		...
Presweetened cereals							
Age	10.01	1.26	9.90	1.28	9.93	1.28	0.67
Net increment	2.01	3.89	2.15	2.80	2.34	2.82	0.73
Caries incidence rate	2.34	4.31	2.70	3.73	2.88	3.50	1.36
Permanent treatment	2.13	3.47	2.13	2.77	2.31	2.91	0.33
Total treatment	3.05	4.29	3.32	3.84	3.33	3.64	0.48
No. children	261		453		265		...
Range of consumption in boxes per year	0-9.8		9.9-21.7		21.8-90.0		...
All types of cereal							
Age	9.99	1.30	9.91	1.27	9.93	1.25	0.40
Net increment	2.02	3.83	2.05	2.80	2.50	2.87	2.12
Caries incidence rate	2.36	4.26	2.55	3.67	3.11	3.62	2.83
Permanent treatment	2.02	3.33	2.18	2.92	2.32	2.80	0.65
Total treatment	2.92	4.04	3.39	3.94	3.36	3.73	1.33
No. children	264		446		269		...
Range of consumption in boxes per year	6-20.7		20.8-39.8		39.9-206		...

*New decayed and filled surfaces.
†New decayed and filled surfaces per 100 surfaces at risk.

Analyses of age, caries increments, and dental restorative treatment needs according to cereal consumption: second year.

	Low consumers		Medium consumers		High consumers		
	Mean	SD	Mean	SD	Mean	SD	F
Regular cereals							
Age	10.91	1.31	10.92	1.26	10.99	1.25	0.32
Net increment*	4.24	4.87	3.84	4.16	3.53	3.93	1.79
Caries incidence rate†	4.30	4.54	3.88	3.86	3.55	3.92	2.26
Permanent treatment	4.38	5.42	3.81	4.72	3.52	4.07	2.23
Total treatment	5.06	5.67	4.36	4.88	4.12	4.30	2.65
No. children	263		451		265		...
Range of consumption in boxes per year	0-7.4		7.5-17.1		17.2-72.0		...
Presweetened cereals							
Age	11.01	1.28	10.91	1.30	10.91	1.21	0.64
Net increment	4.04	5.02	3.68	4.01	4.01	4.04	0.80
Caries incidence rate	3.91	4.56	3.81	3.90	4.07	3.86	0.34
Permanent treatment	4.48	5.95	3.73	4.38	3.57	3.98	2.90
Total treatment	4.98	5.99	4.35	4.64	4.21	4.33	1.89
No. children	263		452		264		...
Range of consumption in boxes per year	0-7.6		7.7-19.2		19.3-68.0		...
All types of cereals							
Age	10.94	1.30	10.95	1.28	10.90	1.24	0.14
Net increment	4.22	5.09	3.82	4.11	3.59	3.76	1.46
Caries incidence rate	4.14	4.61	3.92	3.94	3.65	3.73	0.98
Permanent treatment	4.33	5.81	3.89	4.52	3.45	3.94	2.27
Total treatment	4.90	5.92	4.46	4.74	4.12	4.27	1.68
No. children	263		446		270		...
Range of consumption in boxes per year	2.0-16.2		16.3-35.7		35.8-138.0		...

*New decayed and filled surfaces.
†New decayed and filled surfaces per 100 surfaces at risk.

FIGURE 5.

FIGURE 6. Correlation coefficients of dietary and dental variables for 487 subjects

	Calories	Proteins	Fats	CHO	Calories Snacks	CHO Snack
D.M.F. teeth	0.17	0.14	0.13	0.20	0.16	0.18
Ratio of D.M.F. to erupted teeth	0.09	0.04	0.05	0.13	0.13	0.10
New D/F surfaces	0.06	0.07	0.04	0.06	-0.01	0.14
Caries rate	0.01	0.02	0.01	0.01	-0.02	0.10

Our group has also carried out several clinical studies involving chewing gum. The latter has been suggested as a possible vehicle for caries preventive agents. Subjects were assigned to one of three groups:

1. No gum supplied.
2. Regular chewing gum supplied.
3. The gum of group 2, to which 0.05% stannous EDTA was added.

Subjects chewed twice daily and were given supplies for use during weekends and holidays. After two years, there was a significant increase in caries in the group chewing the regular gum. This result was not anticipated. Daily chewing of two sticks of gum provides two challenges with two grams of sugar (per stick). A teaspoon of sugar weights around four grams — yet this amount in two doses taken regularly between meals in the form of chewing gum will increase caries incidence significantly. This has practical considerations in attempts to reduce caries incidence by means of dietary recommendations. The addition of 0.05% stannous EDTA neutralized the effect of the sugars.

Another study of two years duration involved a sorbitol gum. The conditions were the same as those described for the first study. However, in the second study, after two years there were not statistically significant differences between group mean increments.

In making statements or drawing conclusions concerning the lack of cariogenicity, the acceptance of the null hypothesis is involved, which brings up important statistical problems.

A sloppy study with a small enough number of subjects will provide results that will enable one to accept the null hypthesis.

It is safe to say that relatively few studies of the cariogenicity of foods have been carried out. Most have not been discussed because of time, and some of them have already been covered. The majority of the studies have been sponsored by commercial organizations. These studies are time-consuming and they are expensive. The fact that commercial sponsorship has been available for some of these studies demonstrates concern at least by selected industrial groups regarding the problems under discussion.

Clinical methods do exist to determine relative cariogenicity, although it may be impossible to determine the absolute cariogenicity of foods. Certainly clinical trials are indicated for the evaluation of food additives. The discussions have indicated that certain phosphates may alter the cariogenicity of foods. It is important to recognize that some revisions are needed in existing concepts of cariogenicity of foods. All must realize that the problem is a sticky one.

REFERENCES

Kelly, T.L. The selection of upper and lower groups for the validation of test items. J. Educ. Psychol. 30; 17, Jan. 1939.

Gustafsson, B.E. and others. The Vipeholm dental caries study. The effect of different levels of carbohydrate intake on caries activity in 436 individuals observed for five years. Acta Odont. Scand. 11:232, Sept. 1954.

Finn, S.B. and Jamison, H. The relative effect on dental caries of three food supplements to the diet. Abstracted. IADR Program & Abstracts of Papers No. 667, March 1969.

Rowe, N.H., Anderson, R.H. and Wanninger, D.A. Effects of ready-to-eat breakfast cereals on dental caries experience in adolescent children: A three year study. J. Dent. Res. 53:33-36, 1974.

Glass, R.L. Diet and dental caries. Dental caries incidence and the consumption of ready-to-eat cereals. J. Amer. Dent. Assoc. 88:807-813, 1974.

Glass, R.L. Unpublished.

DISCUSSION

Dr. Bagramian: I would like to raise a couple of issues that Dr. Glass did not touch. Maybe you are familiar with them and are aware of clinical trials and standards for clinical trials. But I think it would be helpful to point out some of the difficulties and some of the issues that need to be considered. The standards and quality of conducting clinical trials are very critical.

Caries trials require at least two and perhaps three years or longer of study, even though conducting this type of study becomes very expensive and time consuming.

We must have controls — proper controls. We must make sure that the groups we are studying are properly controlled. This is very difficult in human studies.

One of the biggest difficulties that we face now is what is called "patient rights" or "freedom of information." It is becoming increasingly difficult to conduct studies such as those we are trying to conduct today.

We must have proper age groups. If we are looking at dental caries, usually we do not want to look at 25-or 30 year-old people. We look at a critical age. If you are studying poliomyelitis, usually you do not look at adults. You look at the age group in which the problem is critical. Therefore, if you are looking at dental caries or preventive agent, you must pick the proper ages.

With respect to levels of dental care, Dr. Glass pointed out a control that they had in their study which was very good; that is, the amount of dental care that a population receives can affect the measurement that you make. We had a large study in Michigan and within several months after the study was initiated, the automobile companies instituted dental care benefits, and many of the children in our study immediately went to private practioners and received a lot of dental care. This had an effect on the study.

How you measure dental caries is very important. Do you look at it as a white spot or do you look at it as a huge cavity? It was pointed out that there were different methods used in the Turku studies; the types of methods used to measure dental caries are extremely important.

Compliance, use of the product, is very important. You give four sticks of chewing gum to children or send the chewing gum to them at home, or you give children free toothpaste and toothbrushes. Do they use them? How do you know that they use them? Maybe they are getting sugar from other sources. Maybe they take the chewing gum and give it to their brothers and sisters. If you deal with a family situation, you know that there will be problems.

I think the environmental impact of sugar is very important. We look at a toothpaste study or chewing gum study and we try to make generalizations from that. What is the total impact of sugar that the subject gets in his environment? Are the four sticks of chewing gum per day making a real difference in terms of what he is getting with the 'Twinkies' or other tasty cakes that he consumes between meals or in the 24-hour period?

The problem of doing studies in schools now is becoming more difficult. Teachers unions can be a problem. Often when you go into a school system and ask to conduct the study, the answer is that the teachers refuse to do it. They are not going to give you time, or they will not conduct the study for you. So you have to hire more people — teacher's aides — to come in and conduct many of the studies.

The ultimate test is what occurs in human populations. Even though it is extremely difficult to conduct human studies, we believe that they are the only way to determine the efficacy of a product, or the benefits that may accrue. You may get an indication from a laboratory situation, but the ultimate test is the effect on the public at large, or what occurs in the normal population.

Dr. Steinberg: One point that should be made in connection with the studies that have been mentioned is that we are measuring only the initiation of carious lesions. I do not know of any studies in which we have been able to study the speed or rate at which caries develops in the tooth. This is one thing about which we have very little information. We had many problems with the Lincoln bottle beverage studies; no one study goes perfectly. Right from the beginning one of the problems was that we were dealing with a mentally retarded population. There were a lot of limitations in dealing with a population like this. It had a lot of advantages because a lot of the standards just alluded to were present. We had a population that was housed in the same area, they had the same diet, and we had good control of these individuals. But there were many limitations. We had a number of patients who had very low IQs. We had to drop a number of them because we could not handle them in making the caries examination. Eating habits in a lot of these individuals were different. In individuals with low IQ's, if it is something like solid food, they may swallow it whole rather than chewing it, so that it would be very difficult to compare this to normal eating. One of the biggest problems that could have biased our study was that the subjects had very poor oral hygiene. It was very difficult to instill good oral hygiene practices in them. When we started the study there was a question as to whether the mentally retarded or mentally subnormal individuals have a caries rate similar to that of normal individuals. None of these studies are perfect; whether studies are done outside or inside an institution, they all have limitations. However, they show trends and I think that is important.

Mr. Lehnhoff: I think most of us believe that we have valid methods for assessing this. I think it has been demonstrated over the past 20 years in oral product-oriented testing. The problem that you face is primarily one of logistics. It seems like a nightmare on the surface, but I am sure that if your studies are carefully planned and well executed, you will have some success.

Dr. Horowitz: Dr. Steinberg just said that none of these studies were perfect and that is very true. But many of them deviate from perfection to the extent that they do not answer any questions at all. I think Dr. Newbrun made the point yesterday that we really cannot determine the impact of cariogenicity of any one food because of the diversity of the American diet. My concern is that a study on breakfast foods, for example, or on soft drinks in an institution, may show negative results but that is to be expected because of the challenge from the rest of the diet. My concern stems chiefly from the point that these data are used frequently by industry to say, "look, my product is safe; it has been tested in one or two studies and we did not find any more decay." No other outcome really can be expected from such an investigation, because of the rest of the diet. I think the data that emanated from the Vipeholm study and from the Hopewood House study in Australia, which has not been mentioned today, in which there was sucrose restriction because the director of that institution believed that decay was only 10% as great as it was in other institutions for orphans in Australia, are more convincing — studies in which one has a total change in diet rather than individual studies where cereals are given, where soft drinks are given or withheld, are more to the point. I do not think that we should rehash any of the deficiencies of some of the individual investigations that have been mentioned today. They do have certain shortcomings, but the biggest shortcoming that I see is that they cannot possibly answer the question of whether a particular food is cariogenic or not cariogenic because of all the other products in the diet.

Dr. Chilton: I think that we might summarize the role of the clinical trial in its relations to all the other phases, and say that the proof of the pudding really is in the eating. It is in the human being who will actually put these substances in his mouth where we will actually find out whether it works or not. Dr. Steinberg commented about the children's groups perhaps not drinking the beverages. Dr. Bagramian also made the point about compliance. So much of our information comes from dietary histories which, as has been pointed out by Dr. Nizel, are not always very accurate. We and many others have been working on a method of putting markers into the agents to see whether they actually are being used; not just by testimonial or statement, but actually in use. We are all familiar with "One Flew Over the Cuckoo's Nest" where they put the pill in the patient's mouth and he spit it out later. We all know this happens in many populations, particularly with people in jail. They make believe they swallow it. You saw them put it in their mouths; 10 minutes later they spit it right up. This is true of other types of agents put into the mouth; the subjects may not comply.

The only real way is to watch them chew it, watch them swallow it, or have some indication by means of a marker.

Dr. Bagramian made a most important comment about the characteristics of the population. Dr. Steinberg also made the point that when you are dealing with institutionalized children who are retarded, the cooperation is not always good. But even in the framework of what Dr. Bagramian said, we recognize that we have to work with the population which has the disease in question.

There is a very famous classical work on headaches by Jellinick. It is in the statistical literature and the author points out that you could not study the effects of an anti-headache medicine in people who do not get headaches. You cannot study a depilatory agent in, say, a Budhist monastery where the people do not have to shave. In the same way, you do not study polio in the wrong population group. But even within the population that does get caries, the children's population, we can see different characteristics of caries: we might get in certain age groups caries essentially of the occlusal surfaces of molars; in other groups you might get caries of proximal surfaces. It is very important to select the population, even within the caries-prone age group.

One factor that is very important now because of restrictions on agents which can be used as control measures is the control comparison. We are having great difficulty in designing a stand-up comparison. The task force on design analysis met in 1967 and, by the way, several members of that panel are on this one. That meeting was sponsored by at least five groups taking part in the present workshop. We have been looking into these problems of statistics and design, and now we have to modify the designs of our clinical trials to agree with our research committees at the universities and consider what the human experiments committee will allow. You cannot do a study against a sugar. Today you cannot do anything about saccharin for any length of time. Today you heard that we have 18 months grace on saccharin. So the whole question of design now has to be done a little differently. Finally, we have to do something about reporting our clinical trials. There are guidelines and literature on reporting clinical trials. Many times the trials are done well, but when they appear in the literature they are reported rather peculiarly.

Dr. Glass: Our clinical techniques are sufficiently sensitive to discriminate. This has been shown over and over again. I am convinced of this and I disagree with Dr. Horowitz. He is an experienced epidemiologist and has used these tools in the evaluation of preventive measures. Some of them are very effective and some of them less effective. If Dr. Horowitz's point of view were correct, this group might as well fold its tent and silently steal away.

Dr. Brin: I would like to speak to the subject raised by Dr. Horowitz, namely, the noise level of the eating regime. I think there is an important differentiation to be made between the design of a clinical trial and its implementation with regard to the eating regime. I think maybe we should look at the medical profession's concept of the prudent coronary diet; namely, an intermittent exposure to cholesterol-lowering materials at various times of the day at which times the products may be entirely different form one another. It is perfectly conceivable that gum testing could be used as an exposure at many times during the day; but cereal testing or confectionery testing may not be appropriate. A more reasonable, so called prudent, anticaries or noncaries diet would perhaps consist of an appropriate cereal in the morning, a xylitol gum after lunch, a non- or anti-cariogenic confection as a snack, a non-cariogenic dessert after dinner, or followed by appropriate gum, a non-cariogenic snack while watching TV and gum again before retiring; all in association with appropriate oral hygiene measures such as brushing and flossing. It is difficult for industry, in general, to implement such testing because of limited product lines, yet it is analogous to a successful program of the prudent diet in medicine. We may have to reconsider and re-evaluate the truly scientific design which we consider optimal, of only a single limiting factor in the clinical trial. Perhaps this is a panacea not achievable with varied products which are appropriate for testing and which the profession would like to see industry manufacture. This would relate caries testing to the real world of consumer health and consumer practice.

Dr. Newbrun: I cannot let Dr. Glass's comments go unanaswered. In the beginning of his talk, he said that there have been several retrospective studies which have failed to show a correlation between snacking of sugar-containing foods and caries frequency. It is not just the studies of Weiss and Trithout and more recently Martenson in Scandinavia, but massive animal data, Stephen studies, König feeding machine, which all have shown very direct, almost linear relationships between the between-meal eating frequency of sugar-containing foods and the amount of caries. Dr. Glass said that in order to accept the study it has to be well designed. Regarding the studies that you had in mind, perhaps Dr. Bagramian may want to comment. If you want to use the Bagramian and Russell study, which did not find that correlation, you cannot use it because it was not one of caries increments; it was of caries prevalence. It was elegant statistics, but the design of that study cannot answer the point that you are trying to make because they took caries prevalence in high school kids who were 14 to 17 or 18 years of age. The amount of caries that developed had accumulated up to 10 years in the older children. And if you are trying to relate it to diet habits, it was based on a 24-hour diet recall; you cannot make that correlation. I think you should apply your own criteria of well designed studies before you say there are other studies that show there are no correlations. I do not think that is true. I think the mass of data supports a direct correlation between the eating frequency of sugar-containing foods and caries.

Dr. Glass: I have failed to make my point that some studies fail to show this correlation. It is a correlation that we would expect to find ordinarily. However, within the dietary questionnaires which are not always as strong and relevant instruments as we would like, we must not focus only on the amount of highly refined carbohydrate intake, but the frequency of eating and the frequency of eating refined carbohydrates not rapidly cleared from the mouth. Of course we all know that when we measure caries prevalence we are thinking in terms of years of accumulated disease. Human recall is completely inadequate to show a correlation. I was merely commenting on the need for revision of ideas of cariogenicity, to get some concept of the factors that Dr. Bibby was discussing yesterday and that's the consistency of the food as well as its highly refined carbohydrate content and when it is eaten. I am not saying that there was no correlation.

Mr. Khan: Dr. Horowitz's point is well taken. It is extremely difficult to evaluate a food for its impact on health while other foods are being eaten. That is what differentiates human from animal testing. At the same time, I think that it is worthwhile to point out that undertaking such testing is very difficult for any food company for any one of its products, because unlike the pharmaceutical industry, in the food industry we have virtually no patent protection. Whatever formulation we develop, our competitors can copy it virtually within hours, and whatever information we may claim to have uncovered in clinical tests is as applicable to the next man as to us. In order to make progress here, much of this must be considered together. We must do in dental health what, to some degree, we have done successfully in food additives and in nutrition. That is, we must approach these problems not on a total food industry basis, but on a subgroup, or a trade association basis. Perhaps we could make a concerted effort by the confectionery industry, by the baking industry, and so forth. Together they might fund large, well balanced, well designed research programs similar to the effort that was expended in the food enrichment program. Enriching one product would not have made any difference, but having a broad base of enriching flour and bakery products has been a tremendous jump forward in public health.

Dr. Horowitz: I understand Dr. Glass's argument. A study that is designed in a way that cannot answer the question should not be used to exonerate or to implicate any food product from being the cause of dental caries. To be more specific, in reviewing the report of the cereal study with which Dr. Glass was associated, I was concerned about using data that were really intended for an entirely different purpose; it was not designed as a sugar cereal study. It started out as a phosphate study. It was sort of a spin-off to use those data to end up with a final end product to show that sugar-containing cereals were not harmful to the teeth. In that study, mothers ordered for an entire family and there was no true indication that the child in question whose dental caries was being assessed actually used that particular or some other product. The study was based only on parents ordering for a family, and it is a huge jump from what a mother orders for six or seven people in her family to what an individual child develops when he may not even use the preponderant product ordered by the mother. It becomes pretty weak data. My main concern is using those data in testimony before congressional groups to prove that a particular product is not harmful to the teeth.

Dr. Smith: I think Dr. Brin's question is a good one. I think it is the reason why were here. Let's not talk about all the things that are wrong with what we did. Where are we going from here? I agree that maybe what we need is a joint program and this is probably the place to iron it out. I would like to hear the panel respond in a positive manner to that suggestion.

Dr. Volpe: Perhaps we have already achieved a major part of that objective by defining the fact that we ought to get together and at subsequent conferences explore in more depth and time exactly the path that we take.

Dr. Horowitz: I think it is a very good idea, and it is the only way we are going to be able to answer questions. We have an analogous situation in fluoride research, where we are conducting or supporting studies in which a variety of methods are being used by schoolchildren; they are taking part in fluoride tablet programs, fluoride mouth rinsing, and maybe using a fluoride dentifrice, and we can identify what any one of those agents or methods is doing individually when we finish the study. We know the total impact of the program. I think analogous studies in the food area also should be carried out.

Dr. Chilton: Dr. Brin, who comes from a company which only recently has become interested in this area, brings up some very interesting points. One of the things we do not have is much in the way of methodological research. This research usually is not sponsored by commercial concerns because they are generally product-oriented and many of the funds for this kind of work are not available through NIH. We do have the Task Force which has been supported individually; this is the area in which all the industrial firms who are meeting see some of the problems as they relate to their products. The methodology of doing these studies may get a start because now we are aware of the problems. We do have some approach to the solution.

Dr. Glass: I pointed out that common sense was necessary because the human diet requires proteins, carbohydrates, fats and other nutrients. One of the outstanding retrospective studies involved demonstations of reductions of caries during wartime because of shortage of flour and sugar. On the other hand, while the studies are well regarded, the war was not designed to demonstrate this.

PLAQUE pH ASSESSMENTS RELATED TO FOOD CARIOGENICITY

W. Michael Edgar, Ph.D.

I shall begin by describing the methods of assessing plaque pH used by us in Newcastle, then try to describe the Zürich Group's approach as best I can and finally try to present to you a reasoned assessment of the pros and cons of the two methods. Although I shall be concentrating on methods, I may not be able to resist the temptation to describe some of our results on foods commonly consumed in the United States and Great Britain.

First, however, a little elementary background which nevertheless needs to be stated to clarify the role of plaque pH assessments as a guide to food cariogenicity.

Figure 1 shows the basic features of the long-held view that caries develops as a result of acid demineralization of the enamel, and is dependent on the pH of the plaque and the presence of calcium and phosphate ions (and other affectors of enamel solubility) in the plaque. Bibby has drawn our attention to factors other than pH which can influence the dissolution of enamel, but it is possible to make the general statement that foods which provoke a large fall in pH in plaque are likely (but not certain) to be more cariogenic than those which do not.

This view of the importance of plaque pH also leads us to the important and generally-accepted concept that foods which are eaten frequently, between meals, will tend to be more cariogenic than foods eaten at mealtime, because the number of times the plaque pH descends toward the dangerous region will determine whether a tooth succumbs to the attack. Thus, it is the frequency of consumption, rather than the quantity consumed, which is important, and snack foods, drinks and confections therefore have received most study. This concept of the importance of plaque pH in relation to caries receives general support from other types of investigation, e.g., animal studies, human clinical studies.

The method we have adopted in Newcastle for studying plaque pH is based on a technique originating here in Chicago with the work of Fosdick's group,[1] and later adapted by Bibby in Rochester, and by Frostell in Sweden. We do not, therefore, claim any rights of paternity for the method and if I use the term "Newcastle method" it is only as a shorthand title. Plaque is sampled from subjects who have accumulated plaque over the preceding 24 hours and have not ingested food or drink for 2 hours. The sampling removes small portions of plaque from all accessible surfaces of all teeth except the lower incisors. This "average" sample of plaque is then homogenized in 20 μl of distilled water in the cup-shaped pH-sensitive portion of a glass "one-drop" electrode, and the pH of the plaque suspension measured with a suitable meter. After food consumption, this process is repeated at timed intervals, so that the composite picture of the pH response of the plaque as it forms acid *in situ* is recorded. A typical set of data is shown in Fig. 2. The response characteristically follows the biphasic curve first described by Robert Stephan in 1940.[2] Later, Stephan

Plaque pH	
Above 6.0	SAFE AREA Low solubility of enamel. Ca, P adequate to saturate environment
6.0 – 5.5	DOUBTFUL AREA
Below 5.5	DANGER AREA High solubility of enamel. Ca, P inadequate to saturate environment

FIGURE 1. The relationship between plaque pH and enamel demineralization.

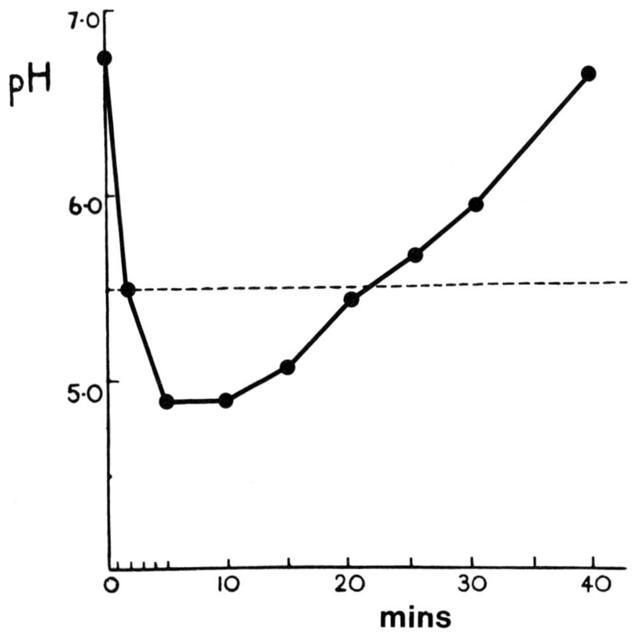

FIGURE 2. "Stephan curve" in plaque pH following a glucose mouthrinse.

showed that the pH range recorded in the curves for different individuals varies — subjects with a low caries experience giving curves in the upper range of pH and vice versa, giving some indication of the validity of the measurement as an index of cariogenicity. To compare the acidogenicity of foods we have employed two measurements: first, the minimum pH recorded in the Stephan curve following food consumption, and second, an assessment we cite as "cH area" which is calculated as the sum of the increments in hydrogen ion concentrations above the resting value ($\Sigma\Delta cH$), and which represents a weighted estimate of the area of the curve under the resting pH. Full details of the method and of the reliability of the results given have been published.[3]

The method has been applied to the assessment of the relative acidogenicity of a range of snack foods commonly consumed in this country,[4] as shown in Table 1. The foods are grouped by category and by their acidogenicity, those in Group 1 being less acidogenic than those in Group 2, etc. "Chewing" candies will be seen to be generally less acidogenic than hard "sucking" candies, we think because they tend to stimulate a higher saliva flow, tend to be neutral in pH, and may dissolve in the mouth to give high inhibitory concentrations of sugars. Sucking candies by contrast may not give rise to such a high flow rate of neutralizing saliva, tend to be acidic (fruit-flavored), thus aiding in the fall in pH, and dissolve more slowly to release optimal concentrations of sugars in the mouth to support bacterial acid production.

TABLE 1. Snack food (U.S.) grouped by category and acidogenicity

Group		Beverages	Fruit etc.	Baked goods	Sweets
Least acidogenic	1	Milk	Peanuts		Sugarless gum
	2	Chocolate milk	Crisps Apple	Bread + buttter Graham crackers	Caramels Sugared gum Chocolate Liquorice
	3	Carbonated beverages	Banana	Cream-filled cakes Sandwich cookies Crackers Bagel	Orange jellies
	4	Apple juice Orange juice	Dates Raisins Sweetened cereal	Doughnut Bread + jam Whole wheat bread Cakes Plain sweet biscuits	
	5			Apple pie Chocolate grahams Angel food cake	Rock candy Clear mints
Most acidogenic	6				Sourballs Fruit gums Fruit lollipops

Other factors possibly influencing the acidogenicity of snack foods are their rate of clearance from the mouth and the method of their use. An example of the latter is given by the differing positions of a well-known carbonated beverage drunk in the normal manner, and the same beverage used as a mouthrinse, swishing it around the mouth for two minues; the rinsing procedure led to a much greater pH fall.

We have also tested a smaller range of foods used in Great Britain,[5] some of which will be self-explanatory and some familiar (Table 2). Some interesting comparisons emerge, such as the similarities between the curves for apple and for chocolate, and the high acidogenicity of sugared coffee in relation to the other foods (Fig. 3). The results for toffees, in Britain (Fig. 4) differ from the position of U.S. toffees, indicating perhaps an interesting difference in their consumption. The effects of sugared and sugarless chewing gums are compared in Fig. 5. Cough syrup, though not a food, is included as a representative of such medications which often contain high levels of sucrose, and are consumed last thing at night when they might be particularly damaging owing to the cut-off during sleep in the flow of saliva with its protective buffering action.

TABLE 2. Acidogenicity of snack foods (Great Britain)

Least acidogenic	1	Sugarless gum
	2	Peanuts
	3	Bread and butter
	4	Potato crisps
	5	Ice lolly (frozen fruit drink)
	6	Unsugared coffee
	7	Cough syrup
	8	Chocolate-covered peanuts
	9	Chocolate/caramel/fondant bar
	10	Apple
	11	Cream filled biscuit
	12	Ice cream
	13	Sweet chocolate
	14	Chocolate covered biscuit
	15	Sugared chewing gum
	16	Plain biscuit (sweet)
	17	Orange drink (sweetened)
	18	Toffee
	19	Sugared coffee
Most acidogenic	20	Boiled sweet (fruit-flavored)

We have also been interested in the interaction between foods, as, for instance, in a meal.[6] Using a four-course "experimental meal" consisting of a sausage roll (sausage meat wrapped in a high fat pastry), half a tinned pear in syrup, a piece (15g) of cheese (Cheddar) and a cup of sweetened coffee, we have noted that the plaque pH tends to follow that of the food being consumed and that the nature of the last item of food is of great importance in influencing

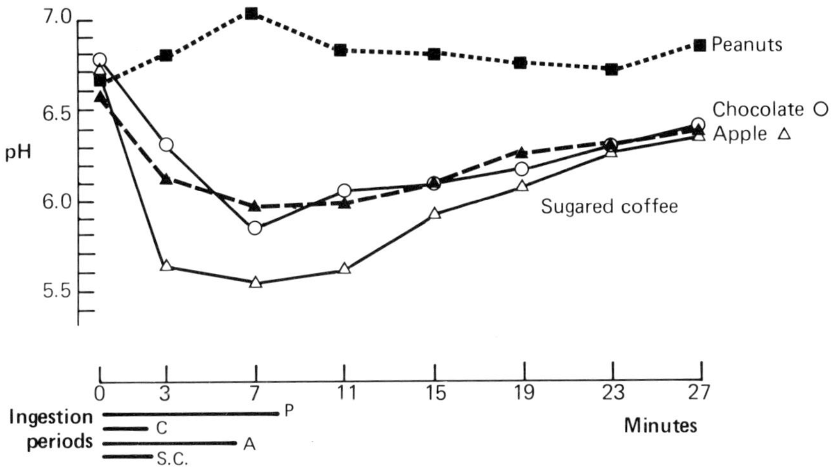

FIGURE 3. Effects of peanuts, chocolate, apple and sugared coffee on plaque pH (by courtesy of the Editor of the British Dental Journal).

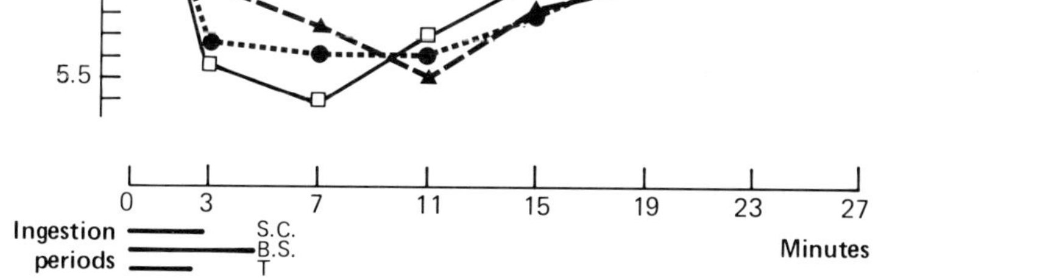

FIGURE 4. Effects of boiled sweets, toffee and sugared coffee on plaque pH (by courtesy of the Editor of the British Dental Journal).

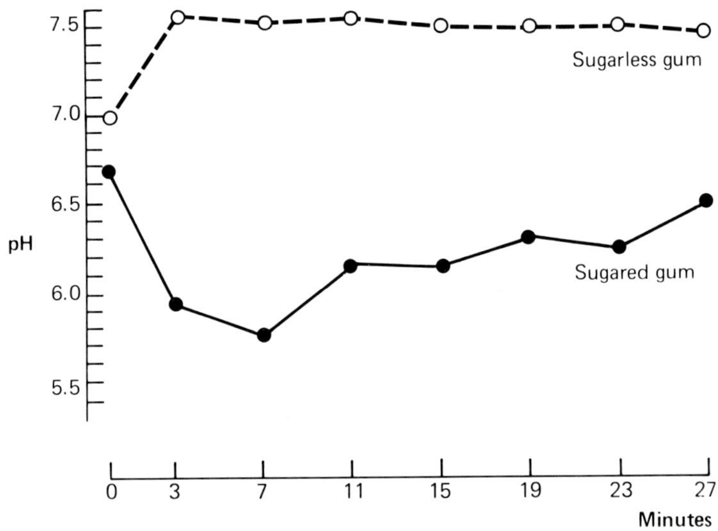

FIGURE 5. Effects of sugared and sugarless gum on plaque pH (by courtesy of the Editor of the British Dental Journal).

the plaque response. In particular, the presence of cheese as the last food item raised the pH of plaque previously lowered by eating the pear (Fig. 6). This effect was less dramatic if there was a prolonged gap (10 min) between "courses." The pH-raising effect was attributed to the flow of saliva, with high pH and buffering power, after cheese consumption.

This finding led us to seek other foods which might have a pH raising effect, nullifying the acidogenic action of previously consumed sugary foods. Apples have been recommended as potentially beneficial in this regard, but we have found[7] that they do not stimulate a rise in pH in plaque when eaten after a sugar lump as convenient sugar challenge, probably because they are themselves acidic and contain sugar (Fig. 7). Peanuts, however, which themselves do not give rise to a fall in plaque pH, almost completely abolish the effect of the sugar lump eaten previously (Fig. 8).

I should like now to turn to the method used by the Zürich group under Professor Mühlemann.[8] This group has developed a method of measuring plaque pH telemetrically, using a partial denture carrying a tooth into which is built a miniature glass pH electrode. The partial denture is worn for up to 7 days, during which plaque accumulates on the intraoral electrode. The pH-sensitive part of the electrode is sited in contact with a healthy tooth surface, so it is believed to record pH at the site where caries often occurs. Using this system, the Zürich group have tested a number of sugary and sugarless candies and beverages in addition to pure substrates and food additives.

By order of the Swiss Office of Health (January 22, 1969) products may be advertized as "Zahnschönend" (safe for teeth) if their consumption does not

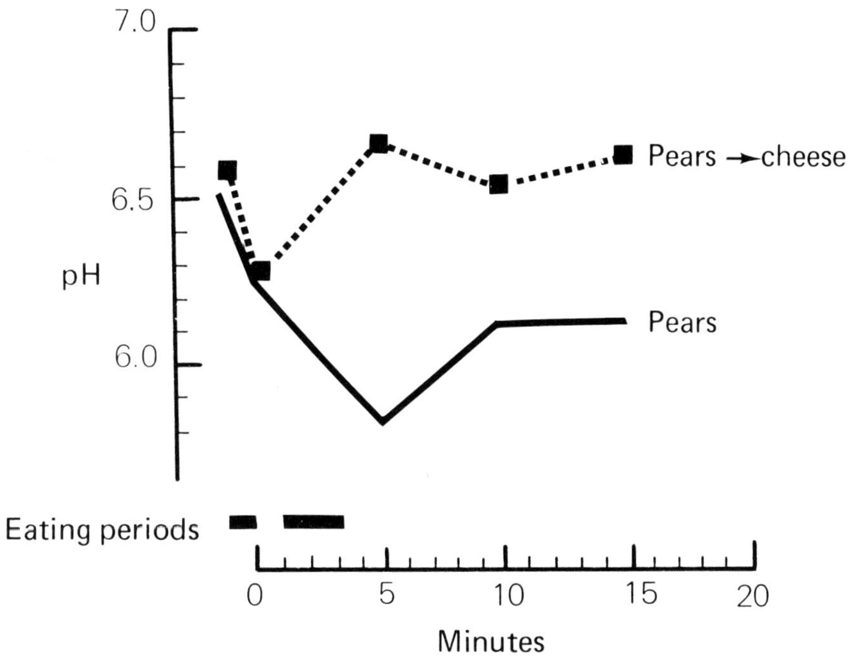

FIGURE 6. Effect of cheese on pH of plaque previously lowered by pear in syrup.

lead to a fall in interdental pH below 5.7 as measured by the telemetric system. The selection of the value of 5.7 is arbitrary. It could be argued that in many areas of the mouth the pH might be permitted to fall below this level without incurring damage to the enamel, but in others it is possible that a level even as high as 5.7 might be harmful.

Attempting to assess the pros and cons of the two methods, I should like first to consider four theoretical and practical aspects.

1. *In the "Newcastle method," an average pH measurement is recorded for all areas of the mouth, in contrast to the single interdental area monitored in the Zürich method.* This latter area is more likely to be the site of caries than the normally caries-free areas sampled with the Newcastle method, which assumes that the data recorded reflect the changes occurring in more caries-prone sites. However, we have some limited information that the pH of plaque sampled from interdental areas and measured by our method does, indeed, parallel the values recorded from more accessible sites, but is about 0.2 pH units lower.

2. *The "Newcastle method" gives a homogenized sample of the plaque, while in the "Zürich method" the electrode is in contact with the inner layer of undisturbed plaque.* However, it is possible that plaque growing on glass differs in a number of important respects from that growing on an enamel surface. It is even possible that the electrode is only correctly functional when not entirely covered with plaque, the plaque-free glass surface responding to the pH of a fluid phase of unknown significance.[9]

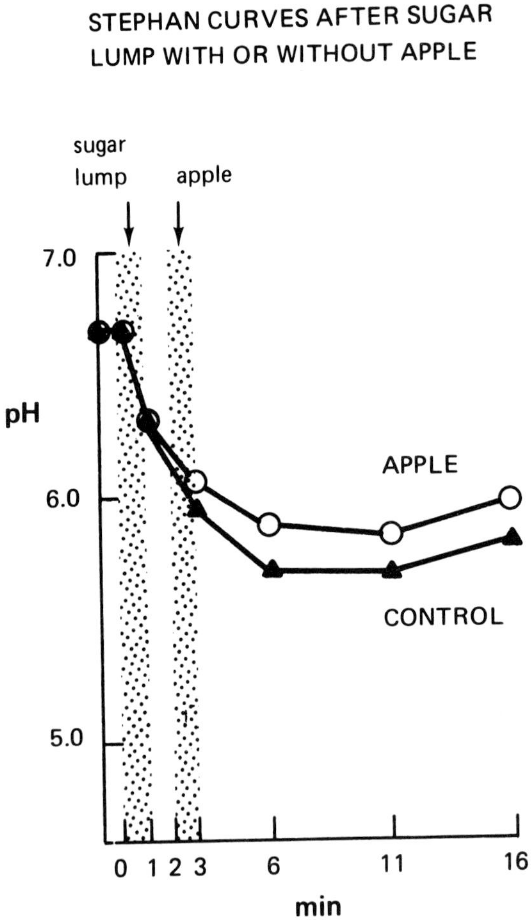

FIGURE 7. Effect of an apple on plaque pH after eating a sugar lump.

3. *Extraoral pH determination is reliable and accurate, while intraoral measurements are prone to errors arising from electrode poisoning and other interferences (e.g., chewing movements).* A wide variety of foods including bread, crackers, cookies and toffees can be studied by the "Newcastle method" which can only be studied with difficulty, or by imposing unnatural conditions on the method of food use (gauze wraps, etc.), when telemetric recording (at least with wires) is used.[8] However, the possibility of contamination of the samples of plaque removed in our method with residues of food should not be ignored, although we believe that this possibility is not a major problem owing to the rapidity with which most foods are cleared from the mouth.[4]

4. *The "Newcastle method" is rapid, flexible and cheap,* and does not require the expenditure of time (subjects and investigators) in the man-

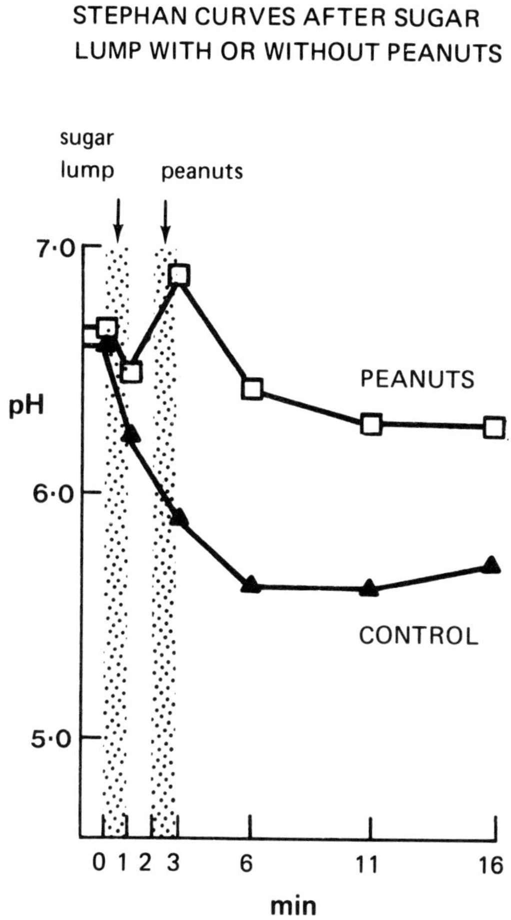

FIGURE 8. Effect of peanuts (salted, roasted) on plaque pH after eating a sugar lump.

ufacturing and testing of the intraoral appliance. Once constructed, however, the Zürich appliance can be reused several times, but may, nevertheless, eventually require replacement. It is clearly easier to study large numbers of subjects (and thus gain data which can be analyzed by powerful statistical tests) if no appliance is required.

Having assessed these advantages and disadvantages, we may compare the results obtained by the two methods.

Imfeld and Mühlemann[8] suggested that a difference of 0.8 pH units may exist between values obtained using the two methods, the "Zürich method" giving the lower values. It is likely, however, that an absolute pH difference of this sort will depend critically upon the design of the intraoral appliance, particularly the relationship between the glass electrode and the abutting tooth. If the electrode is mounted slightly lingually or buccally to the "contact point" with the abutment, it will be exposed to a greater extent to the buffering action of saliva, and will be likely to accumulate a thinner plaque. In the only direct comparison of the two methods simultaneously in the same subject known to me (MacFadyen and Geddes, personal communication), one subject showed a very similar response by the two methods after a sugar rinse, but another showed a normal pH drop (to a pH level of 5.2) by the Newcastle method, while the intraoral appliance did not detect any change in pH, perhaps owing to the electrode being improperly positioned in the appliance.

A further contrast between the results obtained by the two methods is shown in the shapes of the curves obtained in response to a standard treatment (say 10% sucrose rinse). With the Newcastle method, a biphasic curve develops showing a rapid fall followed by a slow recovery, similar to that demonstrated by Stephan. Rarely, however, is a spontaneous recovery phase during the 30-40 minute experimental period given in results using the Zürich method, the pH rise being stimulated by paraffin chewing, or a urea mouthrinse, or both. Whether this demonstrates a crucial difference between the behavior of the interproximal and smooth-surface plaque, or an artifact, cannot yet be decided. In a recent study[10] by the Zürich group which repeated our work[6] on the effect of meal pattern, and notably that of cheese, on plaque pH, the telemetric method was shown to give results which were comparable with our data, but at a pH level approximately 1 unit lower than ours.

Summary

We believe that either method can be used in conjunction with other tests of cariogenicity to give comparative assessments of potential cariogenicity, and thus be useful in giving guidance to patients who seek advice on caries prevention by dietary modification or restriction. They can equally be of value to food technologists in assessing the development of low-caries food products, by, for example, the modification of texture, rate of clearance from the mouth, pH, sweetening agent, etc. We do not, however, feel confident enough to put an absolute value on pH determinations made by either method, and would claim only that they can help us to learn of the relative positions of various foods and drinks in a hierarchy of cariogenicity.

REFERENCES

1. Fosdick, L.S., Campaigne, E.E. and Fancher, O. Rate of acid formation in carious areas. The aetiology of dental caries. Illinois Dent. J. 10:86-95, 1941.
2. Stephan, R.M. Changes in the hydrogen ion concentration on tooth surfaces and in carious lesions. J. Amer. Dent. Assoc. 27:718-723, 1940.
3. Edgar, W.M. The role of saliva in the control of pH changes in human dental plaque. Caries Res. 10:241-254, 1976.
4. Edgar, W.M., Bibby, B.G., Mundorff, S. and Rowley, J. Acid production in plaque after eating snacks; modifying factors in foods. J. Amer. Dent. Assoc. 90:418-425, 1975.
5. Rugg-Gunn, A.J., Edgar, W.M. and Jenkins, G.N. The effect of eating some British snacks upon the pH of human dental plaque. Brit. Dent. J. (In Press)
6. Rugg-Gunn, A.J., Edgar, W.M., Geddes, D.A.M. and Jenkins, G.N. The effect of different meal patterns upon plaque pH in human subjects. Brit. Dent. J. 139:351-356, 1975.
7. Geddes, D.A.M., Edgar, W.M., Jenkins, G.N. and Rugg-Gunn, A.J. Apples, salted peanuts and plaque pH. Brit. Dent. J. 142:317-319, 1977.
8. Imfeld, T. and Mühlemann, H.R. Evaluation of sugar substitutes in preventive dentistry. J. Preventive Dent. 4:8, 1977.

9. Mühlemann, H.R. and De Boever, J. Radiotelemetry of the pH of interdental areas exposed to various carbohydrates. In W.D. McHugh, ed. Dental Plaque. Edinburgh, Livingstone, 1970.
10. Imfeld, T., Hirsch, R.A. and Mühlemann, H.R. Telemetric recordings of interdental plaque pH during different meal patterns. Brit. Dent. J. 144:40-45, 1978.

DISCUSSION

Mrs. Hinkle: I would like to mention perhaps three of four points that have occurred to me, not specifically relevant to the presentation that we just heard, but nevertheless relevant to the thrust of the conference and symposium. I think that it is altogether appropriate that the American Dental Association Health Foundation and Dr. Hefferren requested representation at the symposium by a member of the American Dietetic Association. I cannot imagine anything more appropriate than having a graduate dietitian, a graduate nutritionist, represent all the rest of us in a workshop dealing with cariogenicity of food, beverages and confections. I am more convinced than ever that it is enormously important that we establish and nourish a liaison between dentistry and dietetics and with industry. There are some 23,000 of us trained in nutrition who should have much more awareness of dentistry. We should know a great deal more about dentistry. I consider myself especially fortunate because my husband is a practicing dentist. He is committed to restorative dentistry; thus I am privileged to be in certain situations and circles and am afforded specific opportunities that are not normally available to the trained nutritionist. I think that those of us in nutrition face many of the same problems that you do in dentistry and although I realize that there are home economists and dietitians in industry, we still have a way to go. I believe that our problems and our problem solving should be shared; we should have better understanding between our groups. A suggestion was made to me at a recent ADA Council on Dental Health meeting. Dietetics students should rotate through the colleges of dentistry and other dental facilities just as they now rotate through the medical colleges. More young dietitians and nutritionists should be able to provide better nutritional counseling to the dental students, to the hygienists, dental assistants and to the dentist himself, as well as to dental patients. I cannot think of any group more qualified to help you, at least in this regard, than the trained dietitian. I am certain that we should be participating more visibly and with greater input in the nutrition research projects that were defined yesterday.

Dr. Warnecke: What is the accepted mechanism for the development of dental caries? I don't think we have really explored that subject here yet. Not being a dentist, I will make what I would call a simplistic approach to this and then let my dentist friends correct me. Let us say food is consumed, and at the same time the microflora present in the mouth initiates fermentation which, of course, produces acid. This acid, in combination with the plaque, is held next to the tooth in various areas and causes demineralization. I think Dr. Michaleis commented concerning the actual plaque pH measurements. As we use sucrose or simple sugar as our reference in pH and show dramatic drops, we look at the other aspects of various foods that are low in pH as a beginning. I think particularly of fruit—for example, oranges—I am aware that their pH is below 5.0. A number of foods, soft drinks and many confections have added citric acid to produce a pH below 5. What do you speculate is the difference between the acid produced by fermentation in the mouth and a low pH of food as it is consumed, such as fruit juices, fruits, confections, soft drinks?

Dr. Edgar: A very interesting aspect of these food pH studies is the correlation that we find between food pH and plaque pH. This perhaps is not wholly unexpected. The clinical relationships are a bit more complicated, of course. Dr. Bibby mentioned the difference in demineralization in citric acid and malic acid, and many other examples can be given, such as phosphoric acid. This is the case when our simple measurement of plaque pH may not correlate too closely with cariogenicity. From the clinician's aspect, of course, the effects of food acids are extremely well known and well described. The lesions produced are entirely different in both macroscopic and microscopic appearance, probably because they are not necessarily associated with plaque. They can occur and probably do occur more preferentially on non-plaque surfaces, but the food acids certainly get into plaque, and we believe that a little bit of acid certainly helps the plaque to lower its pH in the presence of sugar.

Dr. Kent Stewart: The techniques now exist in analytical biochemistry, in fact, to analyze quantitatively for individual organic acids at concentrations present in the mouth. Has this been done?

Dr. Edgar: Yes. Beginning a number of years ago, there have been analyses of plaque acids. The most recent one, and probably the best conducted, was done by my colleague, Dorothy Geddes, when she was in Newcastle. She measured the individual acids five minutes after eating a sugar lump and showed with remarkable regularity the enormous production—a 100% increase—in *l*-lactate concentration. The tendency for other acids, volatile acids and *d*-lactate, is to remain the same or go down. The principal metabolic activity which can be correlated with the pH drop is enormous outpouring of *l*-lactate.

Dr. Kreitzman: Many of you may know that several years ago, before Dr. Makinen took up xylitol, his laboratory and our laboratory independently were looking at alternative mechanisms to dental caries related perhaps to the phosphatases. There are certainly no fixed finalities associated with the acid concept. Very likely some other things will be found to occur in terms of the mechanism of dental caries beside the simple dissolution of enamel at pH 5.7.

Dr. Madsen: I might mention our cotton rat caries model. I think we have found something which is of interest. The cotton rat has a very deep fissure in the molar tooth and when we study this model we are really studying fissure caries exclusively. We have been able to feed beverages, soda pops of different kinds, and we also fed or put into the drinking water various of the Krebs cycle acids—citric, malic and fumaric acids. When the animal is drinking the very acidic beverage 20 times a day—he eats and drinks alternately that often—you can see the beverages dissolving away the teeth in a process you might call erosion. Nevertheless, deep within the fissure right behind this flow, caries will develop, and with a sugared solution containing the acid, caries develops in the presence of the acid. However, there is an indication that we get somewhat less caries as a result of the acid being in the sugared solution. We can study the process of caries formation also in the presence of an acidic beverage in this model. It may have some potential for distinguishing between the two features.

I would like to point out that in a study done in children fed malic acid lozenges, there was a borderline significance to a caries protective effect from using the lozenges. The intent was, of course, to stimulate salivary flow which raises pH and the buffer capacity of saliva. But the fact that we were using an acidic material and did not get an increase in caries but rather a potential decrease in caries would indicate that exogenous acid and plaque produced acid at the tooth-plaque interface are two different things.

Dr. Wozniak: Concerning Dr. Edgar's results related to assessment of cariogenic effects, particularly the fact that the pH drops that he observed were affected by the presence of other foods in the oral environment: A pH drop of 5 produced by candy could be altered so the pH would rise again by eating peanuts. The problem we have here, I think, goes back to our efforts to assess a food in terms of cariogenicity when there are other foods present. We should try to assess foods on the basis of their cariostatic behavior rather than their cariogenic behavior. We might be more interested in assessing ingredients of food which lead to a lower caries incidence rather than leading to a higher caries incidence. The effort might be made to alter foods so they will produce a lower caries score.

Dr. Wilson: In your direct comparison between the Newcastle technique and the Zurich technique, there is a difference in the specifications. The Newcastle technique, as I understand it, requires 24-hour plaque, whereas the Zurich technique requires ordinarily a minimum of seven-day plaque to be reliable. In your direct comparisons, which plaque did you use?

Dr. Edgar: This is a slightly awkward situation for me to answer because I did not do the experiment and I just received these results. I can only speculate on the response to this question. It is perfectly possible, of course, to do the Newcastle pH measurements on three-day plaque. It is certainly possible to do the Zurich type measurements on three-day plaque, and I imagine that is what they used. Although in a recent study which may not have been published yet, Professor Mühlemann's group have used one-day plaque and have showed similarities and differences with the kind of results that we have been getting, particularly on the question of interaction of different foods in a meal situation or in a two-food situation as we have had.

Dr. DePaola: Have you assessed the plaque pH drop of selected areas where you did plaque removal, rather than just whole mouth? I understand that one of the problems is that you do not get a lot of plaque; however, have you taken into consideration the selectivity of smooth surface caries and the work of Klineburg, which indicates that there might be a plaque pH differential in different areas of the mouth?

Dr. Edgar: Yes, we have done this but we have never reported it. It is limited, of course, by the amount of plaque that you can study. We have been comparing particularly smooth surface plaque, that is pooled smooth surface plaque with pooled and interstitial plaque and we usually find a small discrepancy in pH—usually the interstitial plaque difference is maybe 0.2 pH units. We have not been able to do individual Stephan curves for different sites because there is not enough plaque there. Certainly on a broad basis interstitial plaque is 0.2 pH units lower than smooth surface plaque.

Dr. Newbrun: Concerning your plaque measurements, first of all I would like to say simply that your extraoral technique is being used by Frostell in

Sweden. It may be appropriate to distinguish it, not as Newcastle or Malmo or Stockholm method versus the Zurich, but as intraoral versus extraoral. You showed a sort of hierarchy of foods, as did Dr. Bibby. I would like to know if they are measured on a unit weight. Do you account for the patient chewing a fixed amount or is it just they bite into an apple and so forth? Is it just per unit weight of food? How do you allow for the fact that patients consume different amounts? I also want to point out that somebody on the panel called it a cariogenicity test. I do not think you or Dr. Mühlemann make that claim. It is, after all, acidogenicity screening only.

Dr. Glass: Professor Edgar, to what extent are the measurements made by the Mühlemann technique dependent on the age of the accumulated plaque and how does this relate to your technique?

Dr. Edgar: We have not studied plaque of such a great age as that of Professor Mühlemann. He has very nicely demonstrated in a group in Adelaide, Australia, the dependence of plaque pH response upon plaque age. You get a nice progressive deepening of the pH drops achieved with the intraoral measurements. In our case, we have not gone beyond three days and we do get a similar kind of drop. We have been much more interested in much younger plaques to see at just what time plaques become potentially cariogenic. We know that we can brush our teeth once every other day and still maintain good gingival conditions. We do not think this is true for caries. We think we have to brush our teeth more often if we want to have some effect on the plaque acidogenicity.

Dr. Baron: I was particularly interested in the combination of foods taken after sugar insult; for example, eating peanuts and seeing the rise in pH. Mühlemann has done similar experiments, of course, and after a pH drop from a sugar insult has shown a rather quick rise after the use of a paraffin tablet, for example. He has also shown an analogous rise with sorbitol, mannitol, i.e., sugarless chewing gum, which I think brings out some very practical implications. Following a sugar-containing snack there are, right now, practical ways of making the pH rise and perhaps lessening the insult from the sugar-containing snack.

Mr. Khan: Dr. Edgar, you have presented an objective measurement technique here. Does it require a dentist to remove little bits of plaque or can this be taught to a skillful technician who could do this and thus give us a tool perhaps to see whether we can make improvements, at least on this one acidogenic factor relating to food? Would you comment on that?

Dr. Edgar: In the United Kingdom—I do not know what the situation is in the United States—it would have to be a hygienist or a dentist. This has been tested in the courts. But we are prudent enough to restrict our plaque collection to a dentist. Maybe that is an aspect of a closed shop coming out, but we always have a dentist collecting plaque, or a hygienist. We do not encourage our technicians to do so. I do not know what the situation is here; perhaps the ADA would have some advice on the subject.

Mr. Khan: Would someone from the ADA respond to my question? Does it require a dentist to remove plaque?

Dr. Hefferren: I think not; dental hygienists do it every day.

EVALUATION OF FOOD CARIOGENICITY BY PLAQUE-pH-TELEMETRY*

H.R. Mühlemann and Th. Imfeld

Introduction

Biotelemetry in general enables direct and continuous measurements of biological phenomena without disturbing the process to be evaluated. Measured data may be conveyed to the recording equipment by wireless transmission (radio-telemetry) or by means of direct connection (wire-telemetry).

In 1965 and 1966 Graf and Mühlemann[4,5] first announced radio-telemetry of plaque-pH from the interdental area. Miniaturized glass electrodes and for a short period also antimony electrodes[6] were used to measure H^+ ion activity with potential freedom from experimental artifacts in otherwise fairly inaccessible places of the oral cavity. Since 1965 valuable experiences and innumerable data have been accumulated. Reviews were published in 1969,[3] 1971[8] and 1977.[7] All these studies have shown the reliability and reproducibility, the quality and accuracy of the pH-telemetric system for the investigation of human plaque-pH behavior.

Thus telemetry has become an important tool for assessing pH-changes both of dental plaque and oral fluid in response to any kind of food or drug.

Materials and Methods

The construction and use of telemetric partial prostheses has been described in detail in 1977.[7] A diagram of the electronic circuitry is given in Figure 1. As shown in Figure 2, the electrodes with their tips are embedded in perforated tooth crowns in the prostheses and the volunteer's abutment teeth.

The test prostheses with clean pH electrodes are inserted and the subjects are asked not to alter their eating habits. With the single exception of water rinses they are to refrain from all oral hygiene measures. The prostheses are not removed during the test period of 3 to 7 days, thus allowing an undisturbed growth of plaque over the tips of the electrodes. pH changes resulting from acids formed in interdental plaque when exposed to fermentable carbohydrates can be recorded with good reproducibility and analyzed statistically when experimenting with 3- to 7-day old bacterial deposits. pH changes of mixed saliva by dietary acids, e.g., citric acid added to candies, also can be measured with the same pH sensor if clean and not covered by plaque.

Some prostheses are equipped with two pH electrodes. Using a prosthesis with an interdentally oriented electrode which is plaque-covered and a plaque-free lingually orientated pH sensor submerged in mixed saliva, it is possible to record simultaneously:

—acid formed by plaque coating the interdental sensor,

—acid formed by the total oral microflora (dental plaques and microorganisms on the dorsum of the tongue, etc.) which lowers the salivary pH at the site of the lingual sensor, and

—dietary acid contacting the clean electrode directly during ingestion.

*Presented at Niagara Falls, N.Y., Caries Conference, 1977. Printed in "Methods of Caries Prediction" and reproduced here with permission of and thanks to the National Institute of Dental Research.

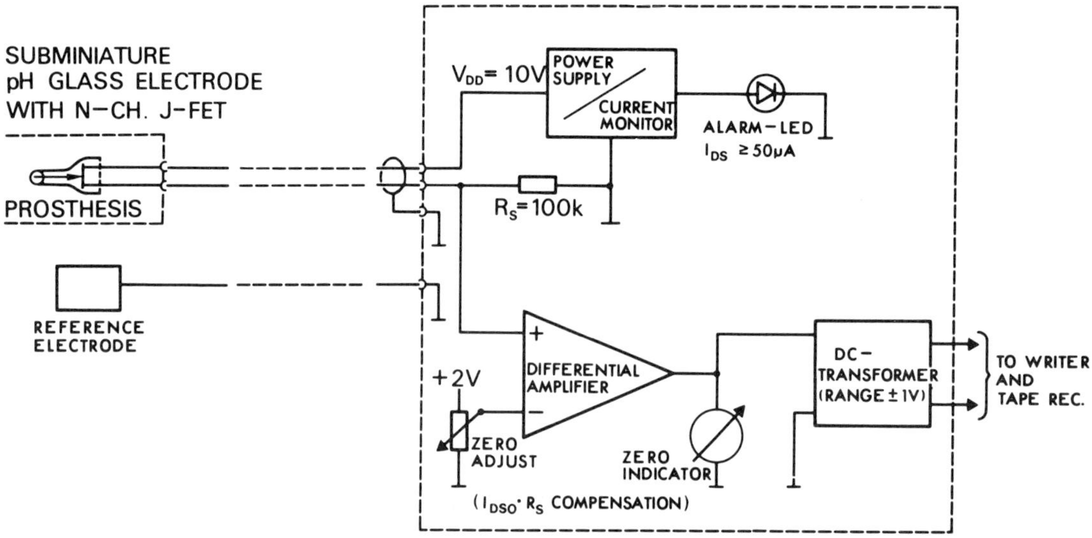

FIGURE 1. Schematic diagram of pH-wire telemetry electronic circuitry with FET-impedance converter.

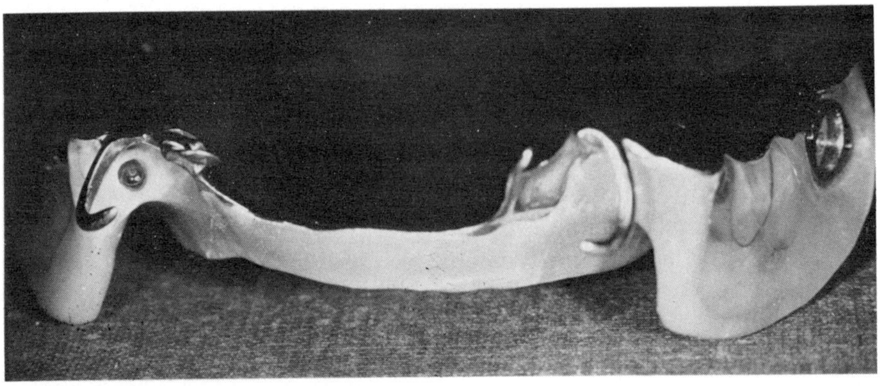

FIGURE 2. Prosthesis with interdental pH-sensor.

Discussion

Another method for the assessment of the glycolytic activity of dental plaque was described by Frostell in 1970.[2] It is mainly used in Great Britain.[9] The pH of plaque samples collected from the teeth before and after the ingestion of carbohydrates is measured *in vitro*.

A reevaluation of these classical *in vitro* plaque pH-studies in the light of plaque pH telemetry reveals that the latter is yielding far more detailed information on pH changes in plaque with regard to the acidogenicity of foods.

Plaque pH is influenced by several factors that are assessed to differing degrees by the two methods. The most significant ones are presented in Table 1.

A final assessment of the acidogenicity and potential cariogenicity of marketed foods, drugs and sugar substitutes[7] should preferentially be performed under *in vivo* conditions with plaque pH telemetry. *In vitro* measurements are only indicators of substrate fermentability.

TABLE 1. Comparison of plaque pH telemetry and pH measurements of collected plaque

Influencing factor	pH telemetry	Collected plaque
- Permeation of plaque by carbohydrates	Adequately assessed	Permeability characteristics destroyed by sampling procedure
- Buffer activity of plaque environment	All dynamic changes adequately assessed	Not assessed
- Dietary carbohydrates containing protein and fat	Effects on pH adequately assessed	Possible contamination of collected plaque and non-physiological interference with pH
- Dietary acids permeating the plaque	Discrimination between dietary and glycolytic acids possible	No discrimination between dietary and glycolytic acids
- Oral clearance time of dietary carbohydrates	Continuous clearance curve possible	Not possible

pH telemetry today is utilized on a statistical base similar to pH measurements on collected plaque.[10] Plaque pH telemetry can be performed only on adults and not on children. Apparently this is only a theoretical disadvantage because it has never been shown that plaques collected in adults and in children behave differently when exposed to fermentable carbohydrates.

REFERENCES

1. Brunner, K., Gabathuler, H., Schneider, Ph. Multi-channel oral wire telemetry. Helv. Odont. Acta 18:83, 1974.
2. Frostell, G. A method for evaluation of acid potentialities of foods. Acta Odont. Scand. 28:599, 1970.
3. Graf, H. Telemetrie des pH der Interdentalplaque. Med. Habil., Zürich 1969.
4. Graf, H., Mühlemann, H.R. Glass electrode telemetry of pH changes of interdental human plaque. J. Dent. Res. (Abstract) 44:1039, 1965.
5. Graf, H., Mühlemann, H.R. Telemetry of plaque pH from interdental area. Helv. Odont. Acta 10:94, 1966.
6. Hassel, Th. M. Construction of micro-antimony electrodes for use in radio telemetry of plaque pH. Helv. Odont. Acta 15:50, 1971.
7. Imfeld, Th. Evaluation of the cariogenicity of confectionary by intra-oral wire-telemetry. Helv. Odont. Acta 21:1, 1977, in Schweiz. Mschr. Zahnheilk. 87:437, 1977.
8. Mühlemann, H.R. Intra-oral radio telemetry. Internat. Dent. J. 21:456, 1971.
9. Rugg-Gunn, A.J., Edgar, W.M., Geddes, D.A. and Jenkins, G.M. The effect of different meal patterns upon plaque pH in human subjects. Brit. Dent. J. 139:351, 1975.
10. Imfeld, Th., Hirsch, R.S., Mühlemann, H.R. Telemetric recordings of interdental plaque pH during different meal patterns. Brit. Dent. J. (in press), 1978.

FOOD CARIES TEST USING ANIMAL MODELS

Juan N. Navia, Ph.D.

Introduction

Approximately seven years ago a workshop to study the role of human foodstuffs in caries was organized by Drs. B. Bibby, R.S. Harris and J.H. Shaw and held at the Eastman Dental Center in Rochester.[1] In the introduction to this conference Dr. Henry Scherp formulated the objectives for the workshop with the following questions: "What in our current knowledge of human nutrition and foodstuffs can be used promptly for prevention of caries? Specifically what research is most likely to produce additional information leading to improved nutritional control of caries?" These questions could be restated today. Many variables in the relationship between food and caries were identified in that workshop, but many questions remained unanswered. Notwithstanding the research efforts made during the intervening years, we still have to work on specific issues critical to the understanding of the food-caries interrelationships. One of these is the evaluation of the caries-promoting properties of foods, particularly snacks containing sugar consumed frequently between meals.

If foods are to be evaluated to determine their posteruptive caries potential in an animal model, it is essential to recognize that the chemical, physical and organoleptic properties of foods can influence the caries test done in animals. Physical properties such as particle size, adhesiveness, solubility of ingredients and texture can influence food impaction in molar fissures and residence time in the oral cavity of animals and, therefore, the severity of caries. The chemical composition of foods can stimulate the implantation, colonization, and metabolism of the bacteria found in dental plaque. Organoleptic properties, particularly smell and taste, may affect the desirability of the test food for the experimental animal, and thus either change the diet intake pattern or determine a rejection of the food being fed. If uncontrolled, these factors may modify the eating behavior or the ecological environment of the oral cavity in such a way that caries results may not be representative of the true effect of this food snack for humans. These experimental considerations have already been pointed out and discussed.[2] Food caries tests ideally should be conducted in clinical trials, but there are ethical, moral, legal and financial reasons that prevent such an approach from being used to evaluate the great number of foods that ought to be tested. The use of laboratory animals, therefore, has become a desirable alternative to such research efforts.

Many different animals have been used in dental research.[3] Three species have been widely used in dental caries research: non-human primates, rats, and hamsters. Non-human primates are excellent laboratory animals used in several types of caries studies which have been particularly useful in immunologic studies.[4] Because of problems related to availability, space requirements, and cost of procurement and maintenance, they have not been used widely in food caries studies in which we need to use large numbers of animals in fairly complicated experimental designs. Hamsters have also been used, but they are more fastidious than rats in terms of dietary needs and adaptability to experimental manipulations. The rat is probably the laboratory animal most frequently used in caries studies involving specific dietary and microbial manipulations. Rats are easily infected with cariogenic microorganisms, they are omnivorous, inexpensive, and a large amount of information is available describing their anatomy, histology, oral flora and the biochemistry and metabolism of oral tissues.[5]

Experimental Characteristics of Animal Caries Models

To evaluate the usefulness of an animal model to test the caries promoting properties of foods, it is important to recognize first that the same three etiological factors for caries have to be present in both humans and animals: a cariogenic flora, a diet providing a fermentable substrate, and an ecological oral environment in the host adequate for caries development. It is also important to realize that nutrients in the diet can affect tooth susceptibility to caries at two distinct developmental stages: (a) preeruptively, as described previously by DePaola, and (b) posteruptively. Preeruptive nutritional effects are important because dietary inadequacies during development may affect enamel or salivary gland development, and thus increase the susceptibility to caries and the variability of results. Experimental animals even marginally deficient during oral tissue development will respond differently when exposed to a cariogenic challenge than control animals fed adequately during development.

Several rat diets have been used to facilitate implantation of cariogenic bacteria and caries development.[3] One diet that has been used extensively to feed rats is known as diet 2000. This diet contains 56% sucrose; it facilitates the implantation of cariogenic bacteria; and carious lesions develop on the buccal, sulcal and interproximal areas of rat molars. Even though it produces caries, it is not nutritionally adequate and the rats fed this diet do not grow and develop healthily. Another frequently used diet is MIT 200, a purified diet which contains 67% sucrose. Nutritionally, this diet is better, but, like diet 2000, it contains large quantities of sucrose, which induce a severe cariogenic stress. We have largely discontinued the use of diets containing high concentrations of sucrose, which may interfere with implantation and metabolic activity of certain cariogenic bacteria. Unless specific experimental requirements demand the use of high sugar concentrations in the diet, we feed rats diets formulated with lower sugar content, such as MIT 305, which contains 62% starch and 5% sucrose, and therefore induces moderate carious lesions on all surfaces of rat molars.[3] In general, all these diets are characterized by a very low fat and water content. Increases in these two dietary components drastically reduce the caries severity in the rat.[2] Caries-promoting diets are usually made up with ingredients pulverized to small particle size. This powdery, dry consistency enhances the implantation of cariogenic bacteria which seem to be dependent, among other factors, on the type of diet fed, salivary components and age of the animal.

Cariogenic bacteria constitute an essential etiological factor for induction of caries in experimental animals. No single organism produces caries in animals; there are numerous bacteria capable of producing caries. *Streptococci, Lactobacilli, Enterococcus* and *Actinomyces* strains have been reported[6] to produce caries in laboratory animals. These different strains of bacteria vary in their biochemical capabilities and virulence and therefore caries severity is determined largely by the flora present in the plaque and their ability to metabolize the components supplied by the test food. Some of these microorganisms have been isolated from humans and implanted in rats and hamsters, where they have continued to express their cariogenic potential, and so it should not be considered that the rat oral flora is totally different from that of humans. Complications could arise from: (a) induction of specific enzymes during the experiment, which might make the bacteria different from the parent strain; and (b) the presence of background flora which could modify the total metabolic activity and the final caries severity. Nevertheless, the important thing to remember is that there is not one, but several bacteria which are cariogenic, and that the rat oral flora can be modified by inoculating a strain of *S. mutans* or some other cariogenic bacteria, and thus obtain caries results which reflect principally the metabolism of such human isolates.

With reference to oral flora and dental plaque, it is interesting to note that abundant plaque formation is not a strict prerequisite to induce severe carious lesions. In rats inoculated with *S. mutans* 6715 the amount of plaque is usually small, yet extensive carious lesions develop on the buccal and interproximal surfaces of molars. However, if you inoculate a hamster with the same *S. mutans* 6715, you will find large masses of plaque covering the crowns and pushing the gingiva in an apical direction. This difference in plaque morphogenesis between rats and hamsters is caused by factors not yet understood entirely, but which do not seem to be related solely to microorganisms.

Caries scoring and type of lesion used to express results are other important aspects of animal experimentation. Several approaches to caries scoring have been described,[7] but we find the one suggested by Keyes[8] the most convenient and widely used method. The only modification to this procedure worth mentioning is the use of murexide staining to disclose the lesions.[9] This staining method is sensitive and not only discloses superficial buccal lesions, but it also indicates, depending on the hue and intensity of the stain, the depth of involvement of the carious attack. Another important aspect of caries scores is the choice of molar surface used to express final results. Buccal scores may not mean the same as sulcal or interproximal scores. Differences in bacteria colonizing these sites, and in accessibility of diet and saliva, might be responsible for the very different results obtained from studies in which cariostatic agents are tested and different molar surfaces are compared. Ideally, an animal model for caries should be able to yield for comparison caries data from all molar surfaces and, in lieu of this, the same surfaces (buccal or sulcal) should be considered when comparing studies done by different investigators.

Experimental Caries Approaches

Several experimental approaches can be used to test the caries promoting properties of foods in laboratory animals such as the rat. Here, attention is focused on two of them. One is called the *conventional system,* in which a rat is either housed in a stainless steel suspended cage or a plastic tub with bedding and a stainless steel top. Rats are offered distilled water and fed a diet *ad libitum.* Diet MIT 305, for example contains 6% cellulose, a fairly inert, caries-promoting ingredient that can be used to make substitutions of different test foods or compounds. Under these conditions, the rat consumes the diet normally, and with it the test compound. The conventional approach is useful, even though there is no control on intake pattern, and diet disappearance and body weight gains are the only parameters available to monitor diet and test material consumption. This approach has been used to test compounds containing fluoride, and there is a great deal of literature concerning animal caries tests in which fluoride was added either to the water or the diet to investigate its cariostatic properties. This conventional procedure has been used also to evaluate phosphates, antibiotics and many other chemical compounds and food ingredients.[2,10] The variability associated with this conventional procedure is fairly low. Highly controlled parallel rat caries studies of the conventional type were run simultaneously in six laboratories which were provided with animals, diet and water from the same source, and which used the same experimental design. A similar pattern of caries developed in the rats from each laboratory, with a range of mean values such that the results of no investigator were significantly different from those of at least two others. Thus, major factors influencing the variability of caries results can be controlled within reasonable limits.

While this conventional approach is useful to test caries promoting or inhibiting properties of certain substances and compounds, caries evaluation of foods becomes a thorny problem. In caries research, it is well known that the frequency with which a food containing a fermentable carbohydrate is consumed represents a major factor in caries development. One of the complications in the use of laboratory animals to study the caries promoting properties of foods, therefore, is that feeding patterns of animals may change depending on the food under investigation. Nutrients in foods may stimulate or inhibit caries development in rats, depending on physical or organoleptic properties of the food, and yet these same properties may not necessarily affect the caries process in humans in the same manner. Thus, it is possible that caries effects obtained with an uncontrolled animal model may be different from the human effects it attempts to simulate.

The conventional approach therefore is not useful to evaluate the caries promoting effect of foods, and a second approach has been developed in which the food is fed via a programed feeding cage. König *et al.*[12] developed a caging system which allows control of the amount and frequency of diet consumption, and we have modified it to control fluid intake.[9] Frequency of drinking and eating, therefore, can be controlled in accordance with a feeding program which includes meals and snacks. We provided a meal at definite intervals to insure that rats grew normally. Most of their nutritional requirements of vitamins and minerals were met with these meals, which consisted of a gel diet which had a very low caries promoting potential. We also introduced the test food under caries evaluation as snacks between meals. The general experimental procedure was as follows: the rats were weaned early, at approximately 18 days of age, and inoculated with cariogenic bacteria such as *S. mutans* 6715; at 20 days of age they were placed in König cages which were connected to rotating feeding plates holding 18 small feeding trays. An eating pattern was set up with a control panel, such that the rats were offered 3 meals and a series of test snacks (4-5) between meals during a 14-hour night period. The purified gel diet used as a meal contributed to their nutritional needs without stimulating caries to any appreciable extent, and the background caries from meals remained low. The amounts of gel diet and snacks test food were increased during the experiment as the rats were growing actively during that time. Initially the food was limited to 85% of the calories known to be required by the weanling rats to force them to eat all meals and snacks, but after a few days the amount of diet needed was accurately controlled to meet their exact caloric needs. In this way, we were able to adjust the amounts of foods offered to avoid having a hungry rat all the time, but rather one that was content with the amount of diet fed. We have also avoided the problem of leftovers and selective eating by allowing adequate time intervals between meals and snacks. The amount of work involved in setting up the meals and snacks was considerable, but this was the only approach that would insure control of eating patterns. At either 49 or 56 days of age, carious lesions on all molar surfaces (buccal, sulcal and interproximal) were scored by the Keyes procedure[8] under a stereomicroscope (30x).

Using this experimental approach, a number of snack foods have been evaluated for caries promoting properties[13]. Some years ago, NIDR issued a contract to study the caries promoting properties of food snacks in which different sugars were used to substitute the sucrose component of the snack food. The foods that were tested were developed in the laboratories of the Foremost Research Company in Dublin, California. With their expertise in food technology, we came up with various formulations which were carefully tested for acceptability. This testing was done by a panel of trained taste experts and also with young children (boy scouts) who accepted or rejected the products. Cakes, cookies, candies, jellies, pies, pop tarts and many other products with normal and reduced sucrose content were formulated, evaluated and manufactured in limited quantities for caries testing.

When these reduced-sucrose foods were caries-compared with identical foods containing sucrose in the described programed feeding approach, we did not find great differences between our experimental foods and the controls. There were some items, such as a sugar cookie, in which decreasing the sucrose concentration was associated with approximately 25% reduction in caries promoting potential, but most foods tested showed no difference. Comparisons between different types of snacks showed significant differences. A lemon pie was found to be much more caries promoting than a sugar cookie, and caramels did not seem to have the caries promoting properties expected of a food known to be chewy. This was an initial study, mainly to develop methodology and to study cariogenicity of sugars such as glucose and fructose versus sucrose, but further research is needed to apply these animal testing approaches to a variety of snack foods. We have also done some preliminary studies with food texture and we feel that this is an important aspect contributing to the cariogenicity of foods, but one very little understood. Further research should explore the contribution of textural parameters to the caries promoting properties of a food.

I believe that animal models are useful to predict the caries promoting properties of snacks. It seems to me that we have only scratched the surface of what we can do. The laboratory rat is useful in the sense that it lends itself easily to manipulative procedures such as programed feeding and drinking regimes. It can be inoculated with human strains of cariogenic bacteria, and it develops carious lesions on all its molar surfaces. The most difficult problem today is ascertaining the validity of extrapolating to humans the data obtained using this controlled animal model. In general, laboratory results obtained by using the rat as a model cannot be *directly* extrapolated to humans, and the same is true for hamsters or non-human primates. However, properly performed tests could allow for ranking of caries-promoting properties of different foods as an indication of their potential threat to human oral health. The most serious limitation at this time is the lack of a reference human study to use as comparison. We have such studies for fluorides and so we can do different types of experiments with animals, knowing that it is cariostatic for both and being aware of the differences in levels of effective concentrations in the rat and the human. A human reference study dealing with cariogenicity of foods would help us in evaluating the animal data. In the absence of such human data, animal studies still can be extremely useful to yield experimental caries information about foods that could be used now in oral disease prevention programs to insure dental health.

REFERENCES

1. "Role of human foodstuffs in caries." Proceedings of a workshop conference. J. Dent. Res. 49, Part 1, Supplement to No. 6: 1970.
2. Navia, J.M. Evaluation of nutritional and dietary factors that modify animal caries. J. Dent. Res. 49:1213-1227, 1970.
3. Navia, J.M. Animal models in dental research. Birmingham, University of Alabama Press, 1977.
4. Bowen, W.H. Relevance of caries vaccine investigations in rodents, primates and humans: Critical assessment in "Immunologic Aspects of Dental Caries." Washington, D.C., Information Retrieval Inc., 1976.
5. Navia, J.M. and Narkates, A.J. The rat in oral biology and dental research. In "Biology of the Laboratory Rat," H.J. Baker, J.R. Lindsey and S.H. Weisbroth, eds. New York, Academic Press, (In press, 1978).
6. Rosen, S. Laboratory animals and their contribution to oral microbiology. In Nolte, W.A., ed. "Oral Microbiology," ed. 2. St. Louis, C.V. Mosby Co., 1973.
7. Van Reen, R. and Cotton, W.R. Methods for scoring dental caries in experimental animals. In "Art and Science of Dental Caries Research," R.S. Harris, ed. New York, Academic Press, 1968, pp. 277-312.
8. Keyes, P.H. Dental caries in the molar teeth of rat. II. A method for diagnosing and scoring several types of lesions simultaneously. J. Dent. Res. 37:1088-1099, 1958.
9. Navia, J.M. Op. Cit. (3), chapter 13.
10. Harris, R.A. "Dietary Chemicals vs Dental Caries." Adv. in Chem. Ser. No. 94. Washington, D.C., Amer. Chemical Soc., 1970.
11. Larson, R.H., Amsbaugh, S.M., Navia, J.M., Rosen, S., Schuster, G.W. and Shaw, J.H. Collaborative evaluation of a rat caries model in six laboratories. J. Dent. Res. 56:1007-1012, 1977.

12. König, K.G., Schmid, P. and Schmid, R. An apparatus for frequency controlled feeding of small rodents and its use in dental caries experiments. Arch. Oral Biol. 13:13-26, 1976.
13. Lopez, H., Navia, J.M. and Hoskins, W.A. Caries evaluation of sucrose substituted snack foods in rats. J. Dent. Res. Special Issue A, No. 150: 112, 1978.

DISCUSSION

Dr. Briner: Dr. Navia, what is the sensitivity of the methods that you described—the cage feeding and the feeding machine? What differences can you detect?

Dr. Navia: I can detect about two units, more or less, between buccal lesions. If I have a 9 and a 7, I could probably discriminate with the system that I have here.

Dr. Briner: Were these rats inoculated with a specific cariogenic organism? Were their flora repressed beforehand?

Dr. Navia: In a series of about 25 different experiments, we did inoculate some of them and others we did not.

Dr. Briner: Would you recommend that somebody who wants to try this use an inoculated animal or a conventional animal?

Dr. Navia: I think it would be much better to have a definition of the flora because it varies so much from time to time. So it would be better if you could in some way control and define your flora. I do not think that it has to be with one organism only, but with several, and I think that would be better.

Dr. Shaw: I think that Dr. Navia has given us a fine background on some of the parameters of what you can do with caries models. I think I would like to stress particularly the need for doing things like this because there are a number of things that we can do very quickly and inexpensively with rats; things that, as Dr. Horowitz pointed out, one cannot at the moment do with human beings. For instance, you cannot take a particular brand of cookies or breakfast cereals and get a valid reading from a clinical population for the simple reason that you usually cannot get enough of that specific item in the midst of the total diet to get a reading, nor can you control the circumstances as to how much is eaten.

I think the average person today is typified pretty well by the first slide with the electrical tracing that Dr. Edgar showed of many different points taken during the day in response to the amount of sugars, the kind of diet, the frequency of diet which showed a plummeting of the pH in the plaque area. Now in the Vipeholm study, the basic diet was one really very low in sugars compared to what we would think typical in the American population today. I am not even sure that their data would be reproducible today even if you could do it, because so many of our foods already have sugars added to them before we receive them. I think there is a figure we should remember in this regard, that of all the sugar used in the typical diet today, about 75% is added in the manufacturing process and there is an election by the consumer only of the other 25%. In other words, only 25% of the sugar that is used in the typical American diet today is sugar that is bought as such for a direct addition by the consumer.

This procedure of using the clinic cages is a fantastically laborious one. It takes one technician almost complete time to operate that and put the new diets in each day; also it is a maddening job and I do not know how you can stay sane and do it. We have used the alternative of feeding a nutritious diet for several hours a day and then feeding the food item that we want to evaluate for another portion of the day, so the food cup in the first cage shown only has to be changed two or three times a day. It makes a lot less labor, a lot less weighing, etc., and on the basis of our cross-checking between the two methods, I do not see that we get any difference.

Dr. Navia: Two people are required.

Dr. Shaw: There are 1,296 cups on one of those machines for 72 rats that have to be weighed, cleaned, and refilled every day and if you add on the drinking water, you have an additional 1,296 tubes.

Dr. Madsen: We, as experimental scientists using the rodent model, cannot readily make products that are marketable in which you have a control and an experimental sample. Dr. Navia has been able to get some of these products. Attempts to standardize the testing systems have been made by the NIDR, but I would like to suggest that the NIDR include manufacturers and consider an alternative way of getting data. If we could have food manufacturers— each of whom have different products but together have all of our snack products represented—provide each person, whether he is doing an *in vitro* testing, testing one or another rodent system, radio telemetry, or whatever, with the same control and experimental products, then we could all see how it responded in our systems. I would love to have these products that Dr. Navia has been testing. Other people are planning right now to do this, but they are going to do it within the strategy of their own laboratory. I would love to see everyone doing any type of experimental testing be able to test control and experimental products that are acceptable at the market level, things that we can cite as safe items to dentists and hygienists. This is our goal, and if we get to the snack vending machines, convenience foods—this is one way I believe it can be done, or get closer to it.

Now the cotton rat system is more limited but it has a certain value that I mentioned when talking about beverages. It is almost a pure fissure caries system. It has one advantage; it is very insensitive to phosphate and is somewhat like the human situation. We ran about 40 phosphate studies, which is quite a bit of work, and out of these we sometimes got phosphate to work, and trimetaphosphate was the best. It was also best when it was incorporated into a product. There are advantages to using the different systems. If we can get these foods available in all the different systems, we would have a better chance of knowing what is really effective at the use level of a real product. I would test the acid idea, with Dr. Navia's lemon pie, whether that is acid or something else in our system.

Dr. Gaffar: Dr. Navia, when you reduce the concentration of sucrose from 67 to 5%, do you see any difference between the progression and severity of carious lesions?

Dr. Navia: Yes. That is why we use it, because it is a milder kind of attack and you get a score of 25 or 20 with a diet 200 which has 67% sucrose and you might get 50% less with 5% sucrose.

Dr. Naleway: I have rather limited experience with animal studies, but it would appear that there is a need for additional studies to be done which would more properly correlate animal studies, clinical studies, and *in vitro* studies. One is the comparison between the cariogenicity produced in an animal study and the pH effect. I would be interested to see studies done in this area, or animal studies designed to compare more of the parameters which would be obvious within clinical studies and within *in vitro* studies.

Dr. Navia: I think this is an excellent suggestion and I mentioned the collaborative study that was done by NIDR and Dr. Larson as an example of a situation in which the same method was taken by five different laboratories and evaluated. I don't see why we cannot do the same kind of thing using the different methods in trying to find agreement or disagreement. We have not done that.

Dr. Horowitz: Dr. Navia, just for clarification, in the data related to the substitute food in which you tried to duplicate the properties of the original as much as possible, there was very little change in caries scores. What was substituted? Were these sugar-free substitutes, or were they substituted with fructose or glucose?

Dr. Navia: There were different kinds of changes. In some cases there was a reduction of sucrose *per se*, and substituting other kinds of thickening agents and things of this sort. In other cases it was mostly addition of fructose to compensate for the sweetness. There we made different kinds of changes, none of which involved any kind of synthetic sweeteners. All were done with the kinds of ingredients that were normally used in the manufacture of those particular foods. As you can see, there was no big difference.

Dr. Hefferren: Is there a way in the animal model to get at the food or clearance situation in the mouth? Can you get at food clearance with the animal model?

Dr. Navia: I do not know. I have not even been able to have a rat chew gum.

Dr. Briner: They will drink beer though. I have tried that.

Dr. Schiff: Will you please elaborate your judgment about hamster studies versus rat studies?

Dr. Navia: I have problems with hamsters in terms of the kinds of manipulations that you can do and keep the animals doing the things you want. The rat is very pliable and flexible and you can make him comply with whatever regime you want; with the hamsters you cannot. The litter size for the rats is very large; the one for the hamsters is very small. The rats will be contained within the space of the tunnel that leads to the food. The hamster just passes through. They have the capability of disappearing from the cage. I would rather work with rats.

Dr. Briner: Dr. Gaffar has done some work with hamsters. Would he comment?

Dr. Gaffar: We use hamsters routinely for screening anticaries agents and we never have any problems such as those Dr. Navia suggested. In our hands they provide very useful information. But we use both animals.

Dr. Navia: My remarks were in terms of the use of the hamster for food testing in the kind of contraptions that I explained. In conventional studies you can use them and have no problems.

Dr. Madsen: Hamster study on caries is really almost entirely on smooth surface caries. I think we would accept that whereas cotton rat caries is almost pure fissure; with the white rat you have a combination of the two. Of course, there are many other variables. That is why it is valuable to have testing in various systems.

Dr. Newbrun: There is now in the literature sufficient data from rodent studies—by Stephan, König, yourself, Shaw, and Madsen—in which various foods have been tested so that one can get a hierarchical ranking of foods based on animal studies. Certainly König has done it and Stephan has done it. How does that hierarchy compare with the sort of data that Dr. Bibby and Dr. Edgar have shown?

Dr. Navia: First, the work of Stephan was done many, many years ago. He was an outstanding investigator, but at that time did not use the same methodology and precautions that we have now. So I will not comment on the relationship between those values and the values that we are finding today. I can say that in terms of, for example, the studies that Dr. Bibby has done, there are certain foods that come surprisingly close. I will mention one thing that was a tremendous surprise to me, and that was caramels. We, in our systems, do not find caramels so cariogenic. Of course, the caramels and toffees that you have heard about from the Vipeholm study—that is another kind of confectionery product. The caramels that are normally sold here have a high fat content and a high protein content and may not be as cariogenic as we think. I think, correct me, Dr. Bibby, if I am wrong, that you do not find them to be so terribly cariogenic. We have certain things that we agree on. Evidently we need a lot more work. We need to get the same kinds of foods, and as it was pointed out here, we need to test them with these different methods and then correlate them with the methodology that we have today.

Dr. Briner: In our process of alternating between a nutritious diet and a snack item or a food of any kind, I would verify what Dr. Navia says in that we compare all of ours with sucrose. In other words, one of the control groups is a low calorie diet, another group is a low calorie diet alternated with sucrose. And with the various foods and confectionery items that we compared, we have gone from things that had a zero rating relative to sucrose to ones that were more cariogenic than sucrose. On our particular rating system, the caramel that we tested ran around 40% that of sucrose. Something like shredded wheat will be around zero.

Mr. Tiematra: The pet food industry has gone to using carbohydrates or different types of products as in the semi-moist foods. I was wondering if you had cats and dogs on your list, but you have not done any laboratory work with them. Has there been any feedback from the veterinary profession, or from laboratory studies on those types of foods and the instances of caries there?

Dr. Briner: We have not looked at that, *per se,* but we work very closely with some veterinarians. The dogs just do not have a cariogenic flora yet. You just cannot find *S. mutans* in dogs. At least I have not, and I have looked at 300 or 400 dogs. Our veterinarian has not seen any caries that he could attribute directly to eating the high sugar type of dog foods. If they are around long enough, I would be surprised if the dogs did not get infected with *S. mutans* if you can implant them. However, I do not know of any studies that have been tried.

Mr. Atkinson: What were the results of any of the studies in the areas of the world, maybe in Texas, where people have very few cavities or no cavities? And what have been the results of the studies of the water in these situations?

Dr. Briner: Are you talking about the people who are immune to caries despite a high sucrose intake, is that your question?

Mr. Atkinson: No. Without regard to the sucrose intake in some areas, in Texas for example, the people in the communities have no caries. Is this just the result of fluoride, or what have been the studies?

Dr. Madsen: My first suspicion would be that this is simply a high fluoride area. You would expect to get a remarkable lack of caries in a high fluoride area.

Dr. Briner: As in Deaf Smith County, Texas. They have something like 2.5 ppm fluoride in the water, and they do not have much tooth decay there. They have a lot of mottling.

Dr. Chilton: You said, with some degree of levity, Dr. Navia, that you have not been able to train rats to chew gum. Do we have any animal model systems in which gum chewing can be used among the higher primates or others?

Dr. Navia: I am not aware of it. Maybe someone else is.

Dr. Baron: No. Personally I have not tried it. Dr. Bowen has tried it and I think he got two of them to do it. The monkeys do, in fact, chew the gum until the sweetness goes out, and then they start sticking it in their ears and noses.

Dr. Chilton: Am I correct in assuming that the reason that dogs do not develop caries or a cariogenic flora is that they don't have salivary amylase-ptyalin and don't do any pre-digestion before sugar gets down to the lower parts of the intestine?

Dr. Briner: Obviously that could play a part in it. I do not think the dog's sugar intake is very high anyway. There are instances in which people have fed their dogs sweets, and then they develop caries. This is well documented.

Dr. Chilton: Is that true caries, or would it be root erosions?

Dr. Briner: It looks like nursing bottle caries. A lot of such dogs just don't have teeth; they are gone.

Dr. Navia: There have been some occasional clinical reports of veterinarians who have seen certain alterations in teeth of dogs when the owners have given them a lot of sweets. But I do not think these have been documented clearly as carious lesions. I think the dog has many differences when compared to humans and rats. The occlusal habits of dogs are quite different. The respiration—they ventilate through the mouth—plus the conical morphology of the teeth and other factors all go against the development of a flora which would be cariogenic.

Dr. Brin: One of the marvels of oral physiology is the ability of the salivary gland to exclude glucose from the mouth. It maintains a gradient of 100 mg percent in the extracellular fluid to virtually negligible levels in the mouth. Dr.

Edgar's data showed that variation in caries activity was related to preexisting plaque pH. Could one then relate the endogenous saliva sugar level to basal caries activity? Because if this relationship holds, one could use the endogenous saliva sugar levels of a child as perhaps predictive of later caries susceptibility.

Dr. Edgar: I think there has been a fair amount of work trying to correlate salivary factors such as salivary glucose concentration with caries activity. About the only thing that comes up with any regularity is a correlation between flow rate or some flow rate-dependent feature such as bicarbonate concentration, buffering power, pH and caries. This is about the only factor in saliva that turns up with any regularity as being associated with caries activity.

Dr. Chilton: I would like to make the point at this Workshop that there are other types of caries beyond enamel dental caries. We are talking mostly about children, but in our epidemiological studies we have found that in some of our populations, over 50% of the people we study have root caries, which apparently have a different microflora, a different age distribution, certainly a different surface distribution and can produce problems of restorative dentistry which are amazingly difficult to handle. The type of caries which affects such a relatively large proportion of our population, particularly the older population, is often just passed over without even a comment. This is particularly important with the use of certain confections, and certain types of sweetening agents which will stay at the necks of the teeth, particularly in those patients who have exposed root surfaces. We see this clinically. They produce periodontial and endodontic problems.

Dr. Navia: The animal model has not been explored sufficiently in terms of caries produced by late infections. A group at Forsyth, for example, has done an interesting study about the fact that *S. mutans* tends to implant in the active very young animals. However, if you try to implant *Actinomyces* you cannot do it. You have to wait until the animal is 45 days of age and then you can implant. Perhaps late studies of caries would be interesting, but they just have not been done. There is something happening in the oral cavity that allows the implantation of different kinds of organisms at different times. This becomes a very important aspect with regard to the interpretation of the sugar studies, because different organisms have different capabilities of fermenting different sugars. Someone can be doing a study with one animal at one time with one kind of organism and get a very different response for a certain sugar for the cariogenicity than someone else who is using different conditions. We need to understand more about that.

Dr. Bibby: As to dog caries, it is interesting that the museums in Hawaii show that the Polynesian dogs had dental caries. The reason for this is apparently, as you know, in the Pacific Islands there were no mammals. The dog was fed poi, a carbohydrate source, as a carnivorous animal and apparently caries was quite common among them. As to the question of correlation of the animal caries to some of the other indices, we have made preliminary correlations with clearance, with demineralization and with an *in vitro* caries system. We find, not consistent, but really encouraging relationships to the enamel demineralization. The same is true of the *in vitro* caries test. I think that there are possibilities for correlating these things. Dr. Madsen and I compared some data from solubility and hamster caries and got correlations. I would like to suggest that investigations go forward in parallel rather than all in the same way.

Dr. Mackay: Dr. Navia, I noticed that your gel diet contains 5% sucrose. Is that right? You characterized that as non- or slightly cariogenic, yet your 305 diet with 5% sucrose was highly cariogenic, of course, because that was your stress diet. This, of course, points out the well known importance of the particle size of the stressing agent, in this case the sucrose. But I wonder, why did you have 5% sucrose in the gel diet in the beginning? Did you not also use a system to show that xylitol was almost as cariogenic as sugar? I believe that was in one of your earlier reports using the 305 diet.

Dr. Navia: Yes, we have 5% sugar in diet 453 because we would like, in some way, to continue to facilitate the implantation of the cariogenic organism. The reason I said it was essentially non-cariogenic was that I had modified the consistency and the moisture of the diet in such a way that I produced very little caries. As you recall, consistency was one of the factors that was responsible for the cariogenicity of the diet.

Dr. Mackay: There is still proof, in a way, that 5% sugar in that gel diet is, as you say, noncariogenic.

Dr. Navia: Yes. I think that Dr. Bibby's comment about the food being cariogenic is very important. As to my studies on different kinds of sugars, under my conditions — partial substitution of the overall cariogenic attack with 5% xylitol, and for that matter 5% mannitol, and sorbitol—I do not find any special contribution to the overall caries level of the animals when I make these limited substitutions in the diet. This makes me believe that unless you do a total substitution of all the cariogenic components, you will not be able to recognize the beneficial or other properties of sugars.

Dr. Mackay: In fact, your work points out the extreme complexity of the situation, particularly your slides showing the substitution of foods, and how easy it is to go wrong even when you think you are moving in the right direction.

Dr. Shaw: I would like to comment on what Dr. Mackay has mentioned because it is terribly important to know what the other materials in the diet are. Dr. Kreitzman gave an example of that yesterday, for example, where he did not see a diminishing amount of dental caries when he went from around 60% of sucrose to a very small amount, but you noticed he did not tell us what replaced the sugar. What was it?

Dr. Kreitzman: Corn starch.

Dr. Shaw: And exactly what specification of corn starch? Because corn starch varies in its composition, the amount it has been cooked, the particle size and so forth. But by and large, if you buy corn starch just as it would be sold to a home for thickening gravy or something like that, it would be a modestly cariogenic material. I presume that is because there has been enough breakdown hydrolysis of the polysaccharide to make it usable in the home. There will be a certain amount of glucose, maltose, various tri- and tetrasaccharides, all of which are cariogenic in the animal system. Now if you have, and this has been done in a number of laboratories, starch that is much less cooked and processed, it is much less cariogenic. If you go one step further back and supply the same amount of starch as a whole grain, it is even much less cariogenic. So it makes a lot of difference what the background materials are in the diet, whether you get little or much caries when you have a small amount or medium amount. If you are replacing your sucrose with fat, the caries reducing influence of small amounts of carbohydrates goes down precipitously.

Dr. Navia: This why it is very important that we understand which organisms are involved in the system, and their biochemical properties. The work that Dr. Brown presented is really fundamental. It is important that we understand what these different organisms are doing biochemically. We must understand whether they ferment sugar, or whether they ferment handled starches or whatever, and we do not have a lot of that information. We need to study that.

Dr. Briner: Dr. Kent Stewart made a very cogent remark regarding the need for detailed analytical evaluation, not only of foods. I think you can extrapolate that to detailed evaluation of such things as corn starch. I think that is extremely important. If you look at dental research, by and large, and the blandness with which we use corn starch—I have done this myself—it is nothing short of ridiculous when we consider today's ability to analyze.

Dr. Brin: Try milk powder; that could be even worse.

Dr. Madsen: On the matter of starch, it is even more complex. We had a sample of cracked corn from the Amazon that we checked because these children's teeth decayed to the point where they died from severe abscesses. This corn was just like feeding sugar, it decayed the teeth rapidly. We have also compared Argo corn starch with Peerless and with Amadex corn starch, a high gritty compact starch. Peerless was midway in cariogenicity. Amadex was just as cariogenic as sugar—sucrose. So you can really detect this easily; it depends on the rodent's system and the model you use.

IN VITRO METHODS OF STUDYING THE CARIOGENIC POTENTIAL OF COMESTIBLES

George K. Stookey, Ph.D.

One of the objectives of this workshop is to review the state of the art with regard to the cariogenicity of food and another objective is to identify additives or measures which may alter the cariogenic properties of foods. Various methodologies, including *in vivo* studies and clinical investigations for assessing the cariogenic potential of foods have already been reviewed. An important first step in such investigations is the use of *in vitro* models.

By definition, or perhaps by convention, *in vitro* models are considered to be laboratory methodologies which do not involve human subjects or animals. They are methodologies which can be performed in the laboratory and which are typically of short duration, requiring relatively little personnel and generally with limited quantities of specialized or sophisticated analytical equipment. As a result, *in vitro* models are relatively inexpensive.

A key factor in selecting and using *in vitro* models is the identification of the objectives and a full appreciation of the numerous limitations of these test procedures. It is not at all appropriate to select a given *in vitro* model and from the results obtained consider or imply that a given food item has greater cariogenicity than another in man. Very likely the greatest abuse, or misuse, of *in vitro* models rests with the manner in which the results are interpreted and particularly the extrapolations made from these findings.

We may then ask "What are the objectives of such *in vitro* models and how may they be used to explore the cariogenic potential of foods?" To answer this question we must first explore the factors related to the cariogenicity of foods. Among the numerous factors thought to be involved are:

1. the amount of fermentable carbohydrate present in the food;
2. the inherent pH of the food when mixed with saliva;
3. the physical consistency of the food when ingested;
4. the amount of intraoral retention of the food;
5. the inherent pH buffering capacity of the food; and
6. the frequency with which a given food is ingested.

And still we have not even mentioned those factors related to the individual who ingests the food item—his age or expected caries susceptibility, his oral hygiene program (toothbrushing, flossing), his dental care program (fluoride treatments, fluoride dentifrice and mouthrinses), the remainder of his diet, etc.

Thus, *in vitro* models have a very limited, but yet very useful, role in studies of this nature. In particular, they are:

1. very useful in providing specific pieces of information which may (or may not) be related to the cariogenic potential of a given food; and
2. extremely helpful in exploring whether or not various additives or food processing methods have altered a selected characteristic of the food which may be related to its cariogenic potential.

We may then ask what types of *in vitro* models are available and what kind of information can they provide? The literature contains numerous reports describing *in vitro* models, and the specific details of these methodologies are not considered appropriate to this discussion. Instead, let us consider a number of *in vitro* methods in a more general manner.

First, a fundamental piece of information relates to the composition of the food item and particularly to the amount of carbohydrate present—even more especially to the amount of mono- and disaccharides contained in the comestible. The presence or absence of relatively large amounts of mono- and disaccharides is a key piece of information to any investigation of the cariogenic potential of any food items—and it is a piece of information which should be readily available to the food manufacturer. However, this information must be kept in the proper perspective. Even though the consumer may not yet appreciate the meaning of these data, the fact remains that there are a number of reports which indicate that the disaccharide content, more precisely the sucrose content, of a given food is not necessarily directly related to the cariogenicity of the food.

A second type of *in vitro* methodology relates to studies of the pH of the food when mixed with water, or preferably saliva. It is generally accepted that the critical pH for enamel demineralization is about 5.3. Thus, if the pH of a food and water mixture is below 5.3, the food might be considered to have potential for enamel decalcification or erosion. Most likely it will be much more appropriate to mix the food with freshly collected pooled human saliva, as saliva has considerable pH buffering potential. Again the results should be interpreted with caution, with due consideration of the other factors involved in assessing the cariogenic potential of foods including the presence of pellicle which is known to be a protective barrier against acid decalcification of enamel.

Another piece of valuable information is related to the physical form of the food and particularly to the amount of intraoral retention. It is well known that comestibles in liquid form are cleared relatively rapidly from the oral cavity and therefore result in less exposure of the food to the tooth surface. Several *in vitro* approaches have been used to explore the rate of oral clearance or the degree of adhesion of foods to tooth surfaces. For example, one group of researchers devised an apparatus which would simulate the chewing process and then determine the relative amounts of different foods retained on extracted teeth which were mounted in the chewing machine. In a similar manner it is possible to determine the amount of sucrose retained on the teeth.

Still another approach has been used to explore the pH buffering capacity of the food item of interest. This is considered of importance as some food constituents have appreciable pH buffering potential and this characteristic may be of particular interest in those foods with greater periods of intraoral retention. One method of studying this characteristic involves a simple pH titration of a food and water mixture with dilute hydrochloric acid. Another method, which provides additional information, involves the incubation of food and saliva mixture and the determination of pH as a function of time.

Somewhat related to such studies are *in vitro* tests designed to determine the influence of the food upon the growth of dental plaque. Here again a variety of *in vitro* methodologies have been utilized. One approach has been to use a device which simulates the mastication of the food, the removal of food debris from the teeth by toothbrushing, inoculation of the teeth with *Streptococcus mutans* or mixed oral flora, and incubation for various periods of time. The dental plaque then may be scored visually or removed and quantitated. The results observed in this procedure represent a combination of several characteristics of the food, including the degree of retention and the availability of fermentable carbohydrate in the food which supports the colonization of bacteria and the formation of plaque. In some instances it may be desirable to use a simpler study design to test only the plaque-supportive capabilities of the particular comestible of interest.

Yet another *in vitro* model involves the assessment of cariogenicity on the basis of caries formation in extracted human teeth using the so-called "artificial mouths." In this procedure clinically-sound extracted teeth are typically mounted in acrylic plates and exposed daily to the particular food of interest, using a simulated chewing apparatus or some other procedure. The teeth then are freed of residual food debris, inoculated with human saliva or a particular microorganism such as *S. mutans,* and incubated for the remainder of the 24-hour period with a continual flow of media over the teeth. The procedure is continued either until evidence of decalcification can be detected microscopically or visually or, preferably, until the teeth show evidence of clinical cavitation; this latter criterion typically requires 15 to 18 weeks.

From this brief overview it should be apparent that there is a wide variety of *in vitro* methodologies that may be useful in collecting information—information which may be useful in helping characterize the cariogenic potential, not the actual cariogenicity, of a particular food or comestible. In a similar manner it should be obvious that these various methodologies may be quite useful in the identification of food processing procedures or chemical additives which may alter or reduce the cariogenic potential of the food.

As noted, however, the use of extreme caution in the interpretation of data from *in vitro* studies is absolutely imperative. While *in vitro* studies play a very important role in providing basic information for characterizing foods relative to their cariogenic potential or for screening additives for anticariogenic potential, they are only a first step in the data collection process. The true significance of *in vitro* data can be known only after the data collection process has been continued through controlled clinical investigations.

DISCUSSION

Mr. Muller: I think the point was emphasized about a need to correlate the *in vitro* studies with the clinical data, as in the animal model. I do not know how much has been done, but obviously it needs to be done.

Dr. Naleway: We have many manufacturers represented here and I think it would be of some interest to enter into some discussion to consider what sort of *in vitro* tests, as well as other tests, might be considered relevant or be suggested to compare products on a volunteer basis. What specific tests could be run in a simple manner in laboratories which are now set up in industrial firms?

Dr. Madsen: As with the rodent study, if we could get the same food products tested by all the different people, using all of the different testing procedures including the *in vitro,* we could compare these data on those food products that are really used—those that are acceptable and marketable. Individuals volunteer to send me their samples, but that is not what I mean. We need some organized effort in which decisions are made about which samples should be studied. These would be between-meal snack items, such as those we are talking about primarily, and to have these available through some central person or agency that will allow everybody to test them in all these different systems.

Dr. Shaw: I would like to sharpen that even more. It seems to me that there is a limited number of things that can be tested to the point where it would stagger the imagination to set up *in vitro* or animal tests to do it. And I think Rachel Larson was due a great deal of credit for the way she got a little group together to plan, not only the cooperative study that Dr. Navia mentioned, but another one that was a sequel to that, and then organized the whole effort. It seems to me that we need to take what some judiciously selected committee might consider to be ten or a dozen kinds of products highly varied with respect to the time and place and circumstances in which they are likely to be used. Among them would be some that, on the basis of the information that we have today, we suspect would probably give the same kind of readings with an animal assay with two or three of the key *in vitro* tests and with the pH measurements in plaque that Dr. Edgar talked about. Then the others would be ones about which there was disagreement in the kind of data that have been collected so far. You would have maybe ten or a dozen products that have been very carefully selected, and with those you would apply a whole series of *in vitro* plus animal caries tests. It should be done in a situation where everything is very carefully designed so that there can be a good computer assisted statistical analysis later.

Dr. Kreitzman: If we take fluoride, for example, because we know that fluoride is effective, we can attribute all kinds of mechanisms to it, and we know that it can change the solubility characteristics of enamel and, *a priori,* make some decisions about how fluoride is working.

I think it would be much more important to be able to take something for which we cannot predict the reaction in different systems, but we know its cariogenicity or we know how it reacts in the *in vitro* systems where we do not know its cariogenicity and see if that can be predictive in the other system. We might be led astray because we know and have selected a half dozen things about the interactions of which we know something.

Dr. Madsen: I think that you are right. I think, however, we can do it the way Dr. Shaw suggests. I think we can set it up the way we think it is going to work out, and then we will find out whether it does or not. We want to get those that we are sure are the most cariogenic, those that we are sure are safe, and get a good range in the middle—a good spectrum, and then see whether our premise is right or not. I think we will probably be surprised on this matter of food retention that we have talked about; no one came up with anything for animal models. There have been some studies in which the writer, in describing his experiment, tells that he fed something because he knew this was sticky and it would be more retentive than something else, and the data were just dropped because the experiment did not turn out at all the way he thought it would in terms of retentiveness.

Dr. Bibby: I think Dr. Stookey gave a good introduction into the subject. Perhaps in thinking about these *in vitro* methods or caries machines, or whatever you want to call them, it should be kept in mind that although we probably could have a lot of fun building the super machine that had everything on it, it is not necessarily the right approach. I think we are satisfied to find out something about one aspect of the bacteriology, the serology, or the machine. We should be prepared, however, to use them to measure retention separately, and other factors separately. I think we should definitely think in the plural rather than in the singular regarding these *in vitro* approaches.

Dr. Stookey: Yes, I agree with that. I think you should keep in mind that *in vitro* tests are really a means of collecting information about a given food or product. Ultimately probably there should be a clinical trial involved. And that kind of information, individual bits of information you can get about retention, or on all the different aspects—composition, plaque supportive capabilities—are going to be very important in helping the clinical group, the biometrician, to design the appropriate clinical trial and control it and execute it.

Mr. Kahn: I assure you, Dr. Madsen and Dr. Shaw, that the food industry would not only be able, but quite willing to provide each and all of the investigators who wish to do collaborative work in comparative studies of the different methods with a uniform and ample supply of food products. Before anybody is going to sit down and do that, however, you would probably have to do it through a trade association, because you should not do it with individual companies for individual products. And secondly, it will be necessary for you to publish your data appropriately. When you report on a company's brand name as being the highest or lowest of something, you are really cutting off further cooperation. We are in a competitive world and I believe it is just as easy to talk about food number such and such, and describe its type, and then report the comparative values that you have obtained by various methods. If that is the game you are willing to play, I am sure we are willing to play with you.

Dr. Hefferren: I would like Dr. Stookey and Dr. Edgar to comment not only on the pH drop or the acidity of an individual test item but on the titratable acidity. Is that a useful parameter? I am talking about total acidity.

Dr. Edgar: You mean of food itself or food after some sort of incubation?

Dr. Hefferren: Well, in your model of pH drop, can you measure the total acidity rather than just pH *per se*, or do you get at that just by duration of pH?

Dr. Edgar: We probably could, but it is a question of the value of this measurement. I think that such a value, such a measurement, could well be of some importance in view of the fact that pH is not the only factor that controls demineralization. One of the other major parameters is buffering powers of the various demineralizing agents. So total titratable acidity would certainly be an adjunct to our measurement of pH, although I think pH still remains the prime parameter that we should be studying.

Dr. Briner: I have used your model and you can do titratable acidity in that. It is difficult, but one can do it. You have to do everything under a blanket of nitrogen to keep the CO_2 from coming out and you have to put it in a standard type of suspension and then titrate it. It can be done, but I would not want to do it again.

Dr. Stookey: Titratable acidity in *in vitro* tests can be done very easily and, furthermore, I think that this has a greater correlation with other *in vitro* tests than does just the pH of the system. You look at this and include the buffering capacity system and its potential to resist the acid changes. It seems to be more related to *in vitro* caries and some other aspects of caries in *in vitro* methodologies.

Mr. Kelly: I think it is essential to approach this task suggested by Dr. Shaw with caution if we are going to do it productively and really solve the problem. What we have here is a microcosm of the total world but not all elements are represented here. This group is very largely supportive, is willing to consider that there is a problem and is willing to consider that there are solutions that can be found and implemented. However, if we trumpet what we are doing or spread it widely and let less responsible parties have the information, it would be extremely counterproductive. This group could not even meet again after something like that happened. So I think it needs to be approached but approached very wisely. I suggest to Dr. Hefferren that this should be something that an ongoing subcommittee could be set up to pursue—the means of getting the job done, because a false start could really destroy it.

Dr. Lockhart: I am not completely familiar with all the methodology that goes on in this field, but I was taken with the rapidity with which acid appeared to be formed in a solution of neutral material like sucrose or glucose. When I questioned Dr. Edgar privately he told me that, in effect, the bacteria and the plaque acted so rapidly that this was a true appearance of acid from glucose or sucrose. I questioned one of my other friends and he assured me that this was the case. A measure of total acidity in this instance would be of no value because the reservoir of acid, of course, would still be the neutral carbohydrate and it would be a matter of whether bacteria were present while you were trying to do your acidity measurement. One does have to be careful with what appears to be a relatively simple kind of thing because of all of the interpretations that can be drawn from the application of one method or another.

Dr. Briner: I might also point out that this is almost a quantitative conversion, usually to lactate. So one can also follow the lactate and get perhaps an even better reading than with total acidity. That won't hold for all cases.

Dr. Baron: We were talking about the *in vitro* and animal studies—carrying them out on candidate items to give you confidence to proceed to a clinical trial, with the clinical trial being the ultimate test of the cariogenic nature of this food or confection. Yet, by the same token, we are restricted because of the protection of the human subjects from testing the unfortified food or the unfortified confection in that clinical experimental design. What is our basis of comparison? With what are we comparing it?

Dr. Madsen: I think that there is an ideal to be sought, although the Mühlemann technique as described, or even the other *in vitro* techniques like plaque pH measurements, only measure acidogenic potential, not cariogenic. Nevertheless, if, with the tests, you find one that did not drop the pH, I don't know why you have to throw out the whole acidogenic theory of caries not to accept that as a dentally safe food. We could, in the ideal, get a list of those foods which do not, in fact, drop the pH. This is one way to do, even *in vitro*, this type of testing which doesn't involve an extensive clinical trial. We could gear to develop those sorts of food. You are going to have a lot of foods containing fermentable carbohydrate that you want to try to put on an acceptable snack list. You might say that some will be excluded by that procedure. At least it would be nice to find which one would not drop the pH and to which, therefore, we could give a clean dental health bill.

Dr. Baron: You would be satisfied with that sort of data instead of clinical trial testing on each individual product?

Dr. Shaw: I don't think that you could ever test an individual product, because it seems to me almost inconceivable that you could say you could provide a biscuit or cookie or whatever along the lines that you formulated. But I think that you need to go back to the kind of suggestion that Dr. Brin made, in which he compared a clinical test like the Mr. Fit centers are doing in connection with heart disease. I don't think I would want to mix the several different things that Dr. Brin suggested.

What I would hope is that you might make the kind of comparison I mentioned earlier, where you would look for a dozen or more different things, then try and see, first what dependability values you could get in several *in vitro* and animal caries tests. The next step beyond that would be to develop a family of products which you would expect on the basis of this combined testing to be low caries, or anticaries, which would be still better. That would be a tougher goal, obviously. Then, go to people like yourself who, like Wilson and others, have done an admirable job in testing on the gums and have a population in which you made no attempt to alter their lifestyle. They eat just the kinds of things that were available on the public market. Then you would have another group comparable in every other regard, in which you would do as close a job as possible in supervising to see that they use the kinds of foods which you have developed.

I don't know if we could ever get to the point of the Finnish people who had up to 100 products available. That's almost inconceivable; I don't know how they ever did it. Perhaps you could have 12 or 20 products which you thought were red hot as snack items for low caries ability, put them in the hands of a clinical investigator like yourself, and then take a population that you don't change and another population that is comparable in every other way, but in which you make every possible substitution that you can with this family of products.

Dr. Mackay: I would like to reinforce the point made by Dr. Baron. It is very difficult to try practically to change products with the hope of getting any recognition on the part of the FDA. You are moving in the right direction. It is not only a question of not being allowed the standard food as a basis of comparison. If you wish to say about a substance, "this food is less cariogenic," that is considered a drug claim. If it is a drug claim, you must go to the FDA Bureau of Drugs. I can say that I have had very clear indications that being "less cariogenic" is not an acceptable drug claim. In other words, even if you have the proof that something is less cariogenic, it is not going to be accepted by FDA, on the basis that you have created an attractive nuisance. You have not done anything that is therapeutic. I have been told "if you make this candy or gum 50% less cariogenic, the children would eat twice as much gum." How could you win in that situation?

Dr. Bibby: Just as a compromise with the FDA and to avoid that difficulty, might it not be possible if an agency within the American Dental Association followed a policy that would parallel the one that the Council on Dental Therapeutics uses, and list acceptable foods. This would not get into advertising, but if caries is important to the manufacturer, and if the dental profession has any effect—and it should have an effect in determining what foods are chosen as caries or noncaries producing—then at least we could go halfway toward a drug claim and perhaps avoid some of the technicalities.

Dr. Mackay: In my outrage at what I have gone through in Washington, I forgot the point that I was trying to make, which was exactly what Dr. Bibby made now. May I propose that if the American Dental Association were to take a position, make up their own lists, this would have a great deal of weight. It's something; it's an inducement for a manufacturer to move in the direction the dental profession desires. At least, they could say the ADA approves, or the ADA disapproves. We are well aware of the fluoride problem, and people don't want to go through that again. Somewhere there has to be an intermediate position that would be an inducement for manufacturers to move in that direction. Almost certainly, anytime you move in the direction toward less caries, the product becomes less acceptable. The products are what they are because they are most acceptable.

Dr. Wilson: Are you asking the ADA to come up with the position that would be equivalent to the Swiss "safe for teeth" thing?

Dr. Hefferren: I believe that might come up next. Mr. Hutt, in his presentation, will provide background for later consideration.

Dr. Briner: What should be the first 1, 2 or 3 *in vitro* tests we should run to start determining a food's cariogenicity, with the ultimate goal of ending up with a clinical trial? I won't go into the fact that we don't have positive control of the clinical trial. I am going to forget about that.

Dr. Kent Stewart: The first thing you need to do is have an analytical breakdown of the food and determine what is in it, chemically.

Mr. Khan: Is there an artificial surface, some mineral composition that could be used as a starting point, as a screening, to see whether a reformulation in a laboratory has done some good rather than to use *in vitro* tests in which primarily extracted teeth were used? These are not generally available in the food laboratory. Is there an artificial surface or a mineral surface that can be used?

Dr. Briner: Do you have an oral surgeon in your town?

Mr. Kahn: Yes.

Dr. Briner: You can get all the teeth you want.

Dr. Hefferren: I think though, realistically, it is a problem. One hopes it will be more of a problem as we keep our teeth longer. There are animal sources of hard tissue that are relatively close to human teeth in a variety of ways. They are always an alternate substrate. I personally like and have been encouraging many people to use primary bovine teeth. I happen to have a local source; a small packing company specializes in veal. But what is nice about it is that these animals are relatively uniform in age and weight and thus their teeth tend to be relatively uniform in characteristics. That is one specific source. There are alternate animal sources. After all, these rats of Navia's are also carrying around hydroxyapatite so that this is what Dr. Briner would like you to look at. That is very important. What kind of sequence do you want to do in your evaluation? I would like to stay with that.

Dr. Bibby: Dr. Hefferren has said most of what I was going to say, but I can say that he is much luckier than we are in having someone who will extract teeth. Our last deal with the union was they were going to charge $5 for every tooth they extracted from the cow's jaw. Alternatively, you can go in there and get the jaws out and pull them out yourself. It is no easy job. Further than that, I think that the compressed apatite pellets have some potential. There are various ways that you can attach apatite to gelatin, cellulose, etc. This new product from outside of Albany seems to give pretty good service. We have used it in demineralization tests and it looks like a substitute that I personally feel gives more reliable results than working from tooth to tooth where there are variations of solubility.

Dr. Briner: You can also buy hydroxyapatite powder from at least one company, and there are hydroxyapatite plates also available for chromatogrphy. So you do have other products that may be usable for certain types of *in vitro* experimentation.

Dr. Kreitzman: From what I understand of the work Dr. Glimsher did a number of years ago, bovine teeth have a layer of dentin on the exterior surface, so therefore you are not dealing with enamel. I think you have to be careful in interpreting this.

Dr. Hefferren: Primary bovine enamel does not have dentin on the surface; other types of bovine enamel do.

Dr. Kreitzman: In looking at *in vitro* tests, comparing them with the animal model, in some of the work that we have done, and Briner has done, and Navia has done, even as discussed in this session, everything has been done with the phosphates. It would be trivial just to increase the phosphate level of the product. By the time we tested the product in the animal model system, I venture to say that the caries activity of that product would be very low in the animal system. The carry-over from that to the human may be very difficult, as we are not sure how effective phosphate is in the human system. So a little caution is indicated. In the modification, I have to emphasize that knowledge of what the product contains is probably the foremost necessity. One cannot just assume because it is sticky or is a snack that it is necessarily cariogenic.

Dr. Stookey: I would like to respond to the question that was raised about which *in vitro* tests should be considered. I think that Dr. Stewart already mentioned that the first thing should be chemical analysis. I identify that as the foremost characteristic, because we really are collecting information about this food product. Secondly, I think we should know something about the pH characteristics of the food item. The third thing that we need to know is something about the oral retention in terms either of total food retention or of fermentable carbohydrates. We need to know something about the degree of oral retention of that food. And finally, in terms of *in vitro* information, I believe we need to know something about the ability of that food to support plaque growth. Retention could be involved, but, particularly, whether that food is or how well it is going to support the colonization and the development of plaque. Whether we go on to *in vitro* caries is debatable. At least, I think that those tests should be considered in developing information about a given food item.

Dr. Briner: I would like to recap now what Dr. Stookey said. The first thing that everyone is agreed on—we need a chemical analysis so we know the starting point and then we run tests such as pH and tritratable acidity, determine the retention characteristics and determine whether it will support plaque growth.

Dr. Newbrun: I would like to share Dr. Socransky's definition. He says, "the first law of oral biology is that no two oral biologists will agree on what is plaque or what typical plaque is when it is collected because of the tremendous problems." I think in cariology we shouldn't fall into the same error as the periodontists and consider that it is only the thickness or the quantity of plaque that is formed. I think at this stage in 1977 we have to recognize that it is not the quantity but the quality of the plaque, the specific microflora. We know very well that there is real danger if you just believe in the nonspecific plaque hypothesis, that you think all plaque is equally cariogenic. It isn't. Anybody in clinical dentistry recognizes that there are patients who have filthy mouths and a tremendous amount of plaque who don't develop caries or even periodontal disease. At least they only have low grade gingivitis. Yet, in periodontosis, there are patients who have barely perceptible quantities of plaque and yet suffer tremendous bone loss. Microbiologically speaking, we recognize the tremendous differences. I still believe that the *in vitro* or *in vivo* plaque pH drop procedures that have been discussed are a good screening and first approach—after food analysis, before you get into animal or human trials.

Dr. Briner: We don't know what plaque really is, so we shouldn't really try plaque growth because it might be meaningless. You are saying that perhaps, instead, a better reading would be something like a Stephan curve or the Zürich equivalent of it.

Dr. DePaola: I would like to expand a little bit on that. I think, as does Dr. Chilton, that this is broadening our purview here at this symposium. I think it is clear in everyone's mind that oral bacteria can ferment carbohydrates and produce acid and that can demineralize the tooth. But I think we have, in all our testing, forgotten about other factors that may mediate cariogenicity. There has been very little work done on the effects of foods, for example on lysozymes, lactoperoxidase, serum IgA, and saliva IgA in terms of the oral cavity. What sometimes appears to me as a controversy in data with one foodstuff in one laboratory producing apparent cariogenicity and in another laboratory, under almost similar conditions or different conditions, producing a different level, may be the consequence of limiting our attention to pH and perhaps not including in the animal work the variety of other parameters.

Dr. Bibby: I would just like to question Dr. Newbrun's statement. When he implied that the quantity of plaque was of little importance compared to the quality of plaque—did I misunderstand that? I would like to register a reservation. The effect that Mühlemann gets on the greater depression of the plaque on

48 versus 24 hour and 3 day versus 2 day plaque is associated with an increased size of plaque. We can suggest that maybe the quality has changed, but it doesn't exclude the fact that the quantity is important. More than that, there are some of the earlier experiments going back to Stephan's work. You can interpret Stephan's results, if you wish, on the basis of the quantity of plaque. There is also work in which there is toothbrushing and mouthwashing which removes some of the plaque. Presumably, you are disturbing the deeper layers and those produce less acid than the big plaques. In my own experience in the past year, I have taken hundreds and hundreds of plaque samples, and one thing that concerns me about the method which I favor, namely the extraoral measurement, is that I do see a relationship between the amount of acid formed and the size of the sample that I take. It worries me—so I think that the quantity is of very great importance.

Dr. Bowen: A lot of the *in vitro* tests which have been proposed take a considerable time. I would suggest one technique which perhaps has not been considered, and which we developed several years ago in the primate; namely, to gastric incubate most, if not all, of the diet, or essential components of the diet, and just feed the test substance by mouth. This enables you to screen substances in something of the order of one to two weeks, relatively inexpensively. Not only that, you can study the microbial composition of the plaque, and measure the pH of the plaque, and the effect of the foodstuff on the pH of the plaque, and you can measure all the components that Dr. DePaola is worried about, also direct collection of saliva, and so on. I would earnestly recommend that to industry if they really want to screen foodstuffs rapidly.

Dr. Navia: The plaque has the ability to lower the pH, depending on its microbial composition. I wonder to what extent people who deal with plaque collections and use of plaque actually determine what other microbial components there are of the plaque. I think that is essential, especially in a situation in which you want to reproduce the results and where you need some kind of precision in the system. You have to know whether you are dealing with a plaque composed mostly of *Streptococcus sanguis* or *S. mutans* or something else.

Dr. Briner: Our clinical trial was designed to have a microbiological basis so that we knew exactly what we were dealing with in the clinical trial.

Dr. Kent Stewart: When you make these measurements, you make them per what amount?

Dr. Edgar: The amount that you could scrape out of the mouth; it is the amount of plaque which is actually sampled at any one time. The plaque is suspended in a small body of water which varies between laboratories, but it is not important. You try to take the same plaque sample and dilute it. It is suspended in either 10 or 100 microliters of saline and there is no difference whatsoever in pH because the buffering power of the plaque sample is so great that the dilution effect on the hydrogen ion concentration does not affect the pH of the sample.

Dr. Kent Stewart: It has always been useful for me when I do analytical work to have units, because of my sampling technique. When I make my sampling technique on the mouth, it might have a fairly high variable characteristic depending on how my hands were working. Is there a possible way to refine the technique?

Dr. Edgar: It is possible. It is not a technique that I would like to use because in the measurement of the small sub-milligram quantities of plaque in terms of nitrogen you may be introducing more problems than you solve. I share your feeling that perhaps we could refine the technique considerably, but it is not doing badly with our fairly crude method.

VI. OUTSIDE AGENCY REVIEW

Walter E. Wisniewski, J.D., Chairman

REGULATORY CONSIDERATIONS*

Peter Barton Hutt

To outline the legal and regulatory framework within which the subject matter of this conference must be considered, I will discuss three areas: (1) the legal difference between a food and a drug, (2) the legal consequences of a determination that a product or an ingredient is a drug, and (3) the legal consequences if it is determined to be a food and not a drug. I will discuss these subjects on an extremely basic and fundamental level because many people have misconceptions about the legal principles that are involved.

I. The Legal Difference Between Foods and Drugs

Federal Food, Drug, and Cosmetic Act contains definitions of both a food and a drug. Section 201(f) of the Act states that food means "(1) articles used for food or drink for man or other animals, (2) chewing gum, and (3) articles used for components of any such article." Chewing gum is specifically mentioned for historical reasons because under the original Food and Drugs Act of 1906 there was an enormous amount of controversy as to whether chewing gum was a food.

The definition of a drug, in section 201(g) of the Act, is a good deal more complex. It includes articles listed in the USP and NF as well as the Homeopathic Pharmacopeia. It includes articles intended for use in the diagnosis, cure, mitigation, treatment, or prevention of disease—including, of course, dental disease. It also includes "articles (other than food) intended to affect the structure or any function of the body of man or other animals."

The important thing to remember about these definitions is the reference in both to the "intended" use of an article. The intended use, and not necessarily the inherent nature of an article, determines the legal status of whether something is a food or a drug under the Act. The following excerpt from the

*Edited transcript of remarks made from notes by Mr. Hutt, a partner in the Washington, D.C. firm of Covington & Burling, who was chief counsel for the Food and Drug Administration during 1971-1975.

1934 Senate Report on the legislation made this quite clear:

> The use to which the product is to be put will determine the category under which it will fall. If it is used only as a food it will come under the definition of food and none other. If it contains nutritive ingredients but is sold for drug use only, as clearly shown by the labeling and advertising, it will come within the definition of a drug but not that of food. If it is sold to be used both as a food and for the prevention of disease it would satisfy both definitions and be subject to the substantative requirements for both. The manufacturer of the article, through his representations in connection with its sale, can determine the use to which the article is to be put. For example, the manufacturer of a laxative which is a medicated candy or chewing gum, can bring his product within the definition of drug and escape that of food by representing the article fairly and unequivocally as a drug product.

A product can indeed be classified as a food, drug, and cosmetic if food, drug and cosmetic claims are made for it. Under the Act, its legislative history, and court interpretations, it is what is claimed for an article that controls the legal determination of its proper classification.

One common claim is that a product or ingredient is anticariogenic—that it prevents dental cavities. That is unequivocally a drug claim. It is not a food claim. That has been the position of the Food and Drug Administration (FDA) for many years. That is obviously why a fluoride toothpaste has been determined by the FDA to be a drug, as contrasted with a nonfluoride toothpaste which is classified as a cosmetic because it is intended for cleansing the teeth and no anticavities claims are made for it.

Another common claim is that a product or ingredient is noncariogenic—that it does not promote tooth decay. FDA has unequivocally stated that this claim is a food claim. It does not represent that the product will prevent disease, as in the case of fluoride. It simply involves the replacement of what is regarded as a cariogenic substance with a substance that does not promote tooth decay (but also is not represented to prevent tooth decay). A food in which sugar is replaced with a noncariogenic substance such as saccharin has been determined by FDA to be a food and not a drug.

It is not possible to give examples of all of the kinds of ingredients and all the possible representations that could be made about them. There is one area I will mention because it is an important category. It is feasible potentially to add an ingredient to food not to replace sugar, but rather to counteract what are thought to be the cariogenic properties of sugar. FDA has suggested that the addition of that kind of ingredient to a food may result in the product being classified as a drug. One way of analyzing this situation would be to conclude that the resulting product is a drug if that ingredient is intended to act on the teeth in order to counteract the sugar, but is a food if it is intended to act on the sugar rather than the teeth.

This is a very complex issue, and we are not going to resolve it today. But it does begin to give you some idea of how the statutory definitions work. And as I will point out, the differences between the legal requirements for a food and a drug are very substantial.

II. The Legal Requirements for a Drug

There are basically two types of drugs under the Act: "old drugs" and "new drugs." A "new drug" is not simply something that was just recently marketed. A "new drug" is a statutory term that has a very precise legal definition, i.e., that the drug is not generally recognized as safe (GRAS) and not generally recognized as effective (GRAE). An "old drug" therefore is the reverse of that, i.e., it is generally recognized as safe and effective, and therefore an "old drug" can be marketed for the indications or the claims for which it is generally recognized as safe and effective without the requirement that FDA first approve a new drug application (NDA) for it.

As you all know, the FDA has established an over-the-counter drug review to determine which OTC (non-prescription) drugs are generally recognized as safe and effective, i.e., "old drugs," and therefore can be marketed with appropriate claims by anyone without any further FDA approval. One of the several OTC drug panels established by FDA for this review deals specifically with OTC dental products.

A drug that is not generally recognized as safe and effective is a "new drug" by statutory definition. To the extent that work to investigate whether a new drug is safe and effective proceeds on animals or *in vitro,* it may be conducted without any notification of or approval by FDA. FDA has no regulatory control over that work if it is conducted only *in vitro* or in animals. FDA does, of course, have regulatory responsibility for any clinical trials of a new drug in humans. At that point the person who is conducting the trials or the commercial sponsor must file an investigational new drug (IND) notice with FDA. The IND must include a full description of the background information on the drug and the proposed clinical trials. It begins the process leading to an approved new drug application.

Anyone who intends to investigate a new drug under an IND with the thought ultimately of having an NDA approved for a commercial product should first consult FDA to make certain that the kind of clinical study that is being run is likely to produce the kind of information that FDA believes is necessary to show the effectiveness of the new drug. There is no point whatever in running a two- or six-year clinical study and then finding out that FDA would never have approved the protocol and regards the results as irrelevant to whether the product is effective. That would be a very frustrating experience, and indeed it has been for more than one company that failed to consult FDA before beginning its work. Prior consultation with FDA avoids unnecessary and unproductive battles with the agency and expedites the approval process.

One problem associated with clinical trials relates to the requirement that they be controlled. The FDA and an advisory committee have been considering what type of control meets both scientific and ethical standards. In October, 1976 the FDA Dental Drug Product Advisory Committee concluded that use of a sugar product as the control was unethical, and FDA concurred. This decision was made in the context of proposed clinical studies on chewing gum. The Committee and FDA stated that the control should be a sorbitol gum rather than a sugar gum. That is where the matter rests at this moment.

One other issue that necessarily arises for products in this area, whether they are new drugs or old drugs, is whether they will be sold over-the-counter or only by prescription. This can be a most important issue. It is possible that a product will start out as a prescription item and be switched to OTC status. That is one of the issues that the OTC drug review currently is considering for all drug categories.

For example, FDA has previously taken the position that there are only two ways that a fluoride product can be sold over-the-counter: through toothpaste and in the water supply. FDA promulgated a regulation that states any other OTC use of fluoride would be unlawful. Some have suggested that fluoride also should be available through an OTC mouthwash, or through the food supply or at least some particular types of food. At the present moment, however, the FDA has said that sufficient safety and effectiveness data are not available to justify any other OTC use of fluoride. This issue of OTC or prescription status is therefore very important, particularly if you are considering the marketing of a food.

III. The Legal Requirements for a Food

As with drugs, there are two types of food ingredients. A food ingredient that is generally recognized as safe (GRAS) for its intended use may be marketed and used in food products without any further notification or approval by FDA.

It is important to note that GRAS status relates to the intended use of a food ingredient. One cannot necessarily take an ingredient that is GRAS for one use and assume that it is also GRAS for totally different food purposes. Questions could be raised about its safety if different uses resulted in vastly increased consumption.

The other type of food ingredient is one that is not generally recognized as safe, which the Act defines as a "food additive." The legal term "food additive" does not include all food ingredients, only those food ingredients that are not GRAS. If a food ingredient is GRAS, then by statutory definition it is not a food additive.

The Food Additives Amendment to the Act clearly provides that the FDA must approve the safety of any food additive by promulgation of a food additive regulation before any product containing the food additive can be marketed. This raises the question whether a food additive can be tested in humans before it is approved by FDA for general food additive use. Very few people realize that the Food Additives Amendment includes a provision for investigational use of food additives in clinical trials, similar to the provision for investigational use of new drugs. Section 409(i) of the Act requires FDA to issue regulations for investigational food additives, comparable to the IND regulations, so that testing of food additives in humans can proceed even before those food additives are in fact approved for marketing.

Although the FDA has not issued regulations under this provision, that has not been a major problem. I am not aware that any company has proposed to FDA to conduct human testing on a food additive prior to food additive approval. Theoretically it could be done. My judgment is that if anyone ever did wish to conduct such human testing, FDA would impose the same type of general requirements for investigational use of food additives as for investigational use of drugs. Anyone who is interested in pursuing this type of investigational use of an unapproved food additive should not be deterred at all by the fact that there are no implementing regulations for that section of the Act. I believe FDA would be very cooperative in trying to proceed on a reasonable basis.

Once it is determined that an ingredient can be used lawfully in a marketed food, the next question involves the type of claims that can be made for it. Certainly, any claims relating to noncariogenicity such as "does not promote tooth decay" must be substantiated by reliable scientific data. The Act prohibits any false or misleading claims in the labeling of a food. No one, indeed, would contend that a food manufacturer should be able to make such claims without adequate data to back them up.

The question then arises as to what kind of data are needed in order to substantiate the claim, for example, that a product "does not promote tooth decay." The Act does not say what kind of data are needed. The consensus of the scientific community will determine the answer to that question. There is no statutory requirement of adequate and well controlled clinical studies to substantiate food claims, comparable to the requirement for proof of effectiveness for drugs. One can hypothesize that, while FDA might not require the same quantity and quality of data to support a food claim that it requires for a drug claim, nonetheless it would not be totally different.

At this moment, there is some doubt in FDA that there are, for example, adequate data to support a claim that a food containing sorbitol as a replacement for sugar does not promote tooth decay. Whether the quantity and quality of supporting evidence is sufficient is a scientific, not a legal, issue.

There are other regulations governing the formulation and labeling of food products that are also relevant. In particular, there are FDA regulations and policy positions dealing with use of nonnutritive sweeteners and other non-nutritive substances in food, which are now under reconsideration.

Saccharin has been used as a non-nutritive sweetener, for example, in chewing gum products which are labeled as sugarless chewing gums and for which the claim "does not promote tooth decay" is made. In addition to the current safety issue, FDA has long been concerned about the admixture of nutritive sweeteners with saccharin or any other non-nutritive sweetener. Years ago this was not considered to be a toxicity problem, but rather an economic adulteration problem. Sugar was so much more expensive than saccharin that a manufacturer could substitute saccharin for sugar as an economic cheat. Over the years the FDA developed a policy prohibiting any admixture of non-nutritive and nutritive sweeteners in food products in order to prevent fraud. As time went on this policy partially broke down because, in addition to the use of saccharin as a non-nutritive sweetener for weight control purposes, it also began to be used for other technological purposes, one of which was for noncariogenic purposes. Thus, FDA did bend its policy in some situations to permit these mixtures with appropriate informative labeling.

The labeling of noncariogenic foods is now being reconsidered by FDA as part of its revision of the regulations governing special dietary foods. A tentative order published on July 19, 1977 would establish new labeling requirements. The new regulations would state that non-nutritive sweeteners can be used for a technological purpose such as in a noncariogenic food, but the label then must state that the non-nutritive sweetener is not being used for caloric reduction. This would result, for example, in a sugarless gum containing saccharin being labeled not only that it does not promote tooth decay but also that the product is not for use as part of a weight control program.

There are many who think that is a bit of regulatory overkill. They contend that additional labeling is inappropriate for that particular category of products. Certainly, it would be unfortunate if products which apparently serve a useful purpose were to be inhibited by unduly burdensome labeling requirements.

IV. Conclusion

The broad outline I have given you is sufficient to show that there are complex and difficult scientific and legal issues that arise. No one should consider clinical trials or the formulation or labeling of a product in this area without sound scientific and legal advice on the proper way to proceed. This expertise is available within companies, from independent experts, and from FDA. You are far better off checking with people and making certain that you are going about it the right way before you begin.

Despite deep concern among scientists, which will undoubtedly persist, the fact is that the FDA rules and requirements can be met. You can test and market products and ingredients. The government is not trying to put scientists or industry out of business or prevent them from conducting useful studies and selling useful products. If you were sitting in FDA, the regulatory requirements might make a little more sense than appears from your current position. There is a law, called the Federal Food, Drug, and Cosmetic Act, and it must be enforced and obeyed. It was not FDA who passed that law. It was Congress, in the form of your elected representatives. If you do not like the law, go to Congress to get it changed, but do not blame FDA for it or expect the agency to ignore it.

Many scientists and companies have managed to comply with the Act and regulations without difficulty. FDA does a reasonable job in trying to implement the Act. I think we will all be better off if we spend our time trying to determine how to develop useful new ingredients and products within the constraints of the law rather than complaining about the current regulatory requirements, which are unlikely to change.

PANEL DISCUSSION

Mr. Stauffer: I think eventually we will get to the point of the discussion that was started earlier, that is, on a food acceptance program with respect to whether or not the foods promote caries. But before we get to that type of thing, I would like to ask Mr. Hutt whether, with the growth of the Food and Drug Administration, he feels that there will be a revision some time, because of the consumer movement and the concern for the use of sugars in the American diet today, and whether he believes that FDA is under a particular pressure at the moment to add new portions to the legislation to offer more control.

Mr. Hutt: I doubt if there would be new legislation specifically aimed at sugars. The Food and Drug Administration, in my judgment, has legal power today to add a declaration of sugar content to nutrition labeling. Now, the way the nutrition labeling works, as you know, is that if anyone wishes to make any kind of nutrition claim or to add any nutrient to a food product, that person is required to put on the label a standard format including all nutrition information that is specified by the Food and Drug Administration. Currently, that does not include sugar content. I see no reason why it could not. It has been suggested that this might be an appropriate step in the future. That does not mean that FDA was taking a position about whether sugar content was too high, too low, good, bad or indifferent. It would simply be information for the consumer so that the consumer who wanted sugar could get it, and the consumer who didn't want sugar could avoid it. That same approach has been adopted by FDA in the polyunsaturated-saturated fatty acid controversy. FDA says it doesn't take sides, but it has included that kind of information in a standard format on the label. Because this can be done without legislation, I have doubts that there would be legislation directed toward that.

Dr. Schrotenboer: Could the FTC require it?

Mr. Hutt: Well, the FTC and FDA both have legal jurisdictions over labeling. Are you talking about labeling or advertising? (Answer: labeling.) The FDA has what we lawyers call primary jurisdiction and the FTC has agreed that basically it would not intervene in labeling. It would leave that to FDA. The FTC has primary jurisdiction over advertising in contrast to labeling. Whether FTC could require it in advertising is currently the subject of a good deal of litigation in the food advertising trade regulation rules proceeding, which is pending before a hearing examiner at the FTC right now.

Dr. Schiff: I happen to be fortunate, or unfortunate, to represent a raw material supplier. I had the pleasure of visiting FDA with different problems with different customers. People made food, people made new drugs, and I came to a paradox. I found we can go to the Food and Drug Administration for a new drug claim and they decide that that new drug is really not a new drug, because it is going to be a food. This decision would be made by the scientist—the dentist expert of the Food and Drug Administration. He is the one who makes the judgment. Then they say it should be brought over to the food people. But the food end of the regulatory agency does not have a dentist, so what they do before they make a decision about whether this food claim is correct, is to ask the dental expert at the new drug regulation group of the Food and Drug Administration. In this swap we have, I think a specific body making this decision over everything that is either coming into food or going into drugs. When you said that there is a fair and equitable hearing being done when things are to be considered for approval, I don't know if you are familiar with these facts. To my knowledge in the last ten years, short of fluorides in a couple of toothpastes, nothing has been approved. Does that mean that industry is not developing things, or does it mean that FDA just isn't being that fair in judging. I know clinical studies which were done by some of our customers, costing millions of dollars, which have not been approved yet.

Mr. Hutt: I cannot speak with specifics in terms of whether the clinical studies were done properly or whatever. I'm not competent to do that. I am not here to defend the Food and Drug Administration as the world's most perfect organization. Nor do I believe that any of you would defend your institution as the world's most perfect organization. The fact is that FDA is concerned across the board that there would be any single person in the agency who would have that kind of control. That is why the agency over the past five to six years has gone toward advisory committees to broaden the base on these kinds of decisions and to allow a forum of outside independent experts who can, in effect, second guess the agency. Currently there are three such dental committees in the Food and Drug Administration—one deals with medical devices, one deals with prescription drugs, and one deals with over-the-counter drugs. If there are problems that arise in dealing with the agency on a dental product, one should go before the advisory committee. Now, if the FDA and the advisory committee agree, we are not saying that they are necessarily right and you are wrong, but it certainly is not any longer any one person who is controlling the entire fate of these issues.

Dr. Horowitz: With regard to the FDA use of the advisory committees, I am a member of one of those committees and Dr. Schrotenboer is a past member and current consultant to the same committee. We are what the name states. We are advisory to the FDA. In a couple of your statements I got the impression that you believe that the FDA always agrees with the advice that is given by its advisory committees. You made particular reference to the current feelings of FDA about study design, and that a sucrose-consuming group is not a suitable control. There was strong sentiment along those lines by the majority or maybe all the members of the advisory committee, but I should point out that does not mean that the Food and Drug Administration will go along with that advice. There is precedent in terms of other advice that we've given the FDA that they have not accepted and have come to a completely opposite decision. The advisory groups do not have as much authority as you seem to imply.

Mr. Hutt: As a general rule, and I've been fairly close to it, more than 90% of the time the FDA has accepted advisory committee advice. I think that anyone would agree that, legally, the commissioner cannot delegate his responsibility for a decision to an advisory committee. On the other hand, when it is in excess of 90% of the time that their advice is followed, I think that is a pretty good record. I think maybe the truth lies somewhere between what you interpreted my earlier statement to be, which I didn't mean, and what you just said. Don't play down the importance of those advisory committees either. They are in my judgment the single most important development in the Food and Drug Administration in the last 30 years in terms of an attempt to get the best scientific judgment from outside independent expertise into the agency, to make the decisions of the agency more realistic and flexible and more current.

Dr. Schrotenboer: How do the opinions of the advisory committee become known to the public? I don't remember the one that we were discussing at the moment as ever being publicized.

Mr. Hutt: I read it in the so-called pink sheet, because it was a summary of what happened at the meeting. The minutes of every meeting are public information. Anybody who wants all the minutes of all the dental advisory committees just has to write and they will send them to you. You can go and actually sit there and listen to the whole meeting if you want; it is 99% open to the public. On occasion, when trade secrets are being considered, they close the meetings, but otherwise they are as open as—more open than—this meeting.

Unidentified speaker: Mr. Hutt, you raise the question—at least I heard Commissioner Kennedy raise it yesterday—that the number of regulations in the Food and Drug Administration has doubled since 1969, at least in number of pages. He would like to see them pared. You are now in private practice and have had time to reflect on all the regulations written while you were the General Counsel. In what areas would you like to see these regulations pared?

Mr. Hutt: I'll give you a very clear answer. I wouldn't like to see them pared. I would like to see them increased, for one reason. There is a bit of interesting history there. Why are those regulations there? They are largely there because the statute itself is written so broadly that it means a hundred different things to a hundred different people. That statute can only be implemented by taking the general directive. For example, it is necessary to get approval for a food additive that is not generally recognized as safe. Who knows what is generally recognized as safe? There has to be a regulation that lists those things that are generally recognized as safe. Otherwise, every different food company would be going in a different direction on that issue. The statute says you can't make any claims that are false or misleading in any particular. That is all it says. Who knows? People come in and ask the question—do you think this claim is false or misleading? If regulations are not developed to give guidance, then the agency is going to spend all of its time in court suing those it thinks are doing something wrong when instead it could be telling them what is the right thing to do. Basically, 99.99% of the manufacturers in the country will follow advice, as long as it is reasonable, and they want regulations that will tell them what it is that the agency thinks is proper under the law.

Now, I was in private practice for 11 years and I remember, for example, at least thirty times when I debated an inspector as to whether the type size on the label for the net quantity of contents or statement of ingredients was large enough, because the statute said it had to be "conspicuous" and FDA had never defined the word conspicuous. It seemed to me a pointless dispute on which FDA, the outside lawyer, and the company were all wasting their time. FDA, when I was there, wrote a regulation that said conspicuous means 1/16 of an inch. Now, you could have chosen it a little higher or a little lower, it really didn't make any difference, but now everybody knows what the rule is. The industry, I think, doesn't care. They have a rule they can follow, and that debate is over; no one ever has to debate that issue again.

So I think regulations are very important, very useful. Sure, there are a few minor ones that perhaps you could eliminate, but there are not many that you could reasonably get rid of, in my judgment. Now I am sure that there is a different point of view that could be reflected here and I would be delighted to hear it.

Unidentified speaker: Mr. Hutt, in view of the fact that some of the manufacturing processes are not very exact and not able to list anything except an approximate amount of sucrose in the product, I would like you to expand on the answer as far as nutrition labeling is concerned and the impact that it would have on various industries—for example, if you labeled a product as having 35% sucrose, and it didn't have 35% sucrose in the product—in the end product.

Mr. Hutt: I may have missed the point. You are saying that they can't tell how much is in it?

Unidentified speaker: The question was asked about nutritional labeling of sucrose and by implication, that there would be no problem in nutritionally labeling this and putting on a package that the product had 35% sucrose. What is your allowable exception?

Mr. Hutt: What is the tolerance? Without question the FDA has recognized this in many other different areas. Any such regulation would have to have a built-in tolerance. I don't know whether it would be plus or minus 10% or 5% or 20%. But, I thoroughly agree with your point that no one could ever have it exactly on the line every time. In fact, it is not even required for the net quantity of contents declaration today. You have the same problem when you have to declare the percent of the RDA of calcium or iron or something of that kind—overages are recognized as well as insufficiencies.

Dr. Wilson: Mr. Hutt, I wonder if you might speak a little further on this matter concerning the adulteration sugar issue. As a dentist, I would be very happy if the snack food manufacturers would put sugar in their products only to the extent that the sugar was there for functional purposes, but bring up the sweetening with saccharin or whatever is available. Now, as far as what's available today, in bending this regulation, could that be done in snack foods?

Mr. Hutt: I have never viewed that as an insoluble problem. It would come down to a matter of very clear labeling. Indeed I have on occasion in private practice advised people on ways of getting around that problem by front panel disclosure of "sweetened with a combination of saccharin, a non-nutritive sweetener, and sugar" or something of that kind. That could be worked out with the agency and that kind of solution, particularly if there were the kind of rationale that you just gave, I am quite confident would gain some advocates in the agency. There are various ways of attacking it. One would be, of course to allow people to do it voluntarily. Another would be to issue some kind of standard of identity which would only permit certain levels of sugar to be used. There are various control mechanisms, but the economic adulteration issue I mentioned was an historic issue. So few people understand it, I wanted you all to be aware that when you hear of reluctance on the part of FDA, it reflects a 70-year tradition of worrying about the economic adulteration issue, which probably never occurred to most of you as an issue; but it can be surmounted.

Dr. Chilton: You commented that the logical position would be for a sponsor to meet with the Food and Drug Administration people at the beginning of their submissions of an IND so that the protocol, if approved and if the study was done properly when they applied for an NDA, that this would meet approval, rather than to go with an unapproved protocol and at the end of the time—2, 4, 5 or 6 years—come in and find the wrong protocol.

This assumes that people at Rockville will make a decision that this is an approved protocol. Suppose they don't do that? They can always say that it is not a good one, that is, not say it's an approved one. Also, there is, as we know, some change in the people who work in these agencies. If there is an approved protocol and several years later one comes back having done the study, and that person who approved it is no longer there and the person who has taken the position says "I never approved this"—is there any legal position which can be taken?

Mr. Hutt: Let me respond to both. First of all, obviously, one could not force the agency to comment on a protocol. I know of no situation where they have flatly declined to do so. I would suggest, particularly in an area where there is an advisory committee, that you have an excellent chance one way or another of getting FDA to comment. I would also suggest that if you ran into a situation where an individual in an agency said, "We will not take a position on that," you then go up the ladder and talk to his supervisor and his supervisor's supervisor, if necessary all the way up to the present Commissioner. Because my own view is that you would in a very short period of time hit people who would realize that was a stupid way for the agency to do business. And there would be an order to get on with it or it would be referred to an advisory committee. One way or another, my judgment is that it may take a little time and a little patience but you can get an answer. It won't necessarily be definitive, but it will be a reasonable approximation of what they feel.

Second, there is a legal doctrine that says the government cannot be topped, i.e., if the government says "X," and later it wants to change its mind, it has a legal right to do so. There is, however much concern in FDA about the type of situation that you described. As a result, when FDA put out procedural regulations, roughly finalized about a year ago, it included a provision in which you can go and ask for an advisory opinion or obtain what is called a guideline, and the clinical guidelines were particularly in mind there. And once the agency has said "yes" this is a valid guideline, anyone who relies on that can do so with confidence that it will only be overturned in what, I think we put in the regulation, are extraordinary circumstances. So that is now in FDA's own regulations and it provides a protection for precisely the reason that you specify, that never before in history has existed with that agency, or indeed with any other. And it was precisely because of that type of problem, and situations where all of us knew it had occurred. Again, that's no gold-plated guarantee, but it is showing that the agency itself is aware that there are problems of that type.

Dr. Chilton: Thank you, that is very informative. The OTC panels, as I understand it, are empowered to or supposed to write monographs. Then these monographs have to be accepted by the Bureau of Drugs and the Commission. Is it possible that parts of these monographs will not be accepted and that various drugs or possibly food additives which are accepted in category 1 as being safe and effecive, will not be accepted by the Bureau of Drugs and then the IND route has to be taken?

Mr. Hutt: You ask "is that possible," and I say "yes, that clearly is possible," because once again the Commissioner cannot and has not delegated his responsibility—his legal responsibility—to make that decision. On the other hand, if you have followed, this is what has happened. First, a decision was made that the panel report would itself, without one comma change, be published in the Federal Register as a proposal. So there is no way as it now works that the Commissioner could surreptitiously take out a paragraph that he didn't like or something of that kind. That decision has been made.

Dr. Chilton: But now who puts it into the Federal Register—does that have to be approved?

Mr. Hutt: FDA puts it in the Federal Register.

Dr. Chilton; Not the panel?

Mr. Hutt: No, it can't. Legally the only person who can put it in is the Commissioner. But he has never changed a word of any report as a proposal. Then there is time for comment on that proposal, and anybody in the world can comment. In view of those comments, the Commissioner revises that proposal. Now as to those that have gone to the second stage, I know of none where there has been any serious overruling, if you would call it that, of one of the advisory panels. That day will come, I am sure, because, after all, some of the issues that are being debated before the OTC review are very judgmental and are subject to enormous controversy. Moreover, on occasion one of those decisions is made in the proposal stage and people go out and do all kinds of work so that by the time you get to the tentative final order or the final order the decision should be changed. Now on top of that, quite frequently—and certainly this was true of the first panel report on antacids—the panel itself reviewed the tentative final order and the final order, and Franz Ingelfinger and his committee went over every word of every change and gave their comments. Again, that doesn't guarantee that there will be no changes, but it is a system in which the Commissioner quite openly has said "we want outside people to second guess the agency." We are not going to agree with them every time, but I think it is a fair and open procedure.

Dr. Chilton: You made the comment that when a decision of the Bureau of Drugs is requested about the appropriateness of a protocol and if an IND is not obtained, one can go to the advisory committee.

Dr. Hutt: One can try to do so, yes.

Dr. Chilton: I wonder if I could put somebody on the spot, we have a member of the advisory committee here; would he care to comment on that?

Dr. Horowitz: Well, as a member of the committee I know that we have our own frustrations. There is an issue with fluorides right now that we would like to have brought to our advisory committee, because certain actions have been taken by the FDA, and some of us feel very strongly that they are ill advised actions. Yet we haven't been successful in having the FDA bring it to our attention. It has been cut off even when we have raised the issue ourselves. For some reason, they seem to have, in our opinion, a closed mind on this issue. So pressure from the outside to bring something to the FDA Advisory Committee doesn't work, at least with regard to the dental panel at this point in time.

Mr. Hutt: It hasn't worked thus far on one specific instance. However, has your panel written a letter to the Commissioner asking for permission to review the subject?

Dr. Horowitz: Not to my knowledge.

Mr. Hutt: Okay, there is a provision in the regulations that allows your panel to request FDA to raise the issue. It is understandable that people on occasion in a government agency, or even in a professional association or a law firm or anywhere else, are going to have their own views and aren't going to want some outsiders to second guess them. That's human nature, but there are procedures intended to avoid that kind of problem. They won't always work, but I think you still have some avenues to explore there.

Unidentified speaker: Would you comment on the applicability of the rules on foods as to whether they include water. I understand there is enormous controversy right now as to whether water is considered a nutrient and when it is considered a food.

Mr. Hutt: It is a food, and there is no question legally but that water is a food. It is quite frequently a food ingredient as well. To my knowledge it is regarded as generally recognized as safe, although I haven't been in Washington in two days, I'm not sure. Maybe, with the chloroform controversy, it is no longer GRAS. The issue did arise about who had jurisdiction over it. Congress, in the Water Act in 1974, said that the Food and Drug Administration would have jurisdiction over bottled water but that the Environmental Protection Agency would have jurisdiction over all other water. Now, still, water as it is in food is subject to FDA's jurisdiction, as is bottled water.

Dr. Mackay: The dental profession would like to see the food industry move toward noncariogenic or less cariogenic foods. The food industry, Life Savers particularly, would love to move in this direction. What advice can you give the food industry and how may its members call attention to the fact that they have indeed moved in this direction? As a matter of fact, we know that in the case of a General Foods product, there is a hidden, a permitted additive for an unstated purpose, and in some of our products we have added things which we believe are doing something about the dental process, but to which we cannot call attention. However, if you really want to move in this direction, there must be a way to call attention to the fact that a food is indeed less cariogenic. If it is going to be less cariogenic, it is less cariogenic than what?

You cannot compare an improved food with the food that existed beforehand; how do we get out of this little box? Because we aren't going to get out of the regulatory box, I thought that possibly the ADA might be willing to step in to perform this public service.

Mr. Hutt: I am fascinated and I did not understand your comment about your concern. You said that one would not be permitted to make a noncariogenic claim if you altered your food and indeed it was noncariogenic—maybe that's not what you intended. Less cariogenic? I see no legal prohibition against that whatever, and I don't understand who possibly told you that.

Dr. Mackay: Am I right in thinking that less cariogenic is a drug claim?

Mr. Hutt: You are wrong. You are quite wrong.

Dr. Mackay: Am I right in saying, of the famous 50 questions that the FTC referred to FDA, that the statement "does not promote tooth decay" is already being reconsidered as to whether that is a drug claim?

Mr. Hutt: To my knowledge, that is not true.

Dr. Mackay: I am delighted to hear that less cariogenic is not a drug claim.

Mr. Hutt: The latest statement on that subject is an internal FDA memorandum which was given to one of the advisory committees and it dates from late last year, from roughly November or December last year—this was signed by Paul Hile, the Associate Commissioner for Compliance, of the Food and Drug Administration, and it states..."we do not view 'does not promote tooth decay' as a drug claim." That is not equivocal, there are no qualifications, that is a flat statement—it is the position that the Food and Drug Administration has taken from 1938 to the present. Now if "does not promote tooth decay" is a food claim, then clearly "is less cariogenic" is equally a food claim. It is the same legal concept as hypo-allergenic, which is not a drug claim; hypo-allergenic food is a food. Hypo-allergenic cosmetics are cosmetics, they are not drugs. It requires substantiation. That was the point I tried to make earlier, whether it is a food or drug you can't make false claims, or unsubstantiated claims.

Dr. Mackay: How can you substantiate less cariogenic?

Mr. Hutt: If the question is, what are you going to use as the positive control from an ethical standpoint? I agree some solution has to be found, but that isn't a drug or food issue. You shouldn't be talking to the Bureau of Drugs about that. That's none of their business, if you are talking about substantiating a food claim. Furthermore, if this has become confused in the agency, then what you have got to do as an industry, as the ADA, is to try to get it straightened out instead of attending meetings and expressing great outrage.

SUMMATION

John J. Hefferren, Ph.D.

I should thank each and every one of you who have come here in the spirit of exchange, trying to find common ground. That has been very nice and it has exceeded my expectations. I am really very, very pleased that things have gone reasonably well.

From the food industry we have a variety of scientists here who show considerable flexibility and, generally, are willing to interact and try to meet on common ground. Today we are using foods differently than we did a few years ago and maybe this is an important variable in this interaction between food scientists, dental scientists and industry.

We have to be careful to avoid oversimplifying the caries process. Rheology and physical properties must be considered. However, we have to avoid overcomplicating methodology, too.

There are several approaches to modifying food. Approaches of putting a substance into a food or taking something out and at the same time trying to hold various rheological properties constant. At present we have a holding pattern on the synthetic sweeteners. I think we have to be a little bit careful with that term. In this program we have called saccharin, cyclamate and aspartame synthetic sweeteners, as contrasted to some of the polyols. Here, as we approach modification and alteration, we should be very careful of nutritional balance and keep in mind dietetic and other aspects of the situation.

A multitude of things could have been talked about in this meeting. I had to make some decisions and perhaps expected that many of the points that I overlooked might be brought out. Many have been, but to provide time on the program for all of them would have resulted in a schedule even tighter than the one submitted to you; I congratulate you on bearing with it. There is little question that clinical trials are the end point that everyone would like to have. They are difficult to conduct, but I submit to you that they are not impossible, whether it be a food or drug-related problem. The plaque models have a nice compromise to them; you can apply them to human beings, look at one parameter of the situation and it really doesn't make too much difference whether you have the pH electrode inside or outside the mouth. They are largely *in vivo* models measuring one aspect of the process. There are a variety of animal and *in vitro* models which may have greater flexibility, perhaps greater potential for misinterpretation, but collectively have a stronger position. Throughout this area, the experimental people were looking for a point of reference. It is nice to have a place on which to build and I think this is something we can address ourselves to.

Mr. O'Connell: Probably one of the most effective things that came about in this conference is the fact that we are here. At least, in my experience it is the first time that the academic community, industry, researchers, government, people in dental research have come together as a group to discuss the cariogenicity of foods. It's something that we would like to avoid at times, but I don't believe we can avoid it in the future.

It would be very helpful from an industry standpoint if some methololology could be developed to determine the cariogenicity of foods—a very effective, simple, accurate system. I am not certain after listening two days that it is here at this time. I hear differing opinions on which would be the best system to determine cariogenicity. I would suggest that a small select steering committee, under the auspices of the ADA made up of competent technical people, including the broad range of people that are here, look into areas of possible studies; maybe areas of definitions. Which is the best approach for research? A multiple product basis? A single product basis? I have heard a couple of comments that the issue is settled, we probably don't need to go any farther. I don't agree with that. Determining first whether we go on a multiple product basis or whether we go on a single product basis would be an issue for this steering committee to decide. I also noted, when we visited the National Institute of Dental Research a couple of years ago, that the modification of foods, if my notes were correct, was the fourth priority on their list in combating dental caries. Drs. Carlos and Bowen were the people with whom we met; if this is not correct, I will stand corrected. They suggested inoculation, protective coatings, oral hygiene and modification of foods. So even though we are talking about the cariogenicity of foods, I hope that if we set up a steering committee that other factors also will be considered.

Dr. Horowitz: Your comment should be put in perspective in terms of NIDR or the National Caries Program. It was not to belittle the importance of food as a causative agent for dental caries in trying to determine what priority it has in terms of alleviating the problem. I'm not sure that the three you mentioned appeared higher on the list. If in fact it did fall fourth on some lists, I think, in terms of feasibility from a public health standpoint, it is for some of the reasons that have been mentioned during this conference. By changing the cariogenicity of only one or two foods, we didn't see it as having a great deal of potential in terms of solving the problem of dental caries in this country because of the ubiquity of challenges that existed in various foods. However, it is not to belittle the importance of trying to make food less cariogenic.

Dr. Bowen: I would like to reiterate what Dr. Horowitz said. The list you saw was in fact a list of our strategies and obviously they have to be given numbers and the fact that modifying the diet was listed number four does not mean that it is in fact priority number four. It is unfortunate that you got that impression. I should also emphasize that we are in fact the largest investors in research seeking alternatives to sucrose. It should not be forgotten that the National Caries Program within NIDR is the largest supporter in this area. The third point I would like to make, of which many people in industry do not seem to be aware, is that the National Caries Program offers a service in which we will test any compound that the submitter believes to be cariostatic or noncariogenic at no cost or no risk to patents by the submitter. Now we have had some response to this program, but not as much as we would have wished. I can understand that some people are, in fact, a little afraid to get involved in government. But there are people in this audience who have "done business" and so far as I know have been totally satisfied with the results. And when I say we would investigate, I mean we will do *in vitro* tests, we will do animal tests, we will do preclinical tests, and if the results warrant, we will even do full-scale trials at absolutely no cost whatever to the submitter.

Mr. O'Connell: This is a classic example, if I may interject here; it isn't what you say, it is how you say it. My intent in mentioning that was only relative to the factors at hand today, and my whole point was to raise the question about the possibility of continuing with this type of group or a small steering committee. What we are all trying to do is to reduce cariogenicity.

Mr. Kelly: I believe that this effective conference has achieved a great deal in bring people together who otherwise would not have gotten together. We have identified some common areas of interest, some common problems. Two of these, to overgeneralize a little, would be how to test foods in reliable, repeatable projectable manners and what to do about the regulatory or approval considerations associated with marketing such products. I think this group has done a very effective job of pointing out these problem areas. I think we bogged down a little bit when we tried to solve the problems right here. So I have endorsed what Mr. O'Connell says—let's put a steering committee together which can develop and formulate a program for dealing with this after giving it more detailed small group consideration. I would look to the ADA to act as a sort of facilitator, of which you have done a marvelous job, and I think it provides an ideal mechanism.

Dr. Schiff: I want to second those comments. Dr. Hefferren has done an extremely capable job in bringing together all the representatives of various groups, breaking down the boundaries of prejudice, and getting them to work together. He deserves congratulations. I agree we should form a small committee to meet soon. We have identified problems and small groups will solve them.

Dr. Hopper: It has been an excellent meeting. Each of us has had the opportunity to express our opinions, although they are different. I hope the opportunity will continue. I know of no better way to do it than a small group doing some of the things you have suggested. In no way are we going to remove all sugars from the American diet, and as has been stated time and again, we must not isolate one part of the body and forget about everything else. It is a complex area, one in which we are all interested. We are eager to get on with the job.

Dr. Hefferren: What I would like to do is use my position as Director of the Research Institute of the ADA Health Foundation to get some of you people together again to talk about the things we might do. We would have, in such a group, a blend of people who can sit down together, constructively disagree, and end up with a course of action that is positive. The obvious line-up of such a committee would include representatives of the industrial trade associations and to have people who could interact with us. We will select academic people, again with a blend, who can interact and come up with a course of action for a couple of years.

I would like now to acknowledge the support I had for this meeting. We passed the hat very shortly before the meeting and many of you were quick to respond. I would like to acknowledge those who were able to respond in the time available. You contributed in a variety of ways—in a very good way by being here. Our special thanks for financial support from:

Chocolate Manufacturers Association
The Coca-Cola Company
The Estee Corporation
Finn-Cal Sweetener Company
General Foods Corporation
General Mills, Inc.
Gerber Products Company
H.J. Heinz Company Foundation
Hoffman-LaRoche Inc.
ITT Continental Baking Company
Kellogg Company
Life Savers, Inc.
M&M/Mars
Monsanto Company
Nabisco, Inc.
National Confectioners Association
National Soft Drink Association
The Procter & Gamble Company
The Quaker Oats Company
Standard Brands, Inc.
The Sugar Association
The Sunmark Companies
Warner-Lambert Company
Wm. Wrigley Jr. Company

There is a small surplus that will help for another meeting. One of the projected costs is to allow us to gather, edit and publish the proceedings of the meeting. We plan to have a detailed summary of the meeting published in *The Journal the American Dental Association*. We also plan to work closely with trade magazines—*Food Technology* and *Food Product Development*—which we have invited to this meeting because we believe there should be a report in the literature of the food scientists and technologists.

PARTICIPANTS IN THE CONFERENCE

Mr. Robert A. Aherne
President of Xyrofin, Ltd.
Baar, Switzerland
Finn-Cal Sweetener Co.
50 California Street
San Francisco, Calif. 94111
415/397-0425

Ray H. Anderson, Ph.D.
Principal Scientist
Corporate Research
General Mills, Inc.
9000 Plymouth Ave. N.
Minneapolis, Minn. 55427
612/540-2311

Robert A. Bagramian, D.D.S., Dr. P.H.
Professor and Chairman
Department of Community Dentistry
The University of Michigan
School of Dentistry
Ann Arbor, Mich. 48109
313/763-2105

Milton P. Baldauf, Ph.D.
Vice President
Technical Services
L.S. Heath & Sons, Inc.
206 S. Jackson Street
Robinson, Ill. 62454

Hazen J. Baron, D.D.S., Ph.D.
Director, Dental Science
Warner-Lambert Company
170 Tabor Road
Morris Plains, N.J. 07950
201/540-2347

Mrs. Vienna Bennett
Bernard Wolnak Associates
75 Wacker
Chicago, Ill. 60601

Basil G. Bibby, D.M.D., Ph.D.
Eastman Dental Center
800 Main Street
Rochester, N.Y. 14603
716/454-7723

Mr. Bendt Bladel
National Confectioners Association
36 South Wabash
Chicago, Illinois
312/372-1492

Robert W. Boggs, Ph.D.
Associate Director
Food Technology Division
Procter & Gamble
Miami Valley Labs
P.O. Box 39175
Cincinnati, Ohio 45239
513/562-9401

G. Norris Bollenback, Ph.D.
Scientific Director
The Sugar Association, Inc.
1511 K. Street, N.W.
Washington, D.C. 20005
202/628-0189

William H. Bowen, Ph.D.
National Institute of Dental Research
West Wood Building
5333 Westbard
Bethesda, Md. 20016
301/496-7716

Myron Brin, Ph.D.
Associate Director, Research
Hoffmann-La Roche Inc.
Kingsland Street
Nutley, N.J. 07110
201/235-2397

William W. Briner, Ph.D.
Toilet Goods Division
The Procter & Gamble Co.
Winton Hill Technical Center
Cincinnati, Ohio 45224
513/977-7712

Albert T. Brown, Ph.D.
Associate Professor
Department of Oral Biology
University of Kentucky
Lexington, Ky. 40506
606/233-5369

Robert M. Busche, D.Sc.
New Business Opportunities
Development Division
E.I. Du Pont De Nemours & Co., Inc.
Central Research & Development Dept.
6003 Du Pont Building
Wilmington, Del. 19898
302/774-7472

Neal W. Chilton, D.D.S.
Research Professor of Oral Medicine
Clinical Research Center
University of Pennsylvania
School of Dental Medicine
4001 Spruce Street
Philadelphia, Pa. 19104
215/243-6627

Joseph D. Clark, Ph.D.
Director Clinical Research &
Regulatory Affairs
American Chicle R & D
Warner-Lambert Co.
170 Tabor Road
Morris Plains, N.J. 07960
201/540-2080

Fergus M. Clydesdale, Ph.D.
Department of Food Science and
Nutrition
University of Massachusetts
Amherst, Mass. 01003
413/545-2281

Mr. W. Horton Corwin
Vice President
Research & Development
Brock Candy Company
Jersey Pike
Chattanooga, Tenn. 37416
615/899-1100

Richard W. Daniels, Ph.D.
Director, Nutrition,
Health & Product Safety
Standard Brands Incorporated
Betts Avenue
Stamford, Conn. 06902
203/348-6401

William J. Darby, M.D., Ph.D.
president
The Nutrition Foundation, Inc.
489 Fifth Avenue
New York, N.Y. 10017
212/687-4830

Dominick P. DePaola, D.D.S., Ph.D.
Nutrition Director
Health Research
Fairleigh Dickinson University
110 Fuller Ave.
Hackensack, N.J. 07601

Basant K. Dwivedi, Ph.D.
Vice President & Director
Research & Development and Quality
Control
The Estee Corporation
169 Lackawanna Avenue
Parsippany, N.J. 07054
201/335-1000

Mr. Thomas Egan
Research Division
Hoffman-La Roche, Inc.
Nutley, N.J. 07110
201/235-5000

W. Michael Edgar, Ph.D.
Department of Oral Physiology
University of Newcastle Upon Tyne,
Dental School
England
and
Markham Laboratories
Upper Claremont Street
Newcastle, NEZ 4AJ, England
0632, 611059

Edward P. Ehmann, Ph.D.
Manager, Technical Information
Services
Pepsi Company, Inc.
Anderson Hill Road
Purchase, N.Y. 10577
914/253-2040

Neil Finley, Ph.D.
Manager
Product Research & Quality Control
The Seven-Up Company
121 South Meramec
St. Louis, Mo. 61105
314/863-7777

E. Eugene Fisher, Ph.D.
Vice President
Research and Quality Control
William Wrigley, Jr. Company
410 N. Michigan Ave.
Chicago, Illinois 60611
312/644-2121

Joseph R. Fordham, Ph.D.
Food Technologist/Nutritionist
Clinton Corn Processing Company
1251 Beaver Channel Parkway
Clinton, Iowa 52732
312/242-1121

Abdul Gaffar, Ph.D.
Research Associate
Research Center
Colgate-Palmolive Company
909 River Road
Piscataway, N.J. 08854
201/463-1212

Robert L. Glass, D.M.D., Dr.P.H.
Forsyth Dental Center
140 The Fenway
Boston, Mass. 02115
617/262-5200

William Hall, Ph.D.
General Foods Corporation
Technical Center
250 North Street
White Plains, N.Y. 10625
914/631-6400, Ext. 478

James Hamsher, Ph.D.
Pfizer, Inc.
Central Research
Groton, Conn. 06340
203/445-5611

John J. Hefferren, Ph.D.
Director, Research Institute
American Dental Association
Health Foundation
211 E. Chicago Avenue
Chicago, Ill. 60611
312/440-2516

Ms. Kathleen Henrick
Research Associate
Monsanto Company
800 North Lindberg Blvd.
St. Louis, Mo. 63166
314/694-1000

Margaret M. Hinkle, M.S., R.D.
American Dietetic Association
Liaison with ADA
4648 Barry Meade Court
Columbus, Ohio 43220

John H. Hopper, M.D.
Senior Vice President
Scientific Affairs
Kellogg Company
235 Porter Street
Battle Creek, Mich. 49016
616/966-2849

Herschel S. Horowitz, D.D.S.
National Institute for Dental Research
Westwood Building
5333 Westbard
Bethesda, Md. 20016
301/496-7032

Peter Barton Hutt, J.D.
Covington & Burling
888 16th Street N.W.
Washington, D.C.
202/452-6000

Mr. Donald J. Jorgensen
Development Manager
Special Chemical Division
Monsanto Company
800 N. Lindbergh Boulevard
St. Louis, Mo. 63166
314/694-1000

Mr. Ray G. Kelly
Vice President, Development
The Sunmark Companies
8155 New Hampshire Avenue
St. Louis, Mo. 63123
314/832-7575

Mrs. Susan C. Kelly
Public Relations
Monsanto Company
800 North Lindbergh Boulevard
St. Louis, Mo. 63166
314/694-1000

Paul Khan, M.S.
Director of Food Protection
ITT Continental Baking Co.
P.O. Box 731
Rye, N.Y.
914/967-4747, Ext. 478

Mr. John B. Klis
Editor and Director of Publications
Institute of Food Technologists
211 N. LaSalle Street
Chicago, Ill. 60601
312/782-8424

Mr. Harry E. Korab
Technical Director
National Soft Drink Association
1101 16th Street N.W.
Washington, D.C. 20036
202/833-2450

Mr. Ajit Kothari
Research Division
Hoffmann-La Roche, Inc.
Nutley, N.J. 07110
201/235-5000

Steven Kreitzman, Ph.D.
Emory University
School of Dentistry
Atlanta, Ga. 30322
404/329-6767

Mr. Robert W. Lehnhoff
The Procter & Gamble Co.
Winton Hill Technical Center
6110 Center Hill Road
Cincinnati, Ohio 45224
513/977-7704

Earl E. Lockhart, Ph.D.
Assistant to Executive Vice President
Corporate Technical Division-
Administrative
The Coca-Cola Company
P.O. Drawer 1734
Atlanta, Georgia 30301
404/897-2274

Mr. Dick McCormick
Editorial Director
Food Product Development
Two N. Riverside Plaza
Chicago, Ill. 60606
312/346-1040

Mr. John McNaught
Lever Brothers Company
45 River Road
Edgewater, N.J. 07020
201/943-7100

Mrs. Laura M. McQuinn
Technical Assistant
Corn Refiners Association, Inc.
1001 Connecticut Avenue, N.W.
Washington, D.C. 20036
202/331-1634

Donald A. Mackay, Ph.D.
Vice President
Research and Development
Life Savers, Inc.
40 West 57 Street
New York, N.Y. 10019
212/489-3100

Kenneth O. Madsen, Ph.D.
Professor
Nutrition and Biochemistry
University of Texas Health Science
Center at Houston
University of Texas Dental Branch
Box 20068
Houston, Texas 77025
713/792-4220

Kauko K. Mäkinen, Ph.D.
Professor of Biochemistry
Institute of Dentistry
University of Turku
SF-20570 Turku, Finland
3355-33

O.E. Michaleis, Ph.D.
U.S. Department of Agriculture-
Carbohydrate
Nutrition Laboratory
Nutrition Institute
Building 307, Room 317 East
Beltsville, Md.
301/344-2396

H. Eugene Miller, Ph.D.
Senior Research Chemist II
Corporate Research
General Mills, Inc.
9000 Plymouth Avenue North
Minneapolis, Minn. 55427
612/540-3428

Edgar W. Mitchell, Ph.D.
Assistant Secretary
Council on Dental Therapeutics
American Dental Association
211 E. Chicago Avenue
Chicago, Ill. 60611
312/440-2526

Ms. Karen K. Moore
Associate Editor
Food Product Development
Two N. Riverside Plaza
Chicago, Ill. 60606
312/346-1040

R.A. Morck, Ph.D.
Vice President - Research
Technical Group
Nabisco, Inc.
Research Center
2111 Route 208
Fairlawn, N.J. 07410
201/797-6800, Ext. 832

Joseph Muhler, D.D.S., Ph.D.
P.O. Box 36
Howe, Indiana 46746

Mr. Tommy P. Muller
Chief, Biostatistics Research
Institute
American Dental Association
Health Foundation
211 E. Chicago Avenue
Chicago, Ill. 60611
312/440-2542

Conrad A. Naleway, Ph.D.
Director, Division of Chemistry
Council on Dental Therapeutics
American Dental Association
211 E. Chicago Avenue
Chicago, Ill. 60611
312/440-2514

Juan M. Navia, Ph.D.
Professor of Nutrition and Dentistry
Institute of Dental Research
University of Alabama in Birmingham
University Station
Birmingham, Ala. 35294
205/934-2288

Ernest Newbrun, D.M.D., Ph.D.
Professor of Oral Biology
Oral Medicine and Hospital Dentistry
University of California
School of Dentistry
San Francisco, Calif. 94143
415/666-1004

Abraham E. Nizel, D.M.D.
Tufts University
School of Dental Medicine
One Kneeland Street
Boston, Mass. 02111
617/956-6840

Ms. Mary O'Brien
Managing Editor
Food Product Development
Two N. Riverside Plaza
Chicago, Ill. 60606
312/346-1040

Mr. Richard T. O'Connell
President
Chocolate Manufacturers Association
7900 Westpart Drive, Suite 514
McLean Virginia 22101
703/790-5011

Thomas Osberger, B.S., M.B.A.
Technical Sales/Service Manager
Midwest Office
Finn-Cal Sweetener Company
50 California Street
San Francisco, Calif.
312/945-6565

Mr. G. Frank Phillips
Manager Research/Quality Control
Dr. Pepper Company
5523 E. Mockingbird Lane
Dallas, Tex. 75206
214/824-0331

G. Subba Rao, Ph.D.
Chief, Pharmacology Laboratory
Research Institute
American Dental Association
Health Foundation
211 E. Chicago Avenue
Chicago, Illinois 60611
312/440-2532

Mr. Walter Reed
National Automatic Merchandising
Association
7 S. Dearborn Street
Chicago, Ill. 60603

Patricia Richmond, Ph.D.
Lab Head, New Products
Food Research
A.E. Staley Mfg. Company
2200 E. El Dorado
Decatur, Ill.
217/423-4411

William E. Riha, Ph.D.
Director, Technical Services
Cadbury Corporation
P.O. Box 340
Humboldt Industrial Park
Hazleton, Pa. 18201
717/384-3271

G.G. Roussos, Ph.D.
Project Officer
National Caries Program
Preventive Methods Development Section
National Institute of Health
National Institute of Dental Research
Bethesda, Md. 20014
301/496-7135

I.I. Rusoff, Ph.D.
Senior Scientist, Technical Group
Nabisco, Inc., Research Center
2111 Route 208
Fairlawn, N.J. 07410
201/797-6800, Ext. 276

James Scala, Ph.D.
Director, Nutrition and Health Sciences
Central Research
General Foods Corporation
250 North Street
White Plains, N.Y. 10625
914/631-6400, Ext. 422

Thomas Schiff, D.D.S.
Head, Clinical Dentist
Monsanto Company
800 North Lindbergh Blvd.
St. Louis, Mo. 63166
314/694-2159

Gordon H. Schrotenboer, Ph.D.
Secretary, Council on Dental Therapeutics
American Dental Association
211 E. Chicago Ave.
Chicago, Illinois 60611
312/440-2522

James H. Shaw, Ph.D.
Professor of Nutrition
Harvard School of Dental Medicine
188 Longwood Ave.
Boston, Mass. 02115
617/732-1375

Mr. Barton H. Siebers
The Nestle Company, Inc.
R.D. #3, Willobob Terrace
Fulton, N.Y. 13069
315/598-1234

Mr. Sheldon Siegel
Vice President
Research & Development
American Chicle
Warner-Lambert Company
201 Tabor Road
Morris Plains, N.J. 07950
201/540-2265

Chakwan Siew, Ph.D.
Chief, Toxicology Laboratory
Research institute
American Dental Association
Health Foundation
211 E. Chicago Avenue
Chicago, Ill. 60611
312/440-2842

Ronald C. Simpson, Ph.D.
Manager, Nutrition Research
Standard Brands Incorporated
Betts Avenue
Stamford, Conn. 06902
203/348-6401

A. Elizabeth Sloan, Ph.D.
Communications Specialist
Division of Nutrition
General Mills, Inc.,
P.O. Box 1113
Minneapolis, Minn. 55440
612/540-7204

Robert E. Smith, Ph.D.
Vice President
Research & Development
Foods Division
Grocery Products Group
The Quaker Oats Company
617 West Main Street
Barrington, Ill. 60010
312/381-1980, Ext. 2025

Arnold Steinberg, D.D.S., M.S.
Associate Professor of Periodontics
College of Dentistry
University of Illinois Medical Center
801 S. Paulina Street
Chicago, Ill. 60612
312/996-7515

Kent K. Stewart, Ph.D.
Chief, Nutrition
Composition Laboratory
Nutrition Institute
U.S. Department of Agriculture
Beltsville Agricultural Research Center
Room 225, Building 308
BARC - East
Belstville, Md. 20705

Robert A. Stewart, Ph.D.
Director of Research
Gerber Products Co.
445 State Street
Freemont, Mich. 49412
616/928-2461

Charles D. Stone, Ph.D.
Senior Research Scientist
Scientific Affairs Department
M&M/Mars
High Street
Hackettstown, N.J. 07840
201/852-1000

George K. Stookey, M.S.D.
Associate Professor of Preventive Dentistry
Oral Health Institute
Indiana University
School of Dentistry
410 Beauty Avenue
Indianapolis, Ind. 46202
317/264-8822

Mr. Delmar Stauffer
Secretary, Council on Dental Health
American Dental Association
211 E. Chicago Avenue
Chicago, Ill. 60611
312/440-2861

Mr. Edward J. Stegemann
General Counsel U.S.
Mars, Inc.
Westgate Park
1651 Old Meadow Road
McLean, Va. 22101
703/893-2210

Mr. John Stroz
Research Co-ordinator
Research & Development
Life-Savers, Inc.
40 W. 57th Street
New York, N.Y. 10019
212/489-4200

Stan M. Tarka, M.S.
Research Laboratories
Hershey Foods Corporation
Box 54
Hershey, Pa. 17033

Mr. Reinie Thiessen
Senior Lab Manager
General Foods Corporation
Technical Center
250 North Street
White Plains, N.Y. 10625
914/631-6400, Ext. 478

Alan Thomas, Ph.D.
M&M/Mars
Scientific Affairs Department
High Street
Hackettstown, N.J. 07840
201/852-1000

Carl E. Vandercook, Ph.D.
Fruit and Vegetable Chemistry
Laboratory
U.S. Department of Agriculture
263 South Chester Avenue
Pasadena, Calif. 91106

Mrs. Violeta S. Velasco
Technical Service Representative
Industrial Division
Corn Products Company
Moffett Technical Center
P.O. Box 345
Argo, Ill. 60501
312/458-2000

Anthony R. Volpe, D.D.S.
Associate Director, Research Center
Colgate-Palmolive Company
909 River Road
Piscataway, N.J. 08854
201/463-1212

Mr. Barney Wander
Monsanto Company
800 N. Lindbergh Blvd.
St. Louis, Mo. 63166
314/794-1000

M.O. Warnecke, Ph.D.
Technical Director, American Home Products
E.J. Brach & Sons
4656 W. Kinzie Street
Chicago, Ill. 60644
312/626-1200, Ext. 414

Philip White, Sc. D.
American Medical Association
535 N. Dearborn Street
Chicago, Ill. 60610

Charles J. Wilson, D.D.S., M.S.
President
Bio-Research Associates, Inc.
6040 West Lisbon Avenue
Milwaukee, Wis. 53210
414/964-6360, 445-4180

Walter E. Wisniewski, J.D.
Associate Counsel
Secretary, Council on Insurance
American Dental Association
211 E. Chicago Avenue
Chicago, Illinois 60611
312/440-2572

Wayne T. Wozniak, Ph.D.
Research Institute
American Dental Association
Health Foundation
211 E. Chicago Avenue
Chicago, Illinois 60611
312/440-2538

Mr. Otto B. Wurzburg
Senior Vice President - Research
Starch Division
National Starch and Chemical Corp.
10 Finderne Avenue
Bridgewater, N.J. 08807
201/685-5234

Mr. John Zemen
Director of Development
Special Chemical Division
Monsanto Company
800 N. Lindbergh Blvd.
St. Louis, Mo. 63166
314/694-1000

Barry L. Zoumas, Ph.D.
Director of Research
Hershey Foods Corporation
Research Laboratories, Box 54
Hershey, Pa. 17033
717/534-4512

SECTION B:

THE ROLE OF SUGAR AND OTHER FOOD IN DENTAL CARIES.

WHAT CAN INDUSTRY DO?

Conference held October 5-6, 1978

VIII. INTRODUCTION

WELCOME

John J. Hefferren, Ph.D.*

I welcome each of you here today on behalf of the American Dental Association. The ADA has a very nice house, and it is good when such a house is utilized for the purpose of this Conference. One of the things that the American Dental Association has done in the past is to provide a forum for interaction so that paths leading to the future can become less tortuous. The officers, trustees, and members of the American Dental Association join me in hoping that this Conference will be useful for each of you, and for your work.

OBJECTIVES OF THE SECOND CONFERENCE

Donald A.M. Mackay, Ph.D.

The theme of this second Conference on Foods, Nutrition, and Dental Health is "Role of Sugar and Other Foods in Dental Caries: What Can Industry Do?" Should it be "What Industry Can *Do*?" or "*What* Can Industry Do?" or, as some of us are inclined to say, "What *Can* Industry Do?"

At the end of this Conference, I hope that there will be a little more clarification of the problems facing the food industry, and I think perhaps there will be a better understanding of problems facing each of us. A year ago we held the first Workshop on the Cariogenicity of Foods, and at that time many people in industry felt they were being punished. There was general recognition that sugar was somehow involved in the caries process. A number of people in industry aren't exactly prepared to admit all the implications of that statement, so we thought that this year it was time that the industry had a chance to give its side of the story at the Conference.

The program is organized with the intent that there will be three overviews of the situation: a contribution from the American Dental Association, one from the National Institute of Dental Research, and the third from The Sugar

---

*Affiliations of all participants are described in the "List of Persons Attending" included in the Appendix.

Association. Thus, there will be a restatement of positions. We will not argue the different points of view, but rather we emphasize that there are different points of view. Dr. Newbrun will make the argument that sugar is somehow involved in dental caries. Dr. Bibby was asked to take the other side and to point out deficiencies in the argument. Then we will move into responses by people representing various industrial viewpoints about what they think they can do about it—with full recognition of the points of view that will have been expressed earlier.

Another objective is to try to decide what we can do about the future; what we can do about trying to bring together the three parties in the dispute. We really want to establish a base in this meeting upon which we can try to reach common understanding of the problems; to reach a common understanding of what actions are possible for the industry and to recognize that industry is not consciously making products designed to rot away the teeth of the nation. If it can be recognized by the regulatory parties concerned, by the professionals, the dentists, by the academicians, and by industry that there are "carrots" available instead of "sticks," that will help us to move in the desired direction; we will have taken a gigantic step forward.

We hope—and the very fact that we are meeting in this building under the auspices of the Research Institute seems to justify that hope—that the American Dental Association may be persuaded to take a more active role in acting as a middleman between the industry and the profession and the regulatory authorities, recognizing that industry is in the peculiar position of trying to bring about regulatory changes that, on their face, might seem to be self-serving. There are no monolithic viewpoints in industry, and there are no monolithic viewpoints in the dental profession, as we will soon see. We need an uncle—a godfather, if I may use that term—in trying to get clarification of the issues and trying to decide on ways we can move forward.

John Hefferren has presented a very nice analysis of the situation and has given us some objectives and the reasons for establishing this program: to foster improved understanding between the food industry, dental researchers in the profession, and the regulatory agencies; to continue the Workshop on an annual basis; to further the development of model systems to measure the cariogenicity of food; and to consider also other aspects of oral hygiene, namely, the plaque question and periodontal disease. (Note: A copy of the article is included in the Appendix.)

REFERENCE

American Dental Association Research Institute. Cooperative program on foods, nutrition, and dental health. JADA 97(2):239-240, 1978.

IX. INTEREST IN NUTRITION AND DENTAL HEALTH

INTEREST IN NUTRITION AND DENTAL HEALTH: AMERICAN DENTAL ASSOCIATION

Wilbert Fletke, D.D.S.

On behalf of the American Dental Association, I take this opportunity to commend the Research Institute of the American Dental Association Health Foundation for its sponsorship of this Conference and to congratulate it on the first anniversary of its food and nutrition program. For more than 25 years, the American Dental Association (ADA) has recommended the voluntary restriction of the consumption of sweetened beverages and confections. We share the Institute's commitment to improving diet for dental health, and are pleased and impressed by its considerable contribution this year to accomplishment of that goal.

Like the Institute, the ADA recognizes that participation of industry is vital to the success of any attempt to assess the cariogenicity of specific foods and solve the problem of modifying diet for improved dental health. We recognize that achievement of these objectives must be based on a cooperative effort involving not only industry, but government, academia, and the health professions. The ADA, of course, through its Council on Dental Health and Health Planning and other agencies is eager to assume a share of this responsibility.

The Association's councils are agencies which, with the advice of expert consultants, recommend policy to the ADA House of Delegates, its governing body, and who interpret existing policy and act as a resource for the profession, public, government, and others who share our interests.

Included in the scope of the Council on Dental Health and Health Planning is prevention of dental disease, and this includes a special interest in nutrition and diet. In addition to the role of the nutrient fluoride, in nutrition and diet, the role of sugars in caries etiology has for years been a major concern. This year, for instance, the Association has established a national task force for the prohibition of the sale of confections in schools; it operates under the auspices of the Council on Dental Health and Health Planning.

However, our interests in the area of nutrition and diet are broader in scope than simply the relationship between sugar and caries. As early as 1953, we expressed our concern for total nutrition in a joint report with the Association's Council on Dental Therapeutics. Today we are continuing our attempts to broaden our understanding of the relationship between diet, nutrition, and dental health and to increase our ability to communicate effectively with other interested groups and with the public.

Lately we have taken a number of steps in this direction. First, we have added a nutritionist to our staff to help us provide needed program direction. Secondly, we have developed liaison with the American Dietetic Association. Its representative, a registered dietician, attends our Council meetings, is a member of the national task force just mentioned, and advises us in a consultative capacity.

Finally, to counsel us on policies and activities related to diet and nutrition and to act as liaison with the Research Institute's food and nutrition program, we have recently established a subcommittee on foods and nutrition. The affiliations and expertise of its members and consultants cover a broad spectrum. The members of that subcommittee are Dr. Sebastian Ciancio, Chairman of the ADA Council on Dental Therapeutics; Dr. Juan Navia, Senior Scientist at the University of Alabama Institute of Dental Research; Dr. Robert Smith, Vice-President of Research and Development for the Quaker Oats Company Foods Division; Dr. Philip White, Director of the American Medical Association Department of Foods and Nutrition; and I as a member of the Council.

The consultants to this group include Dr. Basil Bibby, Senior Scientist, Eastman Dental Center; Dr. William Bowen, Acting Chief of the Caries Prevention and Research Branch, National Caries Program, National Institute of Dental Research; Dr. Hefferren, Mrs. Hinkle and Dr. James Iacono, Deputy Assistant Administrator for Marketing, Nutrition, and Engineering Sciences, USDA, Agricultural Research Service.

The Council hopes that through such excellent sources of advice it will be able to support actively the efforts of the Research Institute's food and nutrition program and to cooperate more effectively with agencies and organizations which share an interest in this subject. We invite you to call on us if we can be of any assistance.

INTEREST IN NUTRITION AND DENTAL HEALTH: THE SUGAR ASSOCIATION, INC.

G. Norris Bollenback, Ph.D.

I suppose it really need not be said that the sugar industry is interested in the foods in the dental caries problem, but if I let it go without saying, each one of you will have his own inference and will go away thinking that you understand what I didn't say. I will define The Sugar Association's position—by describing briefly the current research support policy and the research funding program of the Association.

Up until the early 1970s, worldwide, the sugar industry—and this includes South Africa which I must mention because Dr. Retief is here, and the European Economic Confederation, South America, the United States, Canada—worldwide supported research in food technology, in nutrition and health, and in sucro-chemistry through the medium of the International Sugar Research Foundation. That foundation no longer exists.

In 1970, in the United States, the very severe antagonism toward sugar and the serious attempts to associate it with many diseases resulted in our finding the ISRF a rather inappropriate medium for funding research, and so we started our own research program . The program was designed primarily to gain an understanding and clarification of the role, if any, of sucrose in these many disease states.

In 1973, to help us define the position of sugar relative to these diseases, we formed a Food and Nutrition Advisory Council. This Council is made up of experts from various health fields—heart, obesity, diabetes, dental caries, and pediatrics. The Council acts strictly as adviser to the Association to help clarify scientific matters and to help select research projects for funding. They are particularly independent and they stay quite aloof from any part of the Association activities except the research.

At present, our procedure for funding research has three steps, we solicit proposals; proposals received are screened, primarily by Council members, for scientific soundness and for correspondence to the priority interests of the Association, and then they are evaluated with regard to return on investment in the short and long terms.

It may be appropriate here to tell you some of the statistics about our funding program. Since 1975, when the program started, we have considered more than 200 different research proposals. About 30% of those, 74 to be exact, were considered close enough to the objectives of the Assocation to be put on an agenda for Council deliberation: Can we fund them or can we not fund them?

Of the 74, 37 (50 percent) were project proposals in the field of dental caries. Of the 37, the Council saw enough merit in 6 to recommend to the Association that we fund. Half of those, 3, were funded. There are several reasons for this high mortality rate. One is that our Council members are really very critical. The proposals frequently are much too far to the pure side of the pure to applied spectrum. And technically, there is always the question of methodology. Experimental designs which are extremely faulty are proposed; this is one of the major reasons for rejecting proposals that come to our attention.

Our priority fields of interests are, in order, dental caries—that is number one—obesity, diabetes, heart disease, and miscellaneous topics such as metabolism of sugar. These priority areas have been selected in accordance with the intensity of pressure for the generation of information in the various health and nutrition fields, to help answer questions that arise continuously.

For instance, three years ago we had quite a few projects in heart disease. But over the past couple of years something like 11 prospective studies have been published showing that if there is any association between sugar and the development of heart disease, it is very difficult to find. The situation with diabetes and sugar is fast coming to the same point. This is why they are third and fourth on our ladder of priorities. What causes obesity and how you treat it are other undecided questions. Because sugar happens to be around, we think, it is selected as a cause of obesity. One frequently hears that obese people eat a lot more sugar than the non-obese. Nobody knows the cause of obesity, and there are several studies that show that there is no relationship between sugar consumption and obesity. It has been shown even more consistently that obese people do not eat more sugar than non-obese people.

However, there are a lot of questions in obesity, and we are not reluctant to fund projects that might show sugar up in a bad light. If there is something bad about sugar, let us be the first to find it.

Sugar is associated with dental caries far more than with any other disease and far more than is any other food. We agree that there is an association. We disagree that it is as exclusive an association as several commanding voices would have us believe.

In the manner of transcendental analysis, we appear to be looking for a yes or no answer to a very complex question. We have a very definite feeling that sugar has provided a very easy answer to the complex question of dental caries.

We believe that there are many gaps in the epidemiology, and these will appear during our discussions, in animal and clinical studies which are frequently cited as irrevocably binding sugar to caries development. It is to fill these gaps and put the role of sugar in a very realistic perspective vis-a-vis caries development that we have caries as our number one priority for research funding.

As to the interests of The Sugar Association in studying the cariogenicity of foods, I can assure you that we think such studies are extremely practical. They offer short-term results, and some of the results could help not only to answer the question of the relative cariogenicity of various foodstuffs but to give us leads about the relationship of the results obtained from animal and clinical studies to the actual human experience.

We have not lost sight of the fact that unless something better develops, some government agency will establish possibly unrealistic methods as a standard for establishing relative cariogenicity of foods. We don't want to see that. I think a lot of the sugar user people here don't want to see that either. I am referring to the possibility, for instance, of the Mühlemann technique (which has come under severe fire) being adopted here, or even worse, to have a government agency select the amount of sugar in a given product as the measure for establishing its relative cariogenicity.

These are the major reasons why The Sugar Association, as a representative of the sugar industry and the sugar user industry, has an interest in the role of sugar and other foods in dental caries.

A question has been raised about the amounts of money The Sugar Association has available for funding. We have a research fund which amounts to well over a quarter of a million dollars. It is replenished periodically as projects develop. However, we have never considered that available money would stand in the way of supporting a project if the project seemed appropriate enough, practical enough, and promised to give us results on a short-term basis. We believe that we can get money for expensive programs if the programs are appropriate.

I have referred to the International Sugar Research Foundation (ISRF). One of the projects that arose from ISRF funding was the development of a sweet material called trichlorosucrose. Trichlorosucrose was developed by Leslie Hough under the ISRF aegis in Bristol, England. Incidentally, theoretically there are 56 trichlorosucroses, but some predominate. Those that predominate are some 10 times as sweet as sucrose. They also are not available to enzymatic attack from *Streptoccus mutans,* so they are very possibly cariostatic.

This material is not available for sampling right now, but one hopes that it will become available in the very near future, through Tate and Lyle in England. Tate and Lyle have another material, too. They call it Talin—it is the protein sweetener thaumatin, and it is being evaluated for its cariogenicity or cariostatic properties in Bristol now. Samples of this material are available through Tate and Lyle.

INTEREST IN NUTRITION AND DENTAL HEALTH: NATIONAL INSTITUTE OF DENTAL RESEARCH

William H. Bowen, B.D.Sc., Ph.D.

The National Caries Program, since its inception, has recognized the importance of sugar and sugar-containing snack foods in the etiology of dental caries. We have already heard about the importance of the triad of a susceptible tooth, microorganisms, and diet.

However, much of the experimental work devoted to the studying of diet and dental caries unfortunately has been focused on sucrose *per se*. We all know of the increasing evidence that sugar and sugars as such are not consumed in anything like the same frequency or rate as snack foods. This places us in a difficult position because we are unable to take any single food and say that it is cariogenic of itself, because the vast majority of snack foods have not been tested, although *a priori,* judging by their content, we could reason that many may be cariogenic.

We prefer to speak in terms of cariogenic potential. By cariogenic potential, I mean a substance or a foodstuff which, if eaten with sufficient frequency would without doubt induce or promote the development of caries. We are not in a position to be able to say, as indeed Dr. Newbrun has been at pains to point out, that a particular product eaten once daily will result in the onset of dental caries.

Because of this, we are greatly interested in developing methods for the determination of the cariogenic potential of a wide range of foodstuffs. We are well aware that many techniques have been in existence for several years. Each of them suffers from one or more major deficiencies. Few of the techniques, if any, measure cariogenicity as such. If we look at the deficiencies of some, perhaps we may be in a better position to select a battery or a combination of tests that meets our needs.

Perhaps the most popular and universally accepted cariogenicity test or cariogenic potential test is that developed by Mühlemann and his group, in which groups of subjects wear intraoral pH measuring devices. They chew on a test food, and the pH drop in the dental plaque is measured over a specified period of time. Arbitrarily, they have decided that any foodstuff which lowers the pH below 5.7 should be termed cariogenic or at least potentially cariogenic, or if it does not lower the pH below 5.7, it is labeled as "kind to the teeth."

We do not wish to find ourselves in the position of denigrating any of the work which Dr. Mühlemann has carried out, but who is to say that someone who chews a food several times per day which lowers the pH in dental plaque to 5.75, he too will not suffer from a caries problem?

If we look at results of investigations carried out in animals we find several problems. If the foodstuff is fed *ad libitum,* we know that animals can be extremely selective in the foodstuffs which they consume, and this selectivity has plagued animal research for many years, and no doubt, despite the fact that the literature is replete with such examples, will continue to do so.

We believe that perhaps the best approach is a combination of well-controlled animal studies together with the pH measuring device as described by Dr. Mühlemann, and we are actively pursuing our research in those areas. As some of our recent announcements have indicated, we are encouraging related grant submissions.

We all recognize that, even if we do succeed in identifying snack foods or foodstuffs which have little cariogenic potential, the record of persuading the public to alter its habits for health reasons is not outstanding, although some success appears to have been achieved in curbing of the intake of saturated fatty acids. Nevertheless, I think it is encouraging to observe that the sales of sugar-free drinks and snack foods is increasing substantially, although personally I doubt whether this sales increase is based on the potential dental benefit. I suspect it is probably based on the belief that such habits will reduce the possibility of obesity.

Simultaneously, while trying to identify methods for screening the cariogenic potential of foodstuffs, since 1973 we have supported research to identify alternative sweetening agents and, indeed, for the past several years the National Caries Program has by far been the largest government supporter of such research.

We have supported investigations of aspartame, the dihydrochalcones and monellin. We have also supported and continue to support research into identifying non-cariogenic sweeteners and in the field of nutrition we are carrying out investigations on xylitol and sorbose.

At the end of fiscal year 1978, we were expending approximately a half million dollars on research for new sweeteners. We recognize that even if we are successful in identifying alternative sweetening agents, that these agents will not be universally acceptable, and that many snack foods will have to be reformulated. The problem is that we do not know which snack foods, as I have already indicated, are particularly cariogenic, and we are also lacking information about the patterns of use of potentially cariogenic foodstuffs. We will support research to identify the pattern of use of cariogenic foodstuffs in various parts of the United States.

We are also prepared to support industry in testing the cariogenicity of reformulated snack foods, and we will carry out research in the rat model, completely free of charge and without any obligation by the food industry, to determine the effect of reformulated foodstuffs on caries in the rodents. Let me hasten to add that anyone who expects results from this research in a matter of weeks obviously will be disappointed, and that the more we are asked to carry out, the longer will be the delay.

To reemphasize our role and our interest in this area: We are attempting to develop reliable methods to determine the cariogenic potential of foodstuffs. We are supporting research to develop alternatives to sugar as sweetening agents. We are willing to test the cariogenic potential of foodstuffs in our animal model. And finally, let me emphasize that we are not and we do not regard ourselves in any way in competition with the American Dental Association Health Foundation Research Institute. We have cooperated and we will continue to do so throughout these investigations, and we hope to be able to extend our cooperation to industry.

X. FOODS AND DENTAL CARIES

Donald A.M. Mackay, Chairman

DENTAL CARIES—AN OVERVIEW

Ernest Newbrun, D.M.D., Ph.D.

An overview of dental caries allows free license to discuss any and all aspects of caries. Let me start by making three points concerning caries in general.

1. Caries is a multifactorial disease in which there is an interplay of three principal factors: The host, the microflora, and the substrate.[1] This has become a cliche' so I will spare you the Venn Diagram which, as Basil Bibby says, is just an advertisement for Ballantine's Ale.
2. Caries is potentially preventable using current knowledge and available methods.[2]
3. Caries is not being prevented, in that it affects about 98% of the population in western countries.[3] Furthermore, there has been an alarming increase in the prevalence of dental caries in developing countries.[4]

Caries Preventive Programs

The major strategies currently directed at reducing or eliminating caries are:

1. To combat the microbial agent, by programs of personal oral hygiene, plaque removal or plaque control.
2. To increase the resistance of teeth, by such means as systemic and topical fluoride and occlusal sealants.
3. To modify the diet, through diet control, restricting sucrose-containing foods and beverages, using non-cariogenic sweeteners and phosphate additives.

These strategies can be considered in terms of their applicability and efficacy when used at home by the individual patient, when practiced in the dental office, and when employed at the community level. Oral hygiene *per se*, exclusive of therapeutic dentifrices, has had an insignificant effect on caries increments. There are several explanations for this. In part, it is because caries most commonly occur in fissures which cannot be cleaned properly by any available method. Another important reason is that teeth usually are brushed in the morning and before going to bed, but not as Johannes Arculanus of the 15th century advised:

Mundificet dentes tibi immediate post cibum

(Clean your teeth immediately after eating)

Communal water fluoridation is unquestionably the most practical, the cheapest, and a highly efficacious means of preventing caries.[5] However, because political support is lacking (not because of controversy in the scientific or health community), only about 60% of the United States population using public water supplies are benefiting from this proven public health measure. But even if all communities were fluoridated, caries would not be totally eliminated and we would still have to employ other known preventive methods.

Time does not permit a full consideration of all these preventive measures. If we focus on the efficacy of caries-preventive methods that involve modifying the diet, we are forced to conclude that the observed efficacy of dietary modification is insignificant when conducted at home or in the office, whereas the potential efficacy of dietary modification is excellent. Modifying the diet markedly reduces caries increments, at least over a limited time, in institutional populations such as at Vipeholm[6] or Hopewood House,[7] or in highly selected and motivated populations such as at Turku[8] (Table 1). However, at a community level, dietary modification has not been tested adequately although the potential efficacy is excellent. The discrepancy between the observed efficacy and the potential efficacy is undoubtedly due to inadequate compliance, the early acculturation to foods containing sugar,[9] the persuasiveness of the food industry in advertising cariogenic products, and, finally, but by no means least, the ease and convenience and almost universal availability of cariogenic snack items.

TABLE 1. Comparison of annual caries increments of subjects on sugar-restricted diets with subjects on unrestricted diets

		Diet		
Study	Patient Age	Restricted	Unrestricted	% Caries Reduction
Vipeholm[6]	31 yr	Low sugar, none between meals 0.67 DMFS	24 toffees/day between meals 4.02 DMFS	83
Hopewood House[7]	10-13 yr	Sugar restricted, vegetarian 0.88 DMFT	Unrestricted 1.81 DMFT	51
Turku[52]	Adults and children average 27.5 yr	Sugar substituted by xylitol 0.74 DMFS	Sugar used as sweetener 1.67 DMFS	57

Cariogenicity or Non-cariogenicity of Foods

In order to implement a caries prevention program that includes dietary modification, it would be desirable to have some means of evaluating the cariogenicity or non-cariogenicity of individual foods and beverages. Lest any of you be so sanguine as to expect this Conference to devise or agree upon a single test of cariogenicity of a food or beverage, I regret that I must dispel any such illusions. There is no single test of cariogenicity—especially none that would satisfy a committee. *In vitro* tests have been criticized because they do not adequately measure host factors; plaque pH determinations predict acidogenicity, but not necessarily cariogenicity. Assessing the cariogenicity of foods fed *ad libitum* to rodents or even primates depends on the animal's food preference. The limitations of all these approaches will undoubtedly be amplified here later.

My greatest concern is the frequent misinterpretation of human clinical trials, particularly those in which only one sugar-containing item, such as breakfast cereal,[10,11] soft drink,[12] or candy[13] is the variable. In such trials the intake of other sugar-containing foods is not controlled and, regrettably, is generally frequent and considerable. Consequently there is a high caries activity in the control groups, i.e., a high background "noise" level (Table 2). In the United States and some European countries, sugar consumption is well over 100 pounds per person per year.[14,15] Slight variations in this amount are unlikely to cause a significant difference in caries increments. It is incorrect, therefore, to claim that there is "no association" between the consumption of presweetened cereals and the incidence of caries.[16,17] Rather, the poorly controlled human model will not show statistical differences. Hamsters fed various commercial cereals develop caries proportionate to the sucrose content of the cereal[18,19] (Table 3).

TABLE 2. Annual caries increments of subjects eating "normal" diet and sugar-supplemented diet

Diet		Age	Reference
"Normal" Water 2X/day 3.42 DMFS	Sugar Supplement Sugar soft drink 2X/day 4.05 DMFS	8-21	12
Breakfast cereal non-eaters 2.14 DMFS	Breakfast cereal eaters (60% presweetened) 1.73 DMFS	13	11
Regular breakfast cereal 1.92 DFS	Presweetened breakfast cereal 1.84 DFS	7-11	10
Sugarless gum 5X/day 1.97 DMFS	Sugar gum 5X/day 2.37 DMFS	12.5	Ref. not given 1967

TABLE 3. Influence of commercial cereals on dental caries in hamsters[18]

Cereal[1]	% Sucrose[29]	Caries Score
Frosted Flakes	44	17.14 ± 0.36
Cap'n Crunch	43.3	14.21 ± 0.24
King Vitaman	58.5	14.09 ± 0.27
Quisp	44.9	10.46 ± 0.15
Corn Flakes	7.8	8.95 ± 0.14
Corn Starch	0	8.46 ± 0.19
Cheerios	2,2	7.66 ± 0.12
Life	14.5	6.92 ± 0.12
Special K	4.4	6.85 ± 0.11
Shredded Wheat	1.0	6.07 ± 0.12

[1]Constituted 33% of total diet

Even more misleading are cross-sectional surveys of populations in which investigators attempt to relate dietary habits, based upon a 24-hour recall, to caries prevalence, forgetting that prevalence data measures the cumulative effect of dietary habits of many years.[20,23] It is unreasonable to expect that one 24-hour period or even a week's dietary survey can be related to an indeterminate time, during which dietary habits can change. Caries usually is a chronic disease that takes 18±6 months to develop into a clinically detectable lesion.[24] Clearly, longitudinal measurements of caries increments and repeated diet histories are essential in any study of the association between caries and eating patterns.

Improving Efficacy of Caries Prevention by Diet Modification

The negligible success of dietary modification to date has already been mentioned. However, I do not wish to start this Conference on a pessimistic note, but on a realistic one: "The times they are a-changing."

1. Consumer advocates have markedly increased their efforts to alter our dietary habits. An example is their efforts to influence which food products are available to children in vending machines and school cafeterias.[24a] Popular lay magazines, paperback books and the daily press have repeatedly drawn attention to the high sugar content of many breakfast foods, as well as other food products containing "hidden" sugar.[26–30]

2. The government and its agencies are paying more attention to food matters. The Senate Select Committee on Nutrition and Human Needs has conducted hearings on television advertising of food to children[31–32] and has specifically recommended hearings about the impact of food advertising, especially of sugar-containing foods, on young children, and on possible restriction on such advertisements.[33] The Select Committee has also recommended a 40% reduction in sugar consumption as a national dietary goal.[33]

The Food and Drug Administration is looking into the question of labeling foods—whether the percentage of sucrose should be disclosed and whether a warning label should be included on potentially cariogenic items.[34] The Department of Agriculture also is considering proposed controls on "junk foods" that compete with subsidized school lunches.

3. The food industry itself can—and must—play an important role in introducing and marketing non-cariogenic or less cariogenic foods.[35] The composition and ingredients of many foods and beverages consumed today are determined by the food manufacturer, not by the consumer. Accordingly, caries control by dietary modification on a public health scale requires the help and cooperation of the food industry if it is to have any serious impact. Strict statutory definitions cover claims that products are "anti-cavity," "non-cariogenic," or "less cariogenic." The FDA stringently enforces the 1958 food additives amendment to the Food and Drug Act that requires proof of safety. This means there is considerable regulatory restraint upon the introduction of food additives.

Cost of clinical trials to demonstrate safety and efficacy is very high, often beyond the capability of a single manufacturer. Clearly, research and development of safe, non-cariogenic sweetening agents or other anti-cavity food additives should be done on an industry-wide, shared basis.

It is also high time that some food manufacturers stop deluding themselves and the public by claiming that sucrose or sucrose-containing foods are not important in causing caries. The relationship between eating sugar-containing food and tooth decay has been clouded by labeling it as "controversial" purely because here is no unanimity.[36,37] Unanimity on any issue is rare, but unquestionably there is a consensus that frequent intake of sugary foods promotes caries (Review: see refs. [2,39–44]) Data on sugar consumption and average numbers of DMF teeth of children 10 to 12 years old, have been compiled from 19 countries[45] (Fig. 1). These data reveal a very strong correlation between sugar consumption and dental caries levels. A similar trend of high caries prevalence or low percentage of persons free from caries has been found among teenage South Africans with a high sugar intake. Conversely, rural negroes of similar age eating less sugar had significantly less caries and more caries-free mouths.[36] This interpretation is contrary to the conclusions of the authors but is supported by the overall data (see Fig. 2). Surveys in Europe and Japan have demonstrated a dramatic reduction in caries accompanying periods of wartime food restrictions.[46–48] In Norway during World War II, consumption of sugar, syrup and all sugar products was reduced.

These epidemiological observations on humans are supported by extensive animal experiments that reveal a parallelism between sucrose content of a food and its cariogenicity.[19] The relationship between dietary sucrose content and caries need not be exactly linear. The curve may rise sharply and then flatten out, as shown diagrammatically in Fig. 3, so that increasing the sucrose content of the diet beyond a certain level does not increase caries. In animals, this flattening of the curve may be explained by the fact that when the threshold level of sucrose in the diet is reached, almost all the susceptible surfaces at risk are already affected.

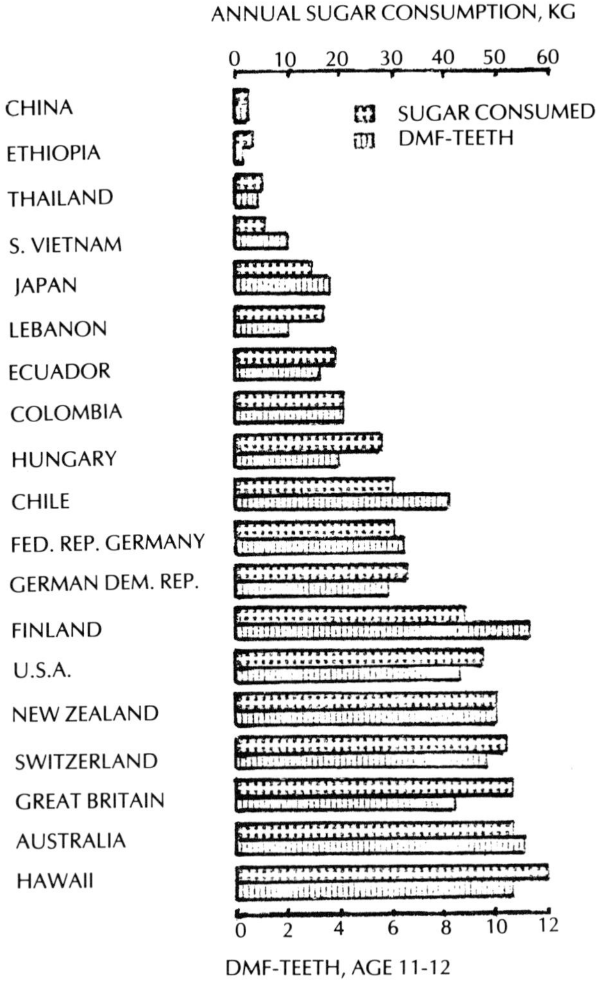

FIGURE 1. Caries score (DMF-teeth) for children (11 to 12 years old) in 19 countries and corresponding annual per capital sugar consumption based on data of 1959. (Courtesy Prof. Dt. T. Marthaler)

Conversely, until the percentage of sucrose in the diet is decreased below a certain level, there is little reduction in caries. This level will depend on the animal model being tested. In one study using gnotobiotic rats, it was as low as 3% sucrose.[49] In conventional rats the threshold level has been estimated at 15% sucrose[50] and 25% sucrose[40] and in the conventional hamster at 20% sucrose (Krasse, unpublished findings). This also may explain why, in some of the human trials in which only one sugary food item was varied, no significant differences in caries were found.

The consensus conclusion that sugar consumption and caries are related is inescapable. It is based not only on epidemiological surveys but on extensive animal experiments and controlled human studies. Bowen has aptly stated: "Evidence incrimiating sugars has continued to accumulate from the results of epidemiological and animal research and has now reached such proportions

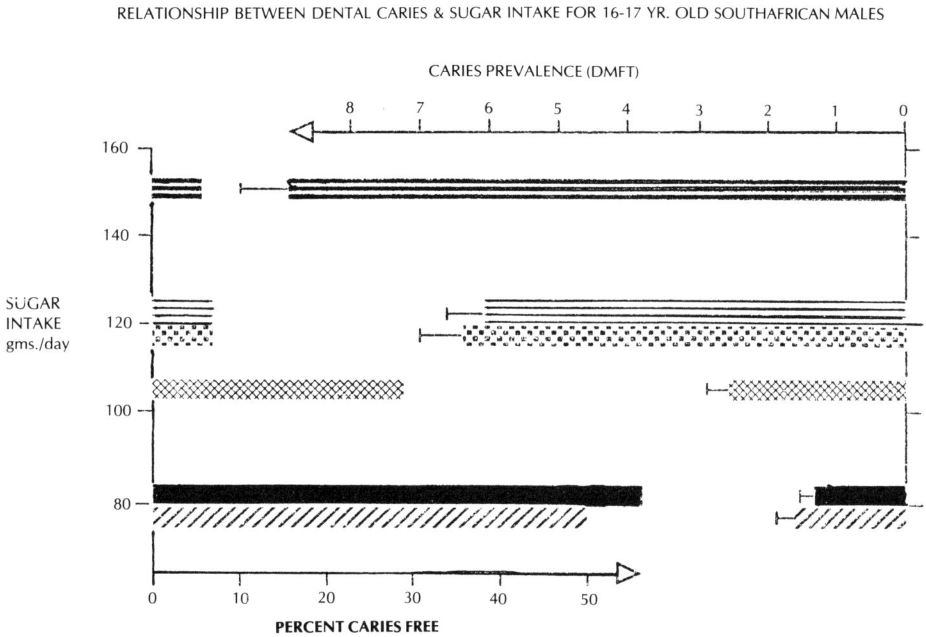

FIGURE 2. Relationship between dental caries and mean sugar intake (gms/day) for South African males (16 to 17 years old) of four different ethnic groups. There is a direct relationship between caries prevalence (DMFT) and sugar intake and an indirect relationship between percent population caries-free and sugar intake. (Drawn from data of Retief *et al.*, Brit. Dent. J. 1975.)

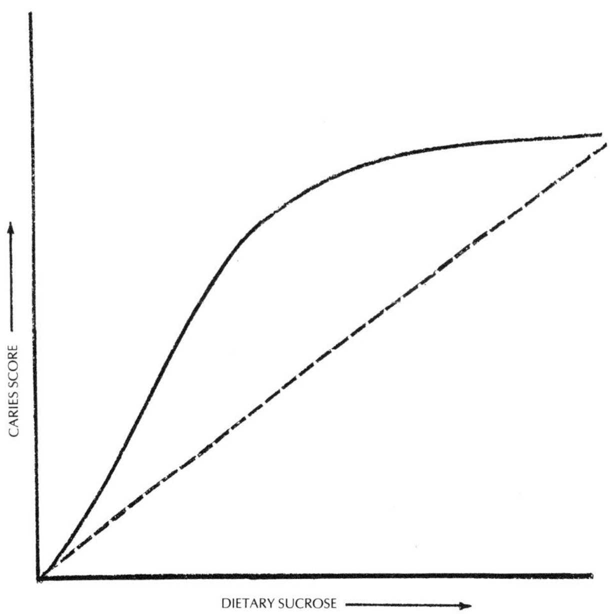

FIGURE 3. Possible relationship between caries score and dietary sucrose intake. Broken line represents a perfect linear relationship, solid line resembles findings with experimental animals.

that no reasonable person would deny that frequent consumption of sugars by caries-susceptible humans will result in the development of dental caries."[51]

Food manufacturers should also cease misinformative advertising, as witnessed last year in response to a television 'expose' on breakfast cereals.[52]

Finally, I am encouraged by the interest and cooperation of food manufacturers in developing reliable methods of measuring cariogenicity of products. Information has been exchanged between some representatives of food manufacturers and the dental profession and dental researchers. In just the last year or two, the participation of industry in such conferences as this one has increased tremendously. It may be hoped that we can work together to develop safe non-cariogenic foods and beverages. Total replacement of sucrose in foods is most unlikely. No doubt there is a hierarchy of foods to be modified, with highest priority given to eliminating sucrose and other readily fermentable sugars from snack foods. Several sugar substitutes may be required to provide a broad range for stability, taste onset, and sweetness intensity. Further development and testing is necessary to provide a sufficient array of non-cariogenic snack foods to the consumer. Such changes could have major public health impact in reducing dental caries.

It would be appropriate to conclude with the words of Isaiah (Chapter 11, verses 6 and 7), in which he prophesies that disparate species--such as candy manufacturers and dentists, breakfast cereal makers and nutritionists, soft drink bottlers and members of the Dairy Council--would one day cooperate with one another. Isaiah even envisioned the possibility of dietary modification:

The wolf shall dwell with the lamb,
and the leopard shall lie down with the kid,
and the calf and the lion and the fatling together,
and a little child shall lead them.
The cow and the bear shall feed;
their young shall lie down together;
and the lion shall eat straw like the ox.

REFERENCES

1. Newbrun, E. *Cariology*. Baltimore, Williams and Wilkins, 1978.
2. Scherp, H.W. Dental caries: Prospects for prevention. *Science* 73:1199-1205, 1971.
3. Carlos, J.P. (ed) *Prevention and Oral Health,* DHEW Publication No. NIH 74-707, Washington, D.C., USGPO, 1974.
4. Barmes, D.E. WHO's accent on prevention. *Scand. J. Dent. Res.* 85:11-15, 1977.
5. Newbrun, E. Systemic use of fluorides: assessment of cost/benefit features and practicality, in *Relative Efficiency of Preventive Procedures in Dental Public Health,* D.A. Burt, ed, Ann Arbor, Mich, University of Michigan, School of Public Health, 1978.
6. Gustafsson, B.E., Quensel, C.E., Lanke, L.S., Lundqvist, C., Grahnén, H., Bonow, B.E. and Krasse, B. The Vipeholm dental caries study. The effect of different levels of carbohydrate intake on caries activity in 436 individuals observed for five years. *Acta Odontol. Scand.* 11:232-364, 1954.
7. Harris, R. Biology of the children of Hopewood House, Bowral, Australia. IV. Observations of dental caries experience extending over five years (1957-1961). *J. Dent. Res.* 42:1387-1398, 1963.
8. Scheinin, A. and Mäkinen, K.K. Turku sugar studies. I-XXI. *Acta Odontol. Scand.* 33: Supplement 70, 1975.

9. King, J.M. Patterns of sugar consumption in early infancy. *Comm. Dent. Oral Epidemiol.* 6:47-52, 1978.
10. Glass, R.L. and Fleisch, S. Diet and dental caries: dental caries incidence in the consumption of ready-to-eat cereals. *J. Amer. Dent. Assn.* 88:807-813, 1974
11. Rowe, N.H., Anderson, R.H. and Wanninger, L.A. Effects of ready-to-eat breakfast cereals on dental caries experience in adolescent children: a three-year study. *J. Dent. Res.* 53:33-36, 1974.
12. Steinberg, A.D., Zimmerman, S.O. and Bramer, M.L. The Lincoln dental caries study. II. The effect of acidulated carbonated beverages on the incidence of dental caries. *J. Amer. Dent. Assn.* 85:81-89, 1972.
13. Ashley, F.P., Naylor, M.N. and Emslie, R.D. Clinical testing of dicalcium phosphate supplemented sweets. *Brit. Dent. J.* 436:361-366, 1974.
14. Page, L. and Friend, B. Level of use of sugars in the United States, in *Sugars in Nutrition,* H.L. Sipple and K.W. McNutt, eds, New York, Academic Press, 1974, pp. 93-107.
15. Wretlind, A. World sugar production and usage in Europe. Ibid, pp. 81-92.
16. Cereal Institute. The role of presweetened breakfast cereals in the American diet. Information from Cereal Institute, Inc., Chicago, Ill., 1974.
17. Hayden, E.B. Breakfast and today's life styles. *J. School Health* 45:83-87, 1975.
18. McDonald, J.L. and Stookey, G.K. Animal studies concerning the cariogenicity of dry breakfast cereals. *J. Dent. Res.* 56:1001-1006, 1977.
19. Newbrun, E. Criteria indicative of cariogenicity or non-cariogenicity of foods and beverages, in *Health and Sugar Substitutes,* B. Guggenheim, ed. Proc. ERGOB Conf., Geneva. Basel, S. Karger, 1978, pp. 253-258.
20. Bagramian, R.A. and Russell, A.L. Epidemiological study of dental caries experience and between-meal eating patterns. *J. Dent. Res.* 52:342-347, 1973.
21. Bagramian, R.A., Jenny, J., Frazier, P.J. and Proshek, J.M. Diet patterns and dental caries in third grade U.S. children. *Comm. Dent. Oral Epidemiol.* 2:208-213, 1974.
22. Kreitzman, S. Human diet and dental caries, in *Proceedings of the Workshop on Carogenicity of Food, Beverages, Confections, and Chewing Gum.* Chicago, Ill. Research Institute, American Dental Association Health Foundation, 1977, pp. 55-59
23. Kreitzman, S.N. New perspectives on diet and dental caries. J. Prevent. Dent. 5:12-17, 1978.
24. Parfitt, G.J. The speed of development of the carious cavity. *Brit. Dent. J.* 100:204-207, 1956.
25. Flor, S. How you can help to ban confection sales in schools. Pharmacy Times 44:48-49, 1978.
26. Consumers Union. Instant breakfast: nutritious junk food? *Consumer Rep* 42:324-327, 1977.
27. Consumers Union. Too much sugar? *Consumer Rep* 43:136-141, 1978.
28. Hess, J.J. Harvard's sugar-pushing nutritionist. *Saturday Rev* 5:10-14, 1978.
29. Lalli, C. The breakfast of chumps: sugar cereals can ruin you. *New West* 2:40-44, 1977.
30. Shannon, I.L. *Brand Name Guide to Sugar,* Chicago, Nelson-Hall, 1977.
31. U.S. Senate. TV Advertising of Food to Children. Hearings before the Select Committee on Nutrition and Human Needs, March 5, 1973, Wahington, D.C., 1973.
32. U.S. Senate. *Edible TV: Your Child and Food Commercials,* prepared by the Council on Children, Media and Merchandising for the Select Committee on Nutrition and Human Needs, September 1977, USGPO, Washington, D.C., 1977b.
33. U.S. Senate. *Dietary Goals for the United States.* Select Committee on Nutrition and Human Needs, USGPO, Washington, D.C. 1977a.
34. Ronk, R.J. Regulation issues, in *Sweeteners: Issues and Uncertainties,* Fourth Acad. Forum. Washington, D.C., National Academy of Sciences, 1975, pp. 45-48.
35. Newbrun, E. The role of food manufacturers in the dietary control of caries. *J. Amer. Soc. Prev. Dent.* 4:33-44, 1974.
36. Retief, D.H., Cleaton-Jones, P.E. and Walker, A.R.P. Dental caries and sugar intake in South African pupils of 16 to 17 years in four ethnic groups. *Brit. Dent. J.* 138:463-469, 1975.
37. Walker, A.R.P. and Cleaton-Jones, P.E. Dental caries and sugar intake. *Lancet* II:765, 1975.
38. Federal Trade Commission. Children's advertising. *Federal Register* 43:17967-17972, 1978.
39. Andlaw, R.J. Diet and dental caries—a review. *J. Hum. Nutr.* 31:45-52, 1977.
40. Hartles, R.L. Sucrose and dental caries, in *Sugar,* J. Yudkin, I. Edelman and L Hough, eds. London, Butterworth's 1971, pp. 221-230.

41. Mäkinen, K.K. The role of sucrose and other sugars in the development of dental caries: a review. *Int. Dent. J.* 22:363-386, 1972.
42. Newbrun, E. Sucrose, the arch criminal of dental caries. *Odont. Revy* 18:373-386, 1967.
43. Nizel, A.E. *Nutrition in Preventive Dentistry: Science and Practice*. Philadelphia, W.B. Saunders, 1972, pp. 27-49.
44. Winter, G.B. Sucrose and cariogenesis *Brit. Dent. J.* 124:407-411, 1968.
45. Marthaler, T.M. Sugar and oral health: epidemiology in humans, in *Health and Sugar Substitutes*, B. Guggenheim (ed), S. Karger, Basel, pp. 27-34, 1978.
46. Sognnaes, R.F. Analyses of wartime reduction of dental caries in European children. *Am. J. Dis. Child.* 75:792-821, 1948.
47. Takeuchi, M. Epdemiology study on dental caries in Japanese children before, during and after World War II. *Int. Dent. J.* 11:443-457, 1961.
48. Toverud, G. Child dental health. Brit. Dent. J. 116:229-304, 1964.
49. Michalek, S.M., McGhee, J.R., Shiota, T. and Devenyns, D. Low sucrose levels promote extensive *Streptococcus mutans*-induced caries. *Infect. Immun.* 16:712-714, 1977.
50. Huxley, H.G. The cariogenicity of dietary sucrose at various levels in two strains of rat under unrestricted and controlled-frequency feeding conditions. *Caries Res.* 11:237-242, 1977.
51. Bowen, W.H. Role of carbohydrates in dental caries. In *Symposium on Dental Nutrition,* S. Wei (ed), University of Iowa (in press), 1978.
52. Kellogg Company. *The Wall Street Journal,* Wednesday, November 23, 1977, p. 21.
53. Scheinin, A. Influence of the diagnostic level on caries incidence in two controlled clinical trials. ORCA Abst. No. 20, p. 65, 1978.

A NUTRITIONAL SURVEY OF CARIES-FREE NAVAL RECRUITS

I. L. Shklair, Ph.D.

The prevalence of dental caries among adult populations in the United States is practically 100% and constitutes a public health problem of great magnitude. Military populations, especially incoming recruits, have always been a favorite target for dental surveys in this country, and justifiably so, because they reflect quite accurately the general dental health status of our nation's youth. From the early studies of Lewis about Federal Army draftees in the Civil War, to recent studies, the results indicate clearly that the dental health of this country's young men and women is deplorable when they report for military duty.

Recently, Wirthlin, of our laboratory, compiled the dental requirements of 1,000 incoming naval recruits (Table 1). Taking the first three figures of decayed surfaces, we see that the average recruit enters the Navy with approximately 6.5 decayed surfaces. In addition, extensive other work is required. Almost every other recruit requires at least one extraction, and almost all require periodontal scaling and prophylaxis.

TABLE 1. Dental requirements of 1,000 incoming naval recruits

Amalgam (1 surface)	3,161
Amalgam (2 or more surfaces)	2,752
Resin Restorations	764
Crown or Bridge	32
Partial Denture	31
Extraction	492
Scaling (periodontal)	728
Prophylaxis	996

These data, together with over 100 years of dental surveys of military populations, have served to remind us painfully of our almost complete failure effectively to stimulate the search for new methods of understanding the carious process.

One approach of our laboratory involves the study of certain individuals who demonstrate no clinical or radiographic evidence of dental caries experience when they join the Navy. They have a DMFT score of 0. We will refer to these individuals as the caries-free group. The question arose as to what we can learn from the individuals who never had a carious lesion. What makes them different from the rest of us mortals who do develop lesions? Definitive studies on caries-free recruits began in the mid 1950's at the Naval Training Center at Bainbridge, Maryland. After Bainbridge closed, studies on the caries-free recruits continued at the Great Lakes Naval Training Center. Extensive epidemiological and laboratory data were collected from the caries-free individuals up to 1972. The caries-free individuals are still being sampled, as specific studies warrant their use.

Table 2 indicates the prevalence of caries-free recruits entering Great Lakes. The mean prevalence for the period from 1960 to 1972 was 3 men per thousand recruits. Starting in 1971 the prevalence of caries-free recruits at Great Lakes has been rising. In 1971 a record rate of 9 men per thousand was observed. Currently we are still seeing this increased rate of about 10 men per thousand.

TABLE 2. Prevalence of caries-free naval recruits at Great Lakes, Illinois, 1960-1972

Year	Total Recruits	Caries-free	Percent
1960	54,439	109	0.200
1961	49,245	84	0.171
1962	47,988	84	0.175
1963	48,839	151	0.309
1964	45,073	94	0.209
1965	69,420	112	0.161
1966	62,617	117	0.187
1967	58,879	77	0.131
1968	68,496	167	0.244
1969	60,493	138	0.228
1970	48,746	184	0.377
1971	43,658	399	0.914
1972	45,601	435	0.953
Total	703,494	2,151	0.306

From 1960 to 1972, a total of 703,494 young men came to Great Lakes for recruit training. Of these, 2,151 were found to be caries-free, for a total prevalence of 3.1 men per thousand (0.306%).

We are not sure why this dramatic increase in caries-free recruits is occurring, but it probably is related to the increase in municipal water supply fluoridation. For example, up to 1970, we never had a caries-free recruit from the New England states--now we do see them; probably in relation to the number of communities that instituted water fluoridation from 1940 to the 1960's.

But certainly everyone in a fluoridated community is not caries-free, and an occasional caries-free individual may be found even in nonfluoridated communities. Many studies have shown that some variance in caries experience within and between populations can be attributed to nutritional factors other than fluoride--which brings me to my major point.

We were interested in the nutritional histories of our recruits prior to their entering the Navy, to see if there were any differences in their food consumption and eating habits. A good deal of our nutritional information about naval recruits was obtained by means of questionnnaires.

1. Name (last first initial)	2. Social Security #	3. Birth date

4. Home Address (street city state)	5. Age	6. Home Phone

7. Birth Place (city county state)	8. Height	9. Weight	10. Blood Type

11. Mother's residence prior to your birth (city state)

12. Places of residence from birth to present: (Circle source of water supply)

A. Birth to Age___ ______ city ______ state well - river - town
B. Age___to Age___ ______ city ______ state well - river - town
C. Age___to Age___ ______ city ______ state well - river - town
D. Age___to Age___ ______ city ______ state well - river - town

---

FILL IN OR CIRCLE THE APPROPRIATE ANSWERS BELOW (QUESTIONS 13 - 24)

13. How much of the following foods did you eat as a child? (only up to age 12)

A. Milk: none little average lots
B. Meat: none little average lots
C. Cooked vegetables: none little average lots
D. Raw vegetables: none little average lots
E. Home preserved vegetables: none little average lots
F. Home preserved fruits: none little average lots
G. Candy: none little average lots
H. Desserts: none little average lots
I. Water: little average lots

14. Before coming into the Navy, did you eat between meals: none little average lots
What did you eat? sweets soft drinks milk fruit sandwiches
15. Before coming into the Navy did you eat Lifesavers? no little lots
16. Before coming into the Navy did you chew gum? no little lots
17. How many cigarettes did you smoke in a day? (Before joining the Navy)
none less than 10 10-20 20-30 more than 30
18. How often did you brush your teeth before going to high school?
never sometimes once a day twice a day more than twice a day
19. Were your parents strict on tooth brushing? yes no
20. Do you ever rinse your mouth after eating? never sometimes always
21. How many times have you been to the dentist (before joining the Navy?) ___
22. Before coming into the Navy, did you drink coffee or tea? ______
How many cups per day___. How many teaspoons of sugar per cup______
23. Before coming into the Navy, how many bottles of "soft drinks" did you consume per day? 0 1 2 3 4 5 more_____
24. Before coming into the Navy, how many pieces of candy did you eat per day?
0 1 2 3 4 5 more______

FIGURE 1. Questionnaire

For this study, three groups of recruits answered a questionnaire (Fig. 1) — the caries-free group (no history of any carious lesions) and, at the other extreme, a caries-rampant group. The individuals in the caries-rampant group had at least ten unrestored lesions. The third group was a randomly selected group of recruits whose caries experience generally fell between the extremes. This latter group we called the controls. The data were collected in 1970-71. We were interested in the age, height, weight, blood type, where the individuals grew up — and the source of their drinking water in order to relate fluoride intake (if any) with tooth development and caries activity. The bottom half of the questionnaire deals primarily with their dietary habits before they entered the service.

For questions 13-A through H, and question 14, four choices were available: none, little, average and lots. In question 15, on Lifesavers, and 16, on gum, three choices were available: no, little and lots. The men were asked to circle the quantity which best described their dietary habits. In questions 13 and 14, scores were given to each response: none = 0, little = 1, average = 2, and lots = 3. In questions 15 and 16, no was score as 0, little = 1, and lots = 2.

The scores for each item were averaged in each group and a χ^2 analysis of the data was made to determine the differences between the three groups.

The remaining questions were of interest for other survey studies. The last three questions, however, could serve as an internal control of the questionnaire. In the last question, about candy eaten, for example, we can compare how many pieces of candy one ate. Some would indicate they ate five pieces, and record that they ate an average amount of candy. To others this would be recorded as lots. So we do have a great deal of subjective answering. However, we could see some definite trends in the large masses of data.

Let us consider nine of these items in more detail. Four of the items we can classify tentatively as non-cariogenic items: milk, meat, and cooked and uncooked (raw) vegetables. Five of the items might be classified as cariogenic: candy, desserts, snacks, Lifesavers and gum.

There were 810 caries-free and caries-rampant recruits and 423 controls. For most of the data to be shown, the greatest differences appear at the extremes. In Table 3, if we look at the "lots" of milk consumed — 54.3% of the caries-free recruits indicated they drank "lots" of milk, compared to 35.6% of the caries-rampant group; the controls with 41.4% fell between the two extremes. Only 8% of the caries-free drank "little" milk as opposed to 17% in the caries-rampant group; the controls were between the extremes at 10.1%. About an equal percentage of the caries-rampant and controls drank an average amount of milk — 46.4 and 47.5 percent. On a group basis, there was a highly significant difference between the caries-free and caries-rampant and the control groups, and to a lesser extent between the caries rampant and the control groups. The caries-rampant group drank significantly less milk than the caries-free or controls.

The differences are most noticeable at the extremes (Table 4). About 48% of the caries-free men indicated they ate lots of meat, compared to 32% of the caries-rampant group. Among the caries-free, only 3.4% indicated they ate little meat whereas 7% of the caries-rampant group ate little meat.

TABLE 3. Nutritional survey on naval recruits: Milk

	Caries Free (A)		Caries Rampant (B)		Controls (C)	
	N	%	N	%	N	%
None	4	0.49	7	0.86	4	0.95
Little	65	8.02	138	17.04	43	10.17
Average	301	37.16	376	46.42	202	47.75
Lots	440	54.32	289	35.68	174	41.13
Total	810	99.99	810	100.0	423	100.0
χ^2	AB = 66.65[3]		AC = 19.67[3]		BC = 11.26[2]	

[1]p = 0.05 [2]p = 0.01 [3]p = 0.001

TABLE 4. Nutritional survey on naval recruits: Meat

	Caries Free (A)		Caries Rampant (B)		Controls (C)	
	N	%	N	%	N	%
None	3	0.37	0	0.0	0	0.0
Little	28	3.46	57	7.06	15	3.57
Average	390	48.21	490	60.64	230	54.76
Lots	388	47.96	261	32.30	175	41.67
Total	809	100.0	808	100.0	420	100.0
χ^2	AB = 49.11[3]		AC = 6.31		BC = 14.17[2]	

[1]p = 0.05 [2]p = 0.01 [3]p = 0.001

The caries-free group, as well as the controls, ate significantly more meat than the caries-rampant group. There were no significant differences between the caries-free group and the controls — which could be interpreted as meaning that the caries-rampant group ate less meat than most individuals.

The pattern again is similar for vegetable eating as with milk and meat (Table 5). The caries-free group tended to eat more cooked vegetables than the caries-rampant or the control group. Fewer of the caries-free group ate "little" cooked vegetables (21.7%) than the caries-rampant (29.8%) or the control group (27.9%). The caries-free group had 23.7% indicating they ate "lots" of vegetables compared to only 16% of the caries-rampant group. The controls fell between those extremes, 19.6%. There was a significant difference between the caries-free and the caries-rampant groups and between the caries-free and the control groups. However, there was no significant difference between the caries-rampant and the control group, indicating the caries-free men ate more cooked vegetables than the rest of the population tested.

As shown in Table 6, 43.7% of the caries-free recruits indicated thay ate an "average" amount of uncooked vegetables, whereas it was about 34% in the caries-rampant and control groups. Fewer of the caries-free group indicated they ate "little" raw vegetables than the caries-rampant or control groups. Again, there was a significant difference between the caries-free and the caries-rampant group and the controls in the amount of cooked vegetables eaten. There was no significant difference between the caries-rampant and control group, both groups indicating they ate about the same in raw vegetables.

TABLE 5. Nutritional survey on naval recruits: Cooked Vegetables

	Caries Free (A)		Caries Rampant (B)		Controls (C)	
	N	%	N	%	N	%
None	9	1.11	11	1.36	12	2.84
Little	175	21.69	241	29.86	118	27.90
Average	431	53.41	422	52.29	210	49.65
Lots	192	23.79	133	16.48	83	19.62
Total	807	100.0	807	99.99	423	100.0
χ^2	AB = 21.48[3]		AC = 12.22[2]		BC = 5.52	

[1]p = 0.05 [2]p = 0.01 [3]p = 0.001

TABLE 6. Nutritional survey on naval recruits: Uncooked Vegetables

	Caries Free (A)		Caries Rampant (B)		Controls (C)	
	N	%	N	%	N	%
None	42	5.20	45	5.60	38	9.07
Little	285	35.27	352	43.84	181	43.20
Average	353	43.69	272	33.87	145	34.61
Lots	128	15.84	134	16.69	55	13.13
Total	808	100.0	803	100.0	419	100.0
χ^2	AB = 17.77[3]		AC = 17.87[3]		BC = 7.19	

[1]p = 0.05 [2]p = 0.01 [3]p = 0.001

To summarize briefly, the "non-carious" foods — milk, meat, cooked and uncooked vegetables — were usually eaten to a significantly greater extent by the caries-free group than by the caries-rampant group and, usually, by the control group.

For candy, the difference between the groups is very apparent (Table 7). Three percent of the caries-free group indicated they "never" ate any candy; 35% ate only "little" candy, compared to 11.5 and 16.3% in the caries-rampant and control groups. A bit less than half of the caries-free group indicated they ate an "average" amount of candy, a rate fairly similar to that of the caries-rampant group. However, only 15% of the caries-free group ate "lots" of candy compared to 37% of the caries-rampant group and 23% of the controls. There were significant differences between the caries-free and caries-rampant and control groups, and between the caries-rampant and controls as well. The caries-rampant group indicated they ate significantly more candy than the caries-free or the control group, and the caries-free group ate less candy than the other groups.

The data on dessert eating (Table 8) is fairly similar to that of the candy consumed. The differences show up most dramatically at the extremes — 2.2% of the caries-free group did not eat dessert, nor did less than 1% of the rampant group or the controls. About 21% of the caries-free group also indicated they ate "little" dessert, compared to 15 and 16% of the caries-rampant and control groups, respectively. The average amount of dessert eaten by both groups is

TABLE 7. Nutritional survey on naval recruits: Candy

	Caries Free (A)		Caries Rampant (B)		Controls (C)	
	N	%	N	%	N	%
None	26	3.22	2	0.25	7	1.65
Little	282	34.94	92	11.94	69	16.31
Average	377	46.72	408	50.94	250	59.10
Lots	122	15.12	299	37.33	97	22.93
Total	807	100.0	801	100.0	423	100.0
χ^2	AB = 192.71[3]		AC = 54.16[3]		BC = 33.49[3]	

[1]p = 0.05 [2]p = 0.01 [3]p = 0.001

TABLE 8. Nutritional survey on naval recruits: Desserts

	Caries Free (A)		Caries Rampant (B)		Controls (C)	
	N	%	N	%	N	%
None	18	2.23	3	0.38	4	0.95
Little	172	21.29	122	15.25	70	16.63
Average	469	58.04	430	53.75	244	57.96
Lots	149	18.44	245	30.63	103	24.47
Total	808	100.0	800	100.0	421	100.0
χ^2	AB = 44.26[3]		AC = 10.47[1]		BC = 6.47	

[1]p = 0.05 [2]p = 0.01 [3]p = 0.001

about the same, but again the biggest difference is between the caries-rampant and the caries-free groups that indicated they ate "lots" of dessert; 30.6% compared to 18.4%.

There were significant differences in dessert eating between the caries-free and caries-rampant groups and the control group. However, there was no significant difference between the caries-rampant and controls in dessert eating, as there was in the candy group; the caries-rampant group ate significantly more candy than either the caries-free or control group.

As with the candy and dessert data, the data on snacks is most noticeable at the extremes (Table 9). About 70% of the caries-free group indicated they had "none" or "little" snacks, compared to about 55% of the caries-rampant group. Notice the difference in those that ate "lots" of snacks — 30% for the caries-free group, compared to 45% of the caries-rampant group and 38% in the control group. The caries-rampant group ate significantly more snacks than either the caries-free or control groups.

These data may not be surprising, when one considers the previous data. That is, the caries-free group drank more milk, and ate more meat and vegetables than the caries-rampant group. As a result, the caries-rampant group subjects may have needed more snacks to reduce their hunger. The relatively low milk and meat scores and the relatively high candy scores in the caries-rampant group may also reflect the socioeconomic-nutritional background of this high caries and dentally neglected group.

TABLE 9. Nutritional survey on naval recruits: Snacks

	Caries Free (A)		Caries Rampant (B)		Controls (C)	
	N	%	N	%	N	%
None	58	7.23	15	1.88	18	4.28
Little	501	62.47	421	52.76	242	57.48
Lots	243	30.30	362	45.36	161	38.24
Total	802	100.0	798	100.0	421	100.0
χ^2	AB = 55.67[3]		AC = 10.28[2]		BC = 10.23[2]	

[1]p = 0.05 [2]p = 0.01 [3]p = 0.001

Parenthetically, it may be noted that the caries-rampant group of recruits generally had lower body weights than the caries-free group or the controls. These data were not significant but the trend is there. There were no significant differences in the heights between the groups.

LifeSaver data (Table 10) also reflects differences in the extremes. There is a significant difference between the caries-free group and the caries-rampant and control groups, but was no significance between the caries-rampant and the controls, again indicating that there were significant differences in the dietary habits of the caries-free group.

Chewing gum was one of the few items where there was no difference between any pair of groups; the data for the three groups are almost identical (Table 11).

TABLE 10. Nutritional survey on naval recruits: Life Savers

	Caries Free (A)		Caries Rampant (B)		Controls (C)	
	N	%	N	%	N	%
None	244	30.20	182	22.55	89	21.14
Little	530	65.59	568	70.38	310	73.64
Lots	34	4.21	57	7.06	22	5.23
Total	808	100.0	807	99.99	421	100.0
χ^2	AB = 16.15[3]		AC = 11.62[2]		BC = 2.10	

[1]p = 0.05 [2]p = 0.01 [3]p = 0.001

TABLE 11. Nutritional survey on naval recruits: Chewing Gum

	Caries Free (A)		Caries Rampant (B)		Controls (C)	
	N	%	N	%	N	%
None	95	11.76	95	11.77	51	12.09
Little	496	61.39	499	61.83	264	62.56
Lots	217	26.86	213	26.39	107	25.36
Total	808	100.0	807	99.99	422	100.0
χ^2	AB = 0.046		AC = 0.32		BC = 0.16	

[1]p = 0.05 [2]p = 0.01 [3]p = 0.001

From all the data (Fig. 2) we see that caries-free men tended to have higher scores for milk, meat and vegetables, but lower scores for candy, desserts and snacks. Conversely, the rampant group scored lower for milk, meat and vegetable items, but much higher for candy, desserts and snacks. In general, the scores for the control group were intermediate between the two extreme caries experience groups. The intensity of the nutritional cariogenic challenge seems to have been quite different in the three groups of recruits, but one cannot conclude from the available data that the caries-free men did not develop caries because of a general lack of exposure to a cariogenic diet, although that seems possible in a few cases.

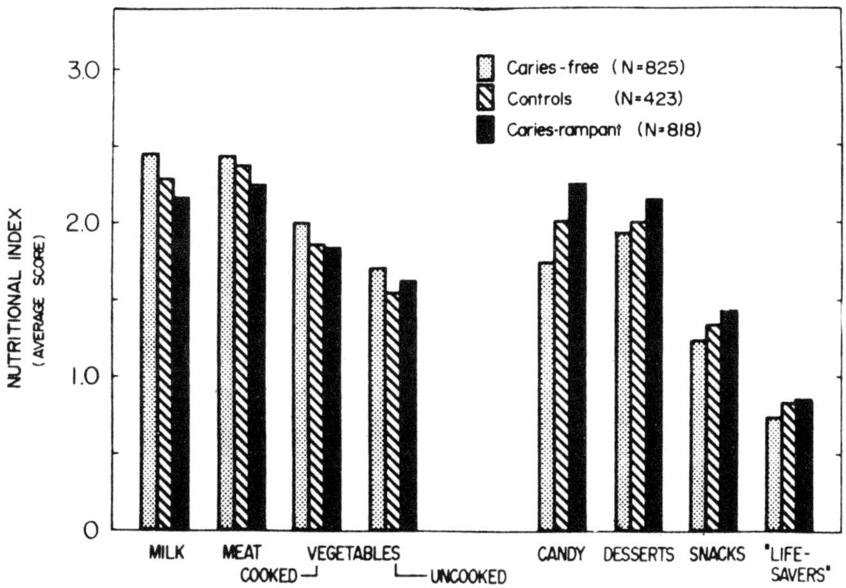

FIGURE 2. Histogram summarizing a dietary survey of these three groups of naval recruits with different caries experience. The tables should be consulted to determine actual scores obtained and methods for calculating scores.

Dental caries is not like other infectious diseases. It is not a one agent, one disease entity. Caries is a multifactorial disease. It can be likened to a constant battle taking place in the mouth (Fig. 3), between the cariogenic challenge of microorganisms and diet (generally sucrose) and the resistance factors such as tooth mineralization, tooth morphology, salivary flow, etc. If the cariogenic challenge is greater than the resistance factors, caries develops; conversely, if the resistance factors are greater, caries does not develop. Why an individual develops caries or does not depends on what is happening within the individual.

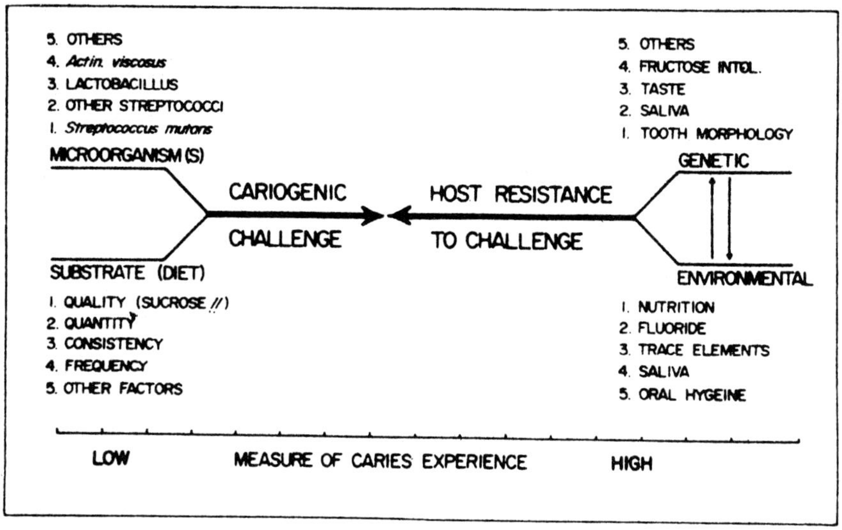

FIGURE 3. Development of a hypothetical population model illustrating the interaction of host resistance and cariogenic challenge in the expression of dental caries experience variation. See text for details.

For that reason, often, in caries research, particularly in the caries-free recruit, trends rather than clear cut differences are noted. These trends, when considered *in toto* account for the caries-free individual's freedom from caries.

The general profile of the caries-free recruit, compiled from many of our studies, shows him to have been reared in areas having relatively high levels of fluoride, producing higher surface-enamel fluoride levels; he has less total infection with *Streptococcus mutans* and fewer tooth sites infected. In addition, the *mutans* in these individuals produced less glucans. The caries-free recruits have higher levels of salivary bicarbonate, with high proportions of basic parotid salivary proteins. They often have a tooth morphology less conducive to bacterial infectivity than is found for the typical caries-susceptible recruit. The caries-free recruit also has greater sucrose taste sensitivity than the average caries-active recruit, i.e., they detect sucrose at significantly lower thresholds than caries-active individuals.

However, individuals within the group do not conform in all the above factors. When comparing the caries-free recruit to others, one finds a great deal of overlapping. It therefore becomes apparent that the particular combination and proportion of factors that protects one individual from developing decay may be quite different from those that protect another.

Sucrose is one of the important factors. Certainly the quantity and consistency of foods containing sucrose can be considered to be one of the prime factors in the initiation and development of dental caries.

CONCLUSION

In this nutritional survey, the cariogenic challenge, on a group basis, was often significantly different between caries-free, caries-rampant and control populations. In general, the caries-free recruit consumed more milk, meat and vegetables, and tended to ingest much less candy, desserts, and other sucrose rich foods than his caries-active counterpart. There was, however, a great deal of overlapping of data. There were caries-free men who indicated they ate "lots" of sucrose, but still remained caries-free, and, conversely, there were some caries-active recruits who indicated they ate very few foods containing sucrose.

Foods containing sucrose are one of the most important factors in the decay process. However, study of the effects of sucrose in the caries process requires consideration of a multitude of other factors involved.

DENTAL CARIES AND SUGAR INTAKE OF 16- TO 17-YEAR-OLD PUPILS IN FOUR SOUTH AFRICAN POPULATION GROUPS

D.H. Retief, D.D.S.

I wish to discuss with you the dental caries and sugar intake of 16- to 17-year-old pupils in four South African population groups. I selected children from this age group for the following reasons: First, being at high school, they were representative of the different socioeconomic classes within a population. We had considered going to universities, but that would exclude particularly the lower economic class group. Second, the caries pattern is well-established in this age group. And third, sugar consumption is maximal at this age, but is reduced after age 30.

South Africa has an area of about a half million square miles, which I believe is about the size of Texas. The total population is approximately 25 million, including 17 million Negroes (Bantu), 3 million Coloureds, 1 million Indians and 4 million Whites.

The Whites, mainly of Dutch, French and British stock, began to settle in the Cape in the middle of the 17th century, at about the same time as the Bantu groups migrated southward from central Africa. The Coloureds largely are Euro-African-Malay admixture. The Malays were brought in early, that is in the 16th and 17th centuries, as slaves from the East Indies. The Asiatic moiety has derived primarily from those who immigrated between 1860 and 1910 as indentured labor for the sugar plantations in Natal.

It is quite interesting that the sugar production exceeds the consumption in South Africa, and I believe that South Africa is one of the major exporting sugar countries; the source is chiefly sugar cane.

The diet consumed by the different population groups varies. Broadly, the rural Negroes consume their traditional diet based on whole or lightly milled cereal products, mainly corn and wheat. Meat is consumed irregularly and milk usually in small quantities. In the urban groups there is a progressive elaboration of diet from urban Negroes, Coloureds, Indians to Whites. The trend is toward increasing consumption of animal proteins and fat and refined carbohydrate foods, principally white bread and sugars.

The pupils studied included all in the particular schools who were 16 or 17 years of age. The schools were the rural Negro high school which is situated in Mabieskraal, 200 kilometers west of Johannesburg in a very sparcely populated region. The urban Negroes attended the Morris Isaacson High School situated in Soweto, a Negro township of approximately 1 million inhabitants adjacent to Johannesburg. The Coloured students attended the Coronationville High School in Johannesburg. The Indian pupils were from Mirvana High School in Lenasia about 30 kilometers south of Johannesburg. The White pupils, of mixed socio-economic classes, attended Sir John Adamson High School in Johannesburg.

The urban pupils lived in an area supplied with piped drinking water from a common source containing on an average 0.2 ppm fluoride; that is why the Mabieskraal area was selected because the drinking water for rural Negroes in this specific area was subterranean, but contained 0.1 ppm fluoride, and this was perhaps the area most closely resembling the fluoride content of that in the other groups.

We did not have all the desirable resources in many of the schools, particularly in the rural area. Dental caries was assessed in good natural light with a mouth mirror and sharp dental probes.

Teeth lost owing to trauma or extracted as part of orthodontic treatment were not included in the DMFT scores. Pupils were examined by two qualified dental surgeons, Dr. Cleaton-Jones and me. To obviate bias in scoring, each recorder studied alternate pupils as they appeared for examination.

Sugar intake was assessed by Dr. Walker of the Human Biochemistry Research Unit of the South African Medical Research Institute, because he has had a lot of experience in this particular field. To secure information on the per capita sugar consumption, three methods may be used:

1. The nationwide approach, in which the total national consumption is divided by the total population. It is the easy way out, but unfortunately this method usually gives much higher sugar consumption values than those obtained with the other methods.
2. The household consumption is determined by questionnaire, and the amount calculated is divided by the number of persons in the household. Such questionnaires usually cover a period of a week, or occasionally a month.
3. Individual questionnaire, as used in this study. We used the individual questionnaire suggested by Bett, Morland and Yudkin.[1]

Basically, in the first part of the dietary questionnaire (Fig. 1), we are interested in detecting any changes in the dietary pattern, and those pupils who did signify that there was a change in pattern were, naturally, excluded from the study. This really affected only a few of the female White pupils, and we had very few pupils that had to be excluded because of changes in their dietary patterns.

The second part of the questionnaire (Fig. 2) is concerned with the numbers of cups of tea and coffee consumed; in South Africa both tea and coffee are consumed extensively by all population groups.

From these sources, by determining the number of teaspoons, etc., the consumption of sugar is calculated (Fig. 3). We work on the basis that a heaping teaspoon is taken as containing approximately 6 g and a level teaspoon as 4 g of sugar.

Figure 4 describes the sweet and cool drinks consumed: note that we were interested only in the non-alcoholic consumption. We assumed that these students did not consume alcoholic beverages.

In the last section (Fig. 5), the sugar consumed with prepared foods is determined. This includes cereals, biscuits, and the amount of sugar taken with cereals or porridge. The calculations of the amounts of sugar in prepared foods and drinks are made from analyses[2] published in food tables or from figures supplied by the manufacturers.

DIETARY QUESTIONNAIRE

Bett, Morland and Yudkin, British Medical Journal 3:153, 1967

Name________________________________ Age______________________

If your weight has increased in the last few years, are you making a serious effort to check or decrease it? Yes/No

If "Yes", are you restricting sweet or sugary foods, or sugar?

____

If you are on a special diet now, why are you on this diet?

____

How long have you been on this diet?________________________

Have you ever been on any other special diet? Yes/No

If "Yes", why were you on this diet?________________________

____

Approximately when did you start on this diet?______________

____

How long did it last?_______________________________________

If your eating habits have permanently changed as a result of being on the diet, in what way?_______________________________________

FIGURE 1.

Go through an average day in your mind, and write down how many cups of tea and coffee you consume:

	Tea	Coffee	Other hot beverages
Before breakfast	______ Cups	______ Cups	______ Cups
At breakfast	______ Cups	______ Cups	______ Cups
Mid-morning break	______ Cups	______ Cups	______ Cups
Midday meal	______ Cups	______ Cups	______ Cups
Teatime	______ Cups	______ Cups	______ Cups
Evening meal	______ Cups	______ Cups	______ Cups
Bedtime	______ Cups	______ Cups	______ Cups
Other	______ Cups	______ Cups	______ Cups

FIGURE 2.

Yudkin and co-workers[3] found that, provided the questionnaires are completed carefully, the results were representative of particular groups, and were also repeatable. Walker and his associates[4] also found that their individual questionnaire gave repeatable results. For example, they initially studied 50 pupils in a population group, repeated the study three months later, and they found that the mean sugar intakes were 85 ± 2 grams at the first visit, and 82 ± 3 grams at the subsequent visit.

We believe that the pupils studied were fairly representative of the population groups. Our results must be regarded primarily as reflections or profiles of sugar intake situations rather than precise features of communities in which all constituent populations are proportionally represented.

How much sugar do you take in tea? __________ teaspoons

Are the spoons level or heaped? ______________

How much sugar do you take in coffee? _______ teaspoons

Are the spoons level or heaped? ______________

Have you always taken the same amount of sugar in these beverages? Yes/No

If "No" how much did you take before? ________________

When did you change? ____________________________

Do you <u>regularly</u> use artificial sweeteners? Yes/No

How long have you used them? ______________________

FIGURE 3.

How much of the following do you eat or drink <u>per week</u>?

Sweets, toffees and fancy chocolates ________________ g

Number of 50g chocolate bars _______________

Fizzy drinks, non-alcoholic ________________ glasses

(including tonic water, ginger-beer, etc.) _____small bottles

Fruit squash ___________glasses

Fruit juice (tinned or bottled) _________glasses

FIGURE 4.

How many a week do you have of the following:

Porridge ________ portions

Plain breakfast cereals _________ portions

Sugar-coated breakfast cereals ________ portions

Jam or marmalade ________ teaspoons

Sweet biscuits _________ number

Pudding or sweets at midday ________ portions

Pudding or sweets for tea or evening meal ____ portions

Individual cakes and slices of cake _______ number

How many spoons of sugar do you take on breakfast cereals?_____

Are they teaspoons or dessert spoons? _________

Are they level or heaped? ____________

How many spoons of sugar do you take on porridge? _______

Are they teaspoons or dessert spoons? __________

Are they level or heaped? ______________

FIGURE 5.

Tables 1 and 2 provide an overview of our subject groups. The numbers of pupils, the mean DMFT scores (±S.E.), the percentage of pupils free from caries and the mean daily sugar intake appears in the Tables.

The general trend for the male pupils was that a progressive increase in sugar consumption from rural Negroes to Whites was associated with an increase in caries incidence and a reduction in the percentage of pupils free from caries. The sugar intake of the urban Negroes (105 g) and the Coloured (118 g) did not differ significantly ($p > 0.05$) but there was a significant difference in the caries incidence of 2.6 and 7.3 respectively ($p < 0.01$) (Table 1).

However, comparable sugar intakes by Coloured (118 g) and Indian (123 g) males resulted in similar caries experience of 6.4 and 6.1, respectively.

The caries incidence in the females of the different population groups was very similar to that of the males in the corresponding population groups (Table 2).

TABLE 1. Males

	Rural Negro	Urban Negro	Coloured	Indian	White
Number	64	67	41	41	54
DMFT	1.2	2.6	6.4	6.1	8.9
± SEM	0.3	0.3	0.6	0.6	0.7
Caries free %	56.3	28.8	7.3	7.3	5.6
Sugar intake g	79	105	118	123	153
± SEM	3.4	4.8	8.4	11.1	9.7

TABLE 2. Females

	Rural Negro	Urban Negro	Coloured	Indian	White
Number	87	62	47	38	50
DMFT	1.2	2.1	5.3	9.4	11.1
± SEM	0.2	0.3	0.7	0.8	0.7
Caries free %	64.4	29.0	14.9	2.6	2.0
Sugar intake g	79	99	117	76	116
± SEM	3.1	4.9	8.8	6.6	12.9

The sugar intake by Coloured females (117 g) was similar to that of their White counterparts (116 g) but the caries incidence in the Whites was twice as high (11.1 vs. 5.3).

The rural Negro and Indian females had a similar sugar intake (79 g and 76 g respectively), yet there is a ninefold increase in the caries experience of the Indian females.

We stratified our male and female groups into upper-third, middle-third and lower-third consumption. Here, naturally, the number of pupils in each group was relatively small.

The sugar consumption of the upper-third of the males was significantly increased (Table 3). In this group it was significantly increased when compared to that of the total male populations, but this has practically no effect; the caries DMFT indices in this group was basically the same as the average of the whole group.

In the lower-third of the males (Table 4), the sugar intake, approximately 45 to 80 g was approximately one-third of that of the upper-third of the males, yet the caries experience was again practically the same as that of the whole class.

Perhaps the most striking feature among the females in the upper-third (Table 5) is that despite the fact that the sugar intake of the Indian females, (117 g — approximately one-half of that of the White females — which was 213 g) — the DMFT scores were approximately the same.

In the lower-third of the females (Table 6), the sugar intakes in the various population groups were of the same order. The progressive increase in caries

TABLE 3. Upper third males

	Rural Negro	Urban Negro	Coloured	Indian	White
Number	21	22	14	14	18
DMFT	1.7	2.8	5.9	6.1	9.4
± SEM	0.9	0.5	0.7	1.3	1.1
Caries free %	52.4	27.3	0	7.1	0
Sugar intake g	115	160	178	206	233
± SEM	4.1	5.5	8.4	13.9	12.4

TABLE 4. Lower third males

	Rural Negro	Urban Negro	Coloured	Indian	White
Number	21	21	14	14	18
DMFT	0.7	2.4	5.9	6.2	8.4
± SEM	0.2	0.7	1.3	1.1	1.3
Caries free %	61.9	33.3	14.3	7.1	5.6
Sugar intake g	45	57	63	57	83
± SEM	3.0	3.8	4.7	4.4	5.8

TABLE 5. Upper third females

	Rural Negro	Urban Negro	Coloured	Indian	White
Number	29	31	16	13	17
DMFT	1.3	2.5	5.8	10.5	11.2
± SEM	0.6	0.7	1.3	1.2	1.1
Caries free %	65.5	22.6	0	0	0
Sugar intake g	88	141	181	117	213
± SEM	2.7	8.0	14.3	11.2	22.7

TABLE 6. Lower third females

	Rural Negro	Urban Negro	Coloured	Indian	White
Number	29	30	16	13	17
DMFT	0.9	1.8	4.4	10.1	11.6
± SEM	0.3	0.5	1.3	1.4	1.5
Caries free %	69.0	33.3	33.3	0	5.9
Sugar intake g	40	63	62	42	43
± SEM	2.1	3.5	4.3	4.6	4.8

experience from the rural Negro to the White persisted, even in this group. The females in the lower-third consumed approximately one-third the sugar as those in the upper group, yet the caries incidence was not significantly affected.

Consider the results for the Indian and the White pupils studied (Table 7). The female pupils in these population groups consumed significantly less sugar than the corresponding males; for the Indians it was 76 g as opposed to 123 g; for the Whites, 116 g as opposed to 153 g. Yet the females had a significantly higher caries incidence than the male pupils.

TABLE 7

	Indian		White	
	Males	Females	Males	Females
Number	41	38	54	50
DMFT	6.1	9.4	8.9	11.1
± SEM	0.6	0.8	0.7	0.7
Caries free %	7.3	2.6	5.6	2.0
Sugar intake g	123	76	153	116
± SEM	±11.1	6.6	9.7	12.9

There was no significant difference between the sugar intake of the female and male pupils, in both the rural Negroes and the urban Negroes, respectively (Table 8); the intake in the rural Negroes was 79 g for males, 75 g for females, and in the urban Negroes 105 g and 99 grams. The caries incidence of both sexes in each group was of the same order, 1.2 and 1.2 in the rural Negroes and 2.6 and 2.1 in the urban Negroes.

TABLE 8

	Rural Negroes		Urban Negroes	
	Males	Females	Males	Females
Number	64	87	67	62
DMFT	1.2	1.2	2.6	2.1
± SEM	0.3	0.2	0.3	0.3
Caries free %	56.3	64.4	28.8	29.0
Sugar intake g	79	75	105	99
± SEM	3.4	3.6	4.8	4.9

There was a significant increase in the sugar consumption of the urban Negroes, which resulted in a modest increase in the caries experience. We were surprised that the caries position of urban Negro high school pupils remained excellent despite a large measure of westernization of diet, including a relatively high total sugar intake.

It has been reported previously that with westernization of diet, dental caries prevalence increased, sometimes rapidly. This has been noticed in diverse regions, for example in the United States among groups of Eskimos[5] in India[6], Nigeria[7] and Ghana[8].

We offer an explanation for this unexpected finding.

In a previous study[9] we determined the effect of water fluoride concentration caries incidence, enamel fluoride concentration and degree of fluorosis. Mabieskrall High School, which is the same school selected to represent the rural Negro population group in the sugar consumption study, was chosen because it is situated in a low fluoride area. The water supply here is subterranean in origin, with a low fluoride content of 0.1 ppm.

Saulspoort High School is situated in a village approximately 20 miles from Mabieskraal. The pupils in both groups are from Tswana ethnic origin with similar socioeconomic backgrounds.

The water supply is also from subterranean origin and the fluoride content of the water sources in this area ranged from 1.0 to 6.0 ppm, with an average of 3 ppm F.

The living conditions of the rural Negroes in both areas of the sparsely populated region are less privileged than in the urban areas such as Soweto.

In Saulspoort, the high fluoride area, the fluoride concentration of the enamel corrected to a depth of 10 μm was three times higher than that of the pupils in Mabieskraal (Table 9). The percentage of pupils with fluorosis in Saulspoort was significantly higher than in Mabieskraal, yet the caries incidence was only marginally reduced.

TABLE 9. Rural Negroes

	Mabieskraal	Saulspoort
Water F (ppm)	0.1	±3.0
Number	79	88
Enamel F PPM		
(10μm)	476 ± 37	1486 ± 143
Fluorosis %	11.4	88
Caries free %	50.6	59.0
DMFT	1.4	1.0
± SEM	0.2	0.2

The daily sugar intake of the pupils in Mabieskraal was found to be approximately 80 g. The total number of pupils examined was 151 and their mean caries score was 1.2 ± 0.2. The mean caries index of 1.4 ± 0.2 found in the same school two years previously indicates that our caries assessment was reproducible. There is no reason to believe that the sugar intake in Saulspoort, although never determined, differs significantly from the sugar consumption in Mabieskraal. The pupils were from the same Tswana ethnic group, of similar socioeconomic status and resided in immediately adjacent, similar geographic areas.

It would appear that the fluoride content of the drinking water has little influence on the caries experience of the pupils from Mabieskraal and Saulspoort and that other influences, such as genetic factors, precluded the

Mabieskraal pupils from the high caries incidence encountered in other population groups. The same influences may be responsible for the moderate increase in caries experience encountered in other population groups and may be responsible for the moderate increase in caries experience in the urban Negro with significantly higher sugar consumption than that of their rural collegues.

CONCLUSIONS

1. There was a trend for the increased sugar consumption from rural Negro, to urban Negro, Coloured, Indian to White pupils to be associated with increased caries experience.

2. The sugar consumption of the lower-third of the pupils in each population group was approximately one-third of that of the upper-third of the pupils in the same population group, yet there was no significant difference in caries experience within each population group.

3. The significantly reduced sugar intake of female pupils, when compared to the male pupils in the Indian and White population groups, had no significant effect on caries incidence.

4. Increased sugar consumption by urban than by rural Negroes resulted in a modest incease in caries experience in the former.

Westernization of the dietary pattern of this population group did not produce the marked increase in caries incidence expected and reported by other investigators in other parts of the world.

5. We were not able to demonstrate a definite relationship between sugar intake and caries experience. We do not wish to imply that the level of intake of sugar and sugar-containing foods is unimportant, but it is apparent that in the various contexts considered in this study, the intake of these products was not the critical influencing factor. Other important factors such as frequency of consumption and the nature of the carbohydrate foods consumed were not evaluated in the study. Additional information about the frequency and manner of application or oral hygiene procedures is required.

I wish to acknowledge the invaluable assistance of my colleagues, Dr. P.E. Cleaton-Jones and Dr. A.R.P. Walker, who were associated with me in this investigation. My sincere thanks are due to the principals, staff and pupils of the schools concerned, whose willing support made this study possible. The investigation was supported by the South African Medical Research Council and the University of the Witwatersrand.

REFERENCE

[1]Bett, Morland, and Yudkin. Brit. Med. J. 3:153, 1957.

Other references available from author on request.

DISCUSSION

Dr. Schiff: Is there a possibility of the influence of different dental habits, such as the use of chew stick, in rural and urban areas?

Dr. Retief: The chewing habit definitely does exist in South Africa, more so in Rhodesia where there is a particular plant that they use to chew and, at the same time, to brush their teeth. But to the best of my knowledge, these sticks are not in the areas that we studied.

Dr. Schiff: I have seen beautiful comparisons in the U.S. Navy studies at Great Lakes of different influences on non-decay populations. However, I didn't see any comparison of their background of dental experiences, number or frequency of visits to their dentists, use of fluoride or non-fluoride toothpaste, or the use or non-use of dental floss. I think these factors are important, and I would like Dr. Shklair to elaborate on these variables.

Dr. Shklair: We have data about the number of times these people went to the dentist, or how many times they brushed their teeth, I don't have it at my fingertips. In general, there did not seem to be much of a difference in dental visits between the caries-free and the caries-rampant or the controls, or in the amount of time that they brushed their teeth.

Dr. Hoerman: One of the most significant things that has appeared today is the fact that the incidence of the caries-free individual, at least in the sample that is being taken among 16- to 19 year-olds at Great Lakes, has gone up to 10 per 1,000 from 2 per 1,000. It is just hard to believe that fluoride alone could account for that. Certainly, if it is true throughout the population, that has shifted the distribution curve of DMF teeth to the left, and that means that we are having less incidence and prevalence of dental caries in the population. Perhaps Dr. Newbrun, I wonder if we could shift that curve further to the left with, say, a drop pf 20% of the sucrose intake in the population in this country.

Dr. Newbrun: I would hesitate to put a value on how much it would shift by reducing sucrose a certain amount. You are aware of the nutritional goals which have recommended a 40% reduction in sucrose ingestion. I would hesitate to put a DMF value on what the effects of that would be, because, as you know, it would depend on how that 40% reduction would occur. If it is only occurring at mealtime, it won't really show up very much. If it is in the between-meal items, it will have a very profound effect on caries increments. So it depends what food and how the sugar is reduced.

Dr. Ross Dr. Shklair, on your questionnaire you did a differentiation of, first, whether they believed they took in none, little, average, or large amounts of the particular food groups, and then later you had a question about how much they actually consumed per day. Was there a difference between the caries-free and the caries-rampant individuals in how they interpreted what an average intake or what a large amount was?

Dr. Shklair: There did not seem to be any differences. There were extremes. Some considered five pieces of candy as a large amount, and others considered that as average. There was nothing overwhelming — the caries-free did not indicate a large amount of candy or a little candy, in contrast to the caries-active. There were some differences, but not large ones.

Dr. Bahn: Dr. Shklair, you indicated that the caries-free group had better nutritional habits in the use of milk, meat, vegetables and other foods, and had a lesser intake of the snacks and sugary foods. Was any study or inquiry made about their motivation? Were those in the caries-free group more tooth-conscious and thus motivated to maintain a proper dietary regimen? If that were true, following through with Dr. Schiff's question, they would maintain different oral habits than would the caries-rampant groups.

Dr. Shklair: We did not do any sociological studies as such to determine if they were motivated more or less. But there was a difference—a tremendous difference in the protein intake between these two groups. The caries-free group really ate much more protein than did the caries-active group. Why? I can't tell you.

Dr. Hoerman: Dr. Retief you showed a difference of 0.4 in the DMFT between the Saulspoort and Mabieskraal data and apparently you had no statistically significant differences. There might be a biological significance. Did you do any sampling of plaque in the two locations? Was there a difference in the distribution of carious lesions by surface?

Dr. Retief: We didn't do either. We did not do any bacteriology in this study. We noted each tooth and particularly where the lesion was situated, but I do not have that information available now. My records are not available.

Dr. Ciancio: Do you have any data on the groups with high caries incidence, with respect to low fluoride areas and high fluoride areas?

Dr. Retief: We published one report and I have just completed another in a high fluoride area which involved the Coloured population. This is an area containing 3.2 ppm. This whole community lived in that part, and the interesting thing is that in this particular group we found that the caries incidence increases with the enamel fluoride concentration, the degree of fluorosis becoming so severe that there is breakdown of the enamel and secondary caries develops as a result.

There is also a White community living in a high fluoride area where the caries incidence was reduced approximately 4 times from that reported here, but I didn't want to discuss too much about fluoride because it didn't enter as part of the discussion of this group. We have that information available.

Mr. Cornell: Dr. Newbrun, you discussed a report by Dr. Retief, and you showed a particular sequence. My interpretation of his report indicates that it was not as drastic or as simplistic as your particular sequence — I would like to get some sort of agreement as to what the situation is.

Dr. Newbrun: Well, I showed you the data on the males, and I think there was no doubt in the male population, 16 to 17 years of age, that there was a clearcut trend. If you saw the standard error of the means in the DMFT scores, there was a direct relationship between DMFT scores and sucrose intake. It is not linear, but it was a direct relationship. As one increased, the other did. Conversely, in the percentage of caries-free students, there was an inverse relationship. There was a group of Indian females that wasn't directly in the line.

One must take data in the whole sense, and in experimental research, very often you get a point that doesn't fit where you would like it to fit on the line.

That doesn't mean you reject the data or you reject the whole interpretation. As Dr. Retief pointed out, where you get smaller numbers, the accuracy of one point is not very great. I think I could elaborate on Dr. Retief's study, too. He pointed out that he had certain limitations. He was not able to use radiographs, he didn't have compressed air, he didn't have artificial lighting. All of these are the sorts of things that are considered by many investigators as necessary for doing survey work.

The questionnaire itself leaves something to be desired, because it was designed in England for the typical English diet, and it may be applicable to the white population in South Africa, and it may not be as valid in estimating the total sugar intake for the Indian population, for example; because, as Dr. Retief told you, their diets are not the same. One of the questions is "How much marmalade do you have?" That may not be the best way of estimating sugar intake in that Indian population. There may be lots of explanations, and I don't want to appear critical of that study, because I know the difficulties of doing field studies on various diverse populations. But I don't look at the Retief study as *the* study. I look at it as part of the whole picture. I showed you the data from 19 countries. I showed you the epidemiological data from the wartime studies. There is abundant epidemiological data as well as that representing controlled institutional groups. Perhaps the interpretation of the data is clouded by what one's viewpoint is, and that, of course, is why we are here together. Perhaps we can persuade you to interpret the data to our way of thinking.

Dr. Retief: I agree with Dr. Newbrun; I don't think we differ. There was a trend for the increased sugar consumption from rural Negro to urban Negro, Coloured, Indian and to White peoples to be associated with the increased caries experience.

We did not pay too much attention to the percentage of caries-free. I mentioned the inadequacies in our study, for example, a lack of sophisticated equipment in some areas. I would like to call it "a study" and not "the study."

Dr. Newbrun: Am I right that the rural children were at a boarding school, and in fact could you comment on all the children in this study — were they at a boarding school, or were the White children living at home and the others in boarding school?

Dr. Retief: It was only in two rural areas that we did have some children in boarding schools because of the distance involved. In all the other schools, the children were not in boarding school.

Dr. Newbrun: Not only in South Africa, but almost in any country where children are at boarding school there has been a trend for lower caries because in boarding schools the availability of food is somewhat restricted compared to children living at home.

Dr. Moss: Dr. Newbrun, if industry were to go through the problems associated with developing a non-carciogenic food, and then they proved its safety, and they did the efficacy study, and then figured out a way of packaging it, how well do you think it would sell?

I ask because of the talk of compliance and the problems we have with fluorides.

Dr. Newbrun: Unfortunately the junk, or the snack foods are readily available to kids when they come home from school. Everybody, even dental students, eats the readily available packaged foods. The problem has been that the sort of things we know are relatively non-carciogenic or have low cariogenic potential, to use Dr. Bowen's terminology — those things that you eat at a cocktail party, like carrot sticks and celery sticks and cheese — are not the things that are marketed and that have a reasonable shelf life. Clearly these items are attractive and people eat them and enjoy eating them; it is a question of availability.

I believe that one can make sweet-tasting snack items without sugar. I know the problems of bulking, etc., but I don't think the problem is one of sweetening agents. One can make food items that consumers will buy and will eat. There are real problems in terms of shelf life, etc., but the food industry has the ingenuity. It is a question of motivation and incentive.

Dr. Zoumas: To my knowledge, Hershey is not producing a colored synthetic chocolate bar that is non-carciogenic. We are looking at some non-chocolate products, but that is a reflection more of the price of cocoa beans than anything else.

Dr. Moss: I think Dr. Newbrun well described the frustration that the dentist, and certainly the pedodontist, feels in his office, in talking about dietary things to parents, and how he feels it is going to be quite hopeless. You mentioned that there was no controversy anymore. I don't think there is much controversy, but maybe there is a lot of confusion. I know that the graduate students in dental school today are very concerned about the relative cariogenicity of food, and they wonder when they see an ADA bulletin suggesting an apple, whether 16% sucrose is indeed potentially cariogenic in comparison with something that has 24%.

Dr. Mackay: I might note that that cream substitute that Dr. Newbrun got on the plane, I think, was cited by Consumers Union as having perhaps one of the highest contents of sugar, around 50 or 60 percent sugar. So it may not have any cream in it, but it has certainly got plenty of sugar — carbohydrates I should say.

Dr. Anderson: You said, Dr. Newbrun, that Dr. Scheinin had reinterpreted the score from the Turku studies and somewhat changed the relationship of xylitol and sucrose. Did he reinterpret the fructose scores too?

Dr. Newbrun: I don't believe so. As you remember, in the Turku studies they used a method of scoring caries which is not the usual method used in this country or elsewhere, where we rely on an actual cavity or a catch by an explorer. They used a dissecting microscope with a strong light source so they detected visual changes in mineralization of the tooth surface. It is difficult to relate these changes to the more commonly used criteria. Because of this, and because of the comments that arose, Dr. Scheinin went back to his data and calculated caries scored in terms of actual cavities or radiographic demineralizations. This has been published (Newbrun ref. 52).

Dr. Clydesdale: I don't think there is any disagreement that certainly sucrose is involved in dental caries, and we see people eating sucrose. I wonder, however, about the concept. Does Dr. Newbrun think it is possible to educate people, to have them stop their consumption of sucrose completely? I believe that this denies some of the reasons why people eat. I don't think that is a possibilty and I wonder whether the question is not an agreement or disagreement about the data. I wonder whether we can stop people from eating sucrose-containing foods, and if we can't, if we continue to propose that, it will only cause confusion. Should we keep on saying, "Don't eat, don't eat, don't eat," or should we be looking for ways to cut down the cariogenicity of foods and perhaps add other agents? Should we be trying to create something that people can eat, or should we continue to confuse them by telling them they shouldn't do something they really want to do?

Dr. Newbrun: I certainly have never said that one should tell people to stop eating between meals. In fact, in growing children that would be foolish. What I am saying, and what I did say, is that one could try to redirect what is eaten between meals.

The question is: can you have a sucrose-free diet? That depends on how strictly sucrose-free you want to be. It is almost like getting a fluoride-free diet. It is almost impossible. You can get a low fluoride diet and you can get a low sucrose diet. We have been doing a study under contract with the National Institute of Dental Research on hereditarily fructose intolerant individuals, their diet, the plaque microflora, and their caries prevalence and plaque scores and oral debris scores. The diets of the hereditary fructose intolerant patients are not strictly sucrose-free. They eat certain vegetables which have very low amounts of sucrose; for example carrots, onions and puffed wheat (as a cereal) have very, very low amounts of sucrose. They do not absolutely lack fructose-1-phosphate aldolase; they have very low levels of the enzyme, and they have practically no caries.

Physiologically, one can certainly manage on a diet free of sucrose or with very low levels. In practice, these patients are very selective about what they eat, because every time they eat something that has fructose, they begin vomiting, they get nausea, and they want to avoid that. Yes, one can do very well on diets low or almost free of sucrose. That time that Isaiah describes will come about only when people in the food industry provide those sorts of alternatives. I think it is foolish in the dental office to advise children, or adults for that matter, to assume diet habits of avoiding pastries and candies and snacks, when there are the social pressures of Halloween and birthday parties, etc.

It is up to the food industry to provide foods with low cariogenic potential. Without that, I don't think we will see a significant change in dietary habits.

Dr. Kabara: Dr. Newbrun, you suggested a direct correlation between the amount of sucrose and dental caries, and then suggested that this curve was not only linear, but was probably convex in shape. Do you think that curve would be the same if you changed the amount and quality of the protein in the diet, the amount and quality of the fat in the diet, the amount and quality of the mineral in the diet?

Dr. Newbrun: I showed two lines. I showed the linear one, which I thought was probably not the straight linear relationship, but that it would be sort of a logarithmic curve, and I did not put any values on it. I think many people in this audience, and Kenneth Madsen in particular, have made the point that frequency is a factor which one has to interpolate into this curve. Any plotting of caries relationship food score requires a frequency factor. I do think that in normal populations, not institutional populations, total sucrose consumption does reflect frequency to a certain extent.

I don't think any hard data answers the question whether proteins and other food components, minerals, influence the cariogenicity of sugar-containing foods. I know there are some studies that show fat may influence cariogenicity, But I know of no protein studies.

Dr. Kabara: Our own studies show that with the same level of sucrose, by simply changing the quality of the protein, one can severely reduce the effects of the high sucrose.

Dr. Newbrun: This is an animal study?

Dr. Kabara: This is in animals. But the literature is resplendent with such examples.

Dr. Newbrun: That is very interesting.

Mr. Jorgenson: Does Dr. Newbrun know of any studies that have ever been made of the dental health of diabetics on low sucrose diets.

Dr. Newbrun: I am sure there have been some studies, but I am not familiar with any significant differences in diabetics. It would depend, of course, whether it is juvenile diabetes or old age onset diabetes. If it is juvenile diabetes, one might anticipate an effect. If it is old age onset, I wouldn't expect much difference.

Dr. Glass: I think Professor Newbrun has noted that once a position is decided, all experience is selectively interpreted to support it. Now, that works both ways, or in many different ways. "In my Father's house there are many mansions."

The Vipeholm dental study, despite its flaws, established that between-meal eating of certain highly refined starches and sugars produced tremendous increases in caries incidence. Meal-time eating of sugars was not a problem. Therefore, we should concentrate our efforts in the field of between-meal snacks. I won't take time to respond to Dr. Newbrun's comments on the noise (uncontrolled variance) in clinical trials caused by individual dietary differences across study groups, because it would take too long, but I don't agree with him.

If cariogenic potential, as Dr. Bowen calls it, of foods is to be equated only against the sugar content of foods, there is no need for the cariogenicity testing program proposed by the Association. I think that Dr. Shklair summed it up very nicely when he said that sugars are a problem in dental caries, but there are multitudes of other factors to be considered.

FOODS AND DENTAL CARIES

Basil G. Bibby, D.M.D., Ph.D.

It is logical to begin any discussion of the role of foods in dental caries with a statement of prevailing beliefs. Informed opinion holds that tooth decay is caused by food undergoing fermentation on the surfaces of the teeth. It accepts the possibility that systemic or nutritional factors can provide some protection for the teeth, but believes that the potential strength of the caries attack that could develop on the tooth surface is so great that it can, and generally does, over-ride any such protective influences. Thus, at a practical level, and for this consideration of dental caries, the important aspect of foods is not whether they have nutritional value, but what they add to, or detract from the strength of the caries attack at the tooth surface. However, before considering that subject, it will be instructive to restate the reasons why there is such general agreement among dental investigators regarding the caries-activating role of carbohydrate foods. Thereafter, consideration will be given to what we know about caries-relevant differences between foodstuffs.

Local Causation

The orgin of the belief that dental decay is related to food deposits on the teeth surfaces cannot be traced. It seems to have sprung up independently among primitive people in several parts of the world, presumably as a result of noticing that the sites on the teeth where caries started were the same as those on which food debris was retained. The claim that sweet foods were particularly blame-worthy can be attributed to the ancient Greeks and Arabians. Aristotle[1] states that the sticking of sweet figs to the teeth causes them to rot. The Arabian Mesu went a stage farther, in the 12th century, writing that dates and "clinging particles of food decompose producing acid moisture that eats (the teeth) away and destroys them."[2]

About the sixteenth century, as increasing supplies of sugar became available in Western Europe, dental decay became more common among the wealthy, who alone could afford to purchase it. Pierre Fauchard[3], who is regarded as the Father of Modern Dentistry, wrote that "all sugary foods contribute not a little to the destruction of the teeth — because there is in sugar a penetrating corrosive acid." A little later, Thomas Berdmore[4] who was dentist to George III, the King who had all the trouble with the American States, reported that in Holland where "sweetmeats are used in excess, the people even at an early age, are remarkable for the badness of their teeth." Anthropological studies offer additional evidence that caries increased several-fold in England, France and Germany as the sugar trade expanded.[5] Unfortunately we have no information about whether like parallels existed between caries activity and the other changes that occurred in diets over the same period.

With the growth of experimental science, information emerged to explain how foods reacted to produce caries. Magitot[6] in France, and Robertson[7] in England, made experiments that demonstrated that carbohydrates, bacteria and acids were involved, but it was left to Miller,[8] an American dentist working in Berlin, to bring the various pieces of information together as a scientifically acceptable explanation of tooth decay. At the end of the last century, he used new chemical and bacteriological methods to demonstrate beyond question that acids produced from carbohydrates by mouth bacteria could destroy tooth enamel. Miller's work has stood the test of time, but one of his conclusions — that flour was the main cause of caries — has been overlooked by those who believe that only sugar is involved. He based this conclusion on his findings that flour produced more acid on fermentation in saliva, that is adhered to the teeth, and that it produced "caries" on one of his own teeth when held on it in an appliance that he wore in his mouth for 10 days.

Recent work supports the chemico-parasitic findings on the nature of the caries attack, and has gone a long way toward excluding alternative possibilities. For instance, it has been demonstrated in animals that the interaction of both bacteria and food on the tooth surface is necessary to produce caries. Experiments that exclude the bacterial component by use of antibiotics[9] (Table 1) or bacteria-free animals [10] show that no caries develops on a diet that produces caries in control animals. That food contact with the teeth is necessary is apparent from experiments[11] in which a cariogenic diet was fed to rats by stomach tube so that it had no contact with the teeth (Table 2). No caries resulted. Also, "Siamese twin"[12] animals got caries only in the twin receiving the caries diet, indicating that blood supply had no effect on tooth resistance or the composition of the saliva that could have modified the caries attack. That bacterial acids formed by fermentation of carbohydrates are part of the carious process is indicated by the caries prevention given in animals, [13] and in some tests in man, [14] by the use of agents that inhibit the acid producing enzymes of bacteria. In addition, the fact that fluorine, which increases tooth resistance to acid, prevents caries may be taken as further evidence that bacterial acids activate tooth destruction.

TABLE 1. Effect of antibiotics on caries in rodents

Animal Study with Penicillin and Tyrothricin				
Level of agent	Source	Duration (day)	Reduction	Worker
75 U/g P	W + D	118	+	McClure & Hewitt ('46)
2-5 U/cc P	W	110	+	Webman et al ('49)
500 U/g P	D	122	+	Stephan et al ('52)
0.05% P	D	100	+	Shaw & Sweeney ('57)
1000 U/g P	Brushing	35	+	Zander & Bibby ('47)
500 U/g P	Brushing	90	+	Zander et al ('51)
0.05% tyrothricin	Brushing	90	+	Shiere ('57)

TABLE 2. Effect of gastric intubation on caries in rats

	Effect of Stomach Tube Feeding*			
	No. of animals	Av. carious molars	Av. no. lesions	Av. extent
Tube-Fed	13	0	0	0
Control	13	5.0	6.7	10.6

*Adapted from Kite *et al.*[11]

Observations in man support the conclusions of these experiments. It has been found that patients who have to be tube fed have low caries and form little acid in their dental plaques.[15] The conclusion that the retention of food on the teeth is an essential part of caries causation can be drawn from the results of a study made in Rochester[16] which can also be interpreted as indicating that nutritional and systemic factors have no observable effects on caries. Table 3 gives figures obtained from examination of over 400 13-year-old boys. The data records the incidence of caries in selected pairs of teeth that developed and erupted at the same time, and thus were subject to the same genetic, systemic, nutritional and salivary influences, both before and after they erupted into the mouth. The caries experience of the these pairs of teeth is vastly different. There is more than 10 times as much caries in the mandibular molars as in the mandibular incisors, and 20 times more in the premolar than the canine. The only explanation for these differences seems to be that it is the teeth with shapes that favor retention of food and bacteria which have high caries. An even more definite relationship between the retention factor and caries location can be found in a comparison of caries in the maxillary and mandibular molars. The maxillary molars that have an extra retention area on their lingual (tongue) surface have almost 20 times more caries in that site than on the lingual of the mandibular molar where there is a smooth, non-retentive surface. The situation is reversed for the buccal (cheek) side, where the lower molars that have the additional retention site have many times more caries than the buccal of upper molars which are non-retentive.

TABLE 3. Caries incidence in relation to times of tooth formation and tooth anatomy—433 Rochester children aged 13 years*

Surfaces	6 ∣ 6	1 ∣ 1	2 ∣ 2	5 ∣ 5	3 ∣ 3	6 ∣ 6
All	1220	123	89	633	33	1448
Buccal	356	---	--	9	--	59
Lingual	24	---	2	---	--	400

*Adapted from Day and Sedwick[16].

The fact that reactions between food and the surfaces of teeth are the dominating factors in caries causation means that the answer to the question of which foods are more or less destructive to the teeth must be sought in an examination of what happens to foods when they are in the mouth.

Carbohydrates and Caries

On the basis of what has already been said, it seems that in looking for differences in the cariogenicity of foods we have to be concerned only with those containing sugar or other carbohydrates. Reasons to doubt this conclusion have not been found, either in observations in man or in laboratory and animal experience. Neither are theories that caries can result from chelation or from acids from non-carbohydrate sources convincing. It is important to mention that enamel decalcification can be caused by the acids that are present in fruits, in acid beverages, and some foods and confections. These produce erosive destruction of exposed non-retentive tooth areas which, although inadequately investigated, is distinct from caries.

The dental literature offers very little guidance in respect to which carbohydrate foods are more or less destructive to the teeth. All but a few of those who have had anything to say on the subject go no farther than distinguishing between sugars and other pure carbohydrates. Even fewer have concerned themselves with the differences between whole foods of the sort that make up the human diet.

Animal experiments have shown that sugars produce more caries than starches, and that sucrose and glucose are more cariogenic than lactose and maltose. While some investigators have found that highly refined flours are more destructive to rat's teeth than less refined meals, others have not obtained the same results.

Test tube fermentation experiments show that unrefined sugars[17] and cereals[18] destroy less enamel than do their refined counterparts (Table 4). They contain substances that offer some protection against demineralization. Actually quite wide differences in decalcifying ability exist between the same types of both refined and unrefined cereals from different geographic locations.

TABLE 4. Difference in enamel dissolution produced by whole and refined flours

Source	Whole flour	Refined flour
Iowa	0.46	0.70
Texas	0.51	2.32
Saskatchewan	0.39	2.51

(From Khanna and Bibby[18])

Studies of caries prevalence in man do not yield clear conclusions about the cariogenicity of individual foodstuffs because, in additon to the effects of the frequency of eating, there are so many variables in human dietary patterns. The marked reduction of caries that occurred in European countries during the two world wars,[19] when sucrose consumption was greatly redued, has been offered as proof that it is the controlling factor in caries. However this very suggestive assocation has probably been over-interpreted because factors such as the reduced frequency of eating and the absence of refined flours undoubtly enter the picture.

Observations on two human study groups have been used to buttress claims regarding the specificity of sucrose in caries causation. The best known is the Vipeholm Study[20] that showed that high sucrose consumption caused increased caries. However, it is seldom pointed out that the effect of sucrose was also raised by the addition of flour and reduced by addition of chocolate, or by dilution in liquid. In the other study, the Hopewood House Study,[21] virtually no caries was found in children on a sugar-free diet, but it is not known to what extent the findings were the result of the absence of sucrose, or that of all refined cereals, the use of a "nature type" of diet, or no between-meal eating.

Obviously there is much to be learned about what makes human diets, or individual foodstuffs, more or less destructive to the teeth. Some attempts to cast light on the problem have been made by studying what happens to pure sugars and starches in situations resembling those of the human mouth. The more logical approach, of finding out what happens in the mouth to complete foodstuffs of the sorts actually eaten by man, has seldom been followed. Our research group seems to have done as much in this area as anyone else. However, the amount of solid information produced is not impressive yet. One way to assemble pertinent information on this subject is to consider separately the characteristics of foods that have been claimed as important in caries causation, to find out whether methods used for studying them have produced information that can be equated with the cariogenicity of the tested foods.

Dental opinion is in almost complete agreement that among the characteristics of food that determine their importance in caries causation are:

a. the sugar or carbohydrates content,
b. the amount of acid they form on fermentation by mouth bacteria,
c. the resultant amounts of enamel dissolved,
d. the amount and duration of food retention on the tooth surfaces,
e. the extent to which they promote the formation of dental plaque,
f. the amount of acid formed in dental plaque by foodstuffs.

These will be discussed in the order given.

a. The sugar and carbohydrate content of foods It has been assumed tacitly both by practicing dentists and by too many dental investigators that the cariogenicity of individual foodstuffs is directly proportional to their content of sucrose or other fermentable carbohydrate. There is no quantitative data to support this belief.

Some findings in man, as in the Vipeholm Study,[20] give contrary indications when human foods are used (Fig. 1). Animal tests, and our *in vitro* work which will be mentioned later do likewise. Actually, the effects of high sucrose concentrations in increasing the rate of food clearance of some foods from the mouth (Table 5), and in inhibiting fermentation processes (Table 6), make it seem improbable that high sugar contents of themselves would be particularly damaging to the teeth. While we must accept the belief that sugar directly or indirectly is a major cause of caries, it has been a common mistake to oversimplify this relationship. It is probable that for different types of foods, there are critical sugar concentrations that are particularly destructive — or possibly safe. As yet, we have no guidance as to what these may be.

TABLE 5. Effect of sugar content of breakfast cereals to retention on mouth

Cereal	Soluble CHO%	Amount retained (mg) 5 min.	15 min.	30 min.	Acid
Corn Flakes	29.8	33.9	12.2	5.9	1.53
(SE)		(7.47)	(1.49)	(1.07)	
Frosted Flakes	60.1	23.0	10.2	5.3	1.31
(SE)		(3.19)	(1.39)	(0.73)	

TABLE 6. Relation of sucrose content of solutions and mixed food on acid production by oral bacteria

Substrate	Sucrose content	Final pH	Titrated acid (ml 0.5 M NaOH)
Lab Cake*	25%	4.75	2.04 ± 0.13
Sucrose Sol.	25%	5.31	0.58 ± 0.09
Sucrose Sol.	10%	4.97	0.85 ± 0.07
Sucrose Sol.	2%	4.95	0.91 ± 0.08

*Contains 40% wheat flour.

b. Acid formation from foods As mentioned earlier, measurements of acid production from foods fermented in saliva were used by Miller[8] in what seems to have been the first attempt to differentiate between the cariogenicity of human foods. A number of other investigators, including ourselves, have measured acid production from foods using a variety of techniques. Our work, which has been reported elsewhere,[22] demonstrated wide differences in acid production. Many food, such as legumes, formed much more acid than like quantities of sucrose or glucose over the 6 hour incubation period we used (Fig. 2). There are obviously many variables such as substrate concentrations,

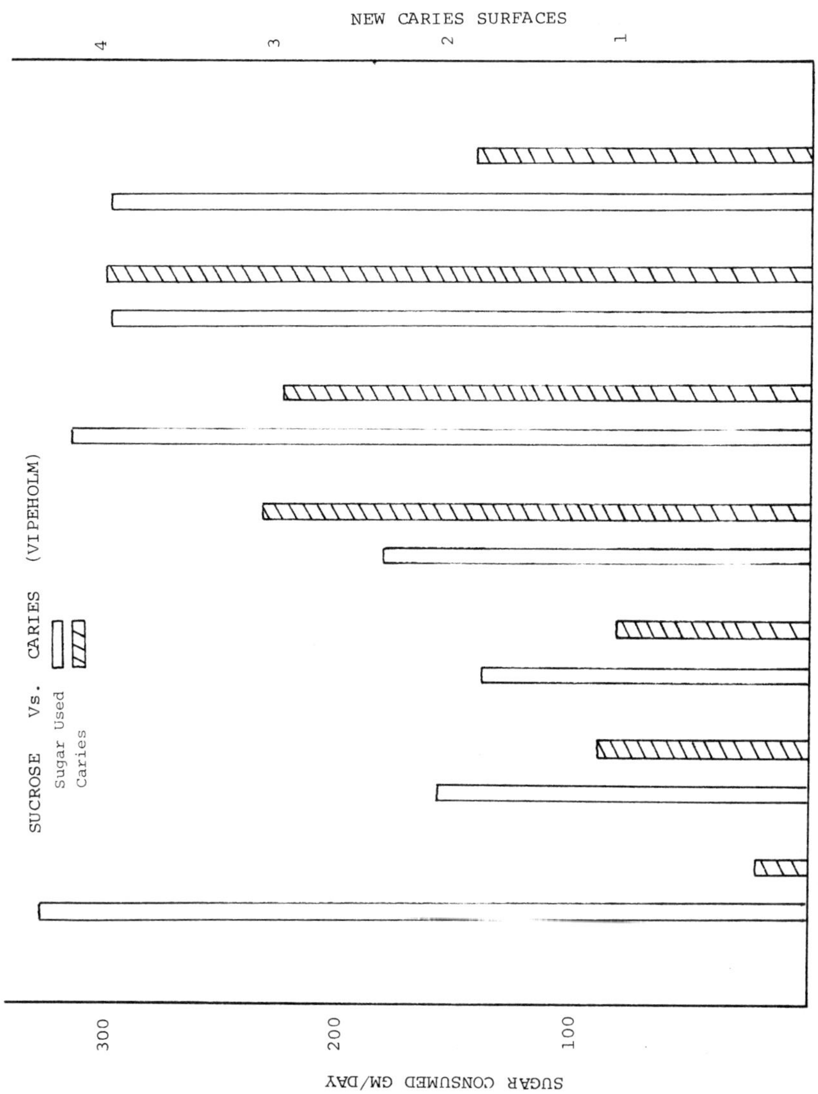

FIGURE 1. Amounts of sugar consumed per day and new caries surfaces per year in groups of patients in the Vipeholm Caries Study. (Gustafsson et al.[20])

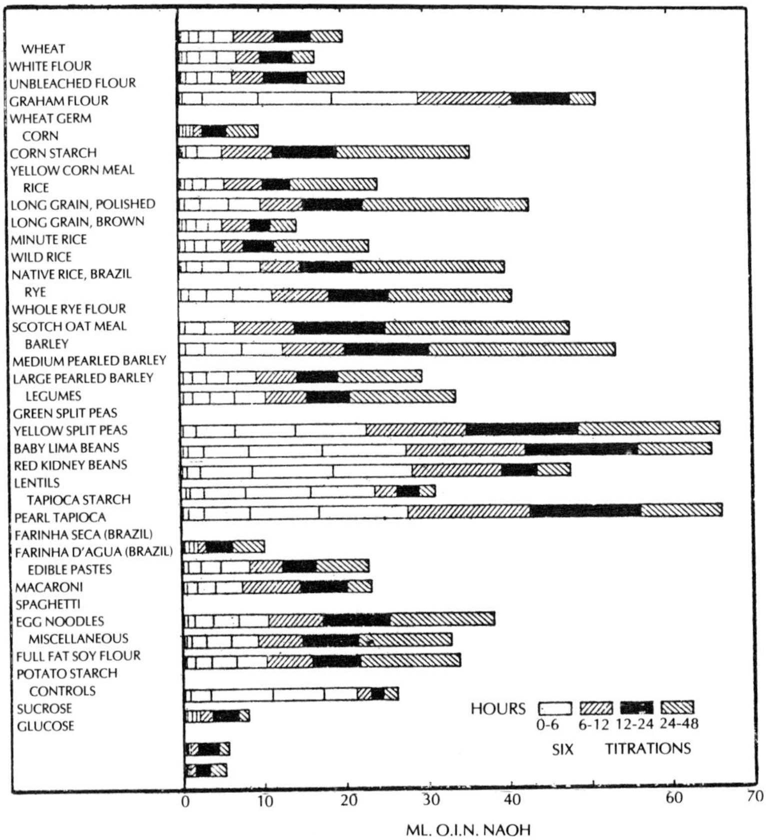

FIGURE 2. Amounts of acid formed during various time periods from various carbohydrate foods fermented in human saliva. (From Beck and Bibby[22])

bacterial density, and nutrients for bacterial growth that modify acid production from foods. The significance of acid production as an index of the cariogenicity of foods can be questioned because we [18,23,24] have shown, in several types of tests, that the total amount of acid (titratable acidity) produced by a food does not parallel the amount of enamel it will dissolve (Table 7).

c. Enamel dissolution by foods On testing the amount of enamel dissolved from teeth incubated in mixtures of food and saliva, or bacterial cultures, it was noted that the amounts of enamel dissolved did not parallel the amounts of acid formed in the fermentation mixtures. [18,23,24] As enamel dissoution is more closely allied to the process of caries than is the presence of acid, we decided that it was a more significant index of cariogenicity and have developed several different methods for measuring the amounts of enamel destroyed when it is exposed to foods that are undergoing fermentation by salivary bacteria.

TABLE 7. Acid formation and enamel demineralization inversely related in cereal products and candies

Food	Acid formed 0.05 *M* NaOH ml	Enamel dissolved mg
Whole Wheat bread	11.0	0.2
White Bread	8.4	0.4
Corn Flakes Cereal	4.3	0.5
All Bran Cereal	16.2	0.1
Chocolate Coconut Bar	11.1	1.1
Milk Chocolate	13.2	0.1
White Flour	4.9	1.0
Graham Flour	5.1	0.2

While a number of investigators have in one way or another indicated that fermenting carbohydrates, generally sucrose, will dissolve enamel, we alone seem to have measured the enamel dissolving potential of a range of foodstuffs.[24] The method we generally use for this purpose is to incubate, for 4 hours, a mixture of food and saliva into which granules of radioactive enamel have been added. A measurement of the radioactive phosphorus going into a solution is used to calculate the amount of enamel dissolved. We have tested several hundred foods. Some of the more interesting results are shown in Figs. 3 and 4.

d. Food retention in the mouth From earliest times it has been accepted that the retention of food on the teeth was a cause of caries. From that it has been assumed that foods that were retained in large amounts, or over long periods would be more destructive to the teeth than those that did not adhere to the teeth. Although few efforts have been made to assess food retention in the mouth, one project carried out in conjunction with the Vipeholm Study demonstrated a fair degree of parallelism between oral retention of the diets used and the resultant caries in the several study groups.[25] This, incidentally, is the only instance in which laboratory measurements of a food characteristic have been related to caries causation in man.

Shreds of supporting evidence of a relationship between food retention and caries causation can also be gleaned from animal experiments, such as those which showed that caries declined with progressive liquefaction of the cariogenic diet,[26] and that much more caries was caused by a dry sugar diet than when the sugar was in solution.

There is no agreed method for measuring food retention. Measurements can be made of the carbohydrate present in the saliva at various time intervals after eating a single test meal, or systems of tooth cleansing can be used and estimates made of the food recovered at times after a series of several meals. The latter is the method we have used. The variations in oral anatomy and physiology and in eating habits mean that it is very difficult to obtain satisfactorily reproducible results in such tests. We have been able to obtain somewhat

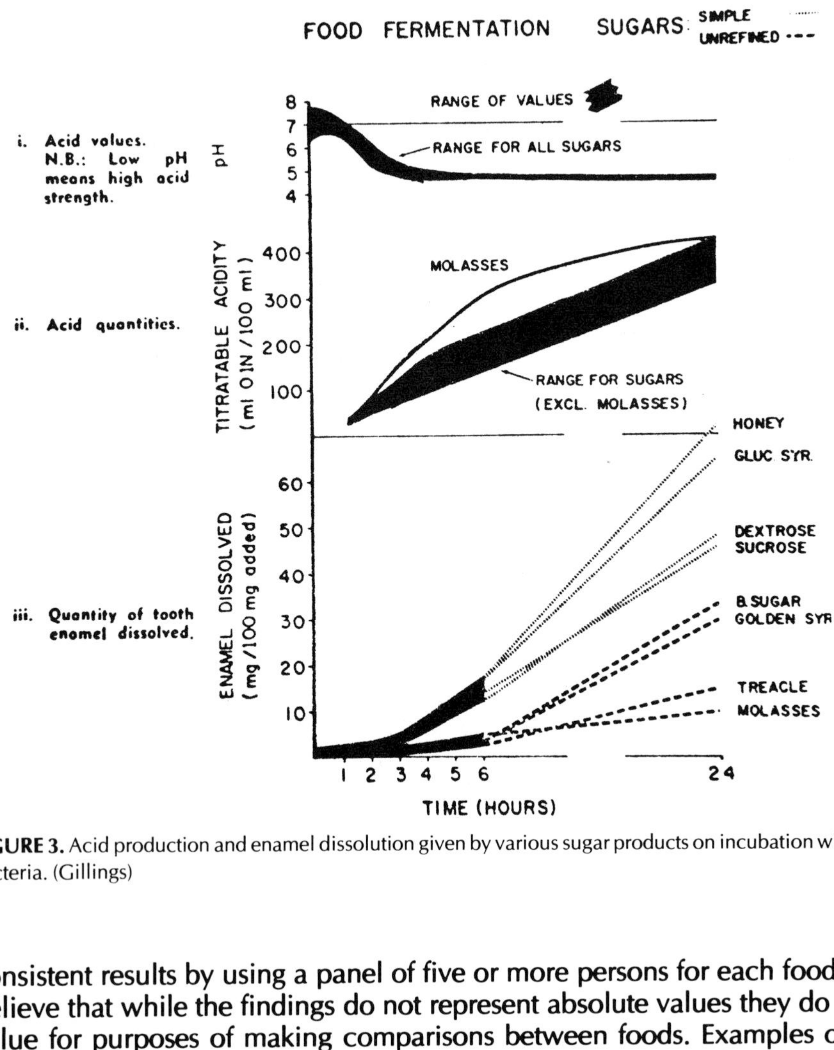

FIGURE 3. Acid production and enamel dissolution given by various sugar products on incubation with oral bacteria. (Gillings)

consistent results by using a panel of five or more persons for each food. We believe that while the findings do not represent absolute values they do have value for purposes of making comparisons between foods. Examples of the types of results we have obtained on the hundred or so foods we have tested are given in Table 8. An *in vitro* system we have developed gives somewhat similar results.

e. The promotion of dental plaque formation by foods Current dental belief, about which I have some reservations, is that dental decay does not occur until after a dental plaque has developed on the tooth enamel. This plaque can be defined as a gelatinous layer of bacteria and polysaccharides that is firmly enough attached to the tooth surface that it is not removed, either by the chewing of tough or detergent foods, or by rinsing with a stream of water.

Some experiments in man and animals show that growth of a certain type of plaque is stimulated by sucrose, but not other carbohydrates, and some evidence exists of inhibition by maltose. The effects of ordinary foodstuffs does not seem to have been studied. Nor has the possibility been investigated that food deposits on the teeth could produce enamel demineralization without the intermediary action of plaque. It is not known whether polysaccharides in food compete with those from bacteria and saliva for the place on the tooth surface, or whether sugar exerts a polymerizing effect on the salivary constituents. In short, our knowledge on the relationship between foodstuffs and plaques is so inadequate that it would be risky to draw conclusions.

Tests of effects of agents on plaque growth have been made in fluids inoculated with bacteria. In some such tests sucrose has been shown to be particularly conducive to the formation of gelatinous deposits on glass or metal rods. Plaque formation has occasionally been compared in animals on different diets, but no systematic study has been made. Tests[27] in man have shown that hourly use of tablets of sucrose or glucose over a period of a few days produces a heavier, more gelatinous plaque with sucrose than glucose. But whether these more gelatinous deposits are more conducive to caries is not known. Technical difficulties, particularly in relation to quantitation of observations reduce the value of plaque measurements as an index of the cariogenicity of foods.

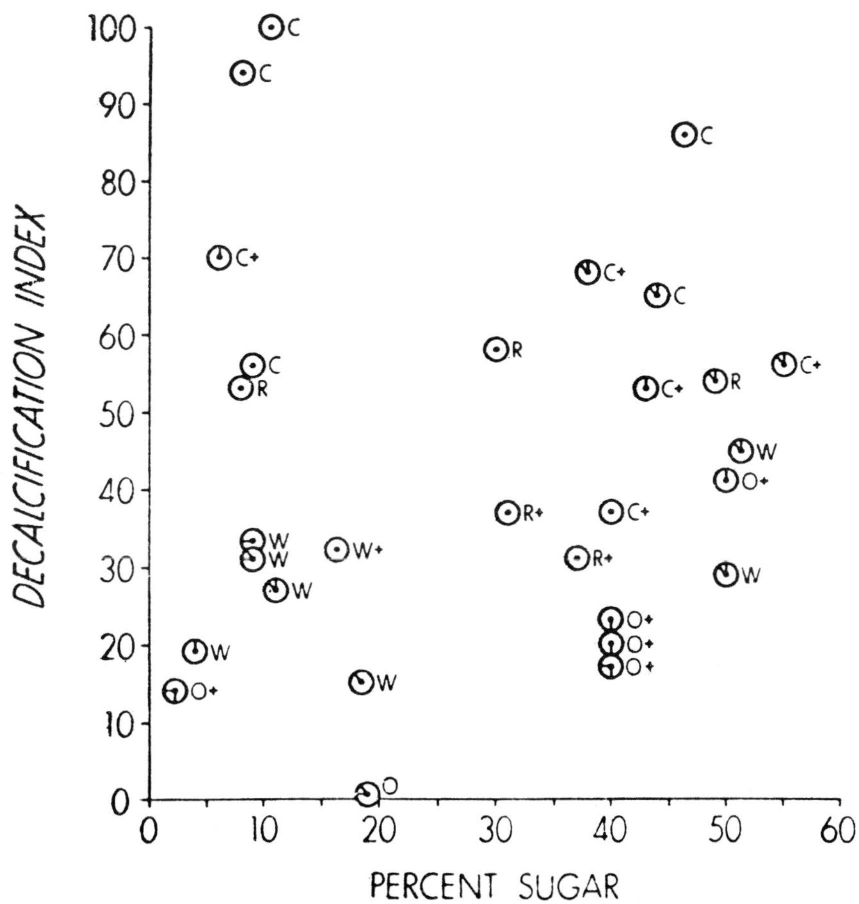

FIGURE 4. Relationship between sugar content of breakfast cereals and enamel dissolved on fermentation with oral bacteria. (Weiss and Bibby)

TABLE 8. Representative figures for food retention in mouth after eating

Food	CHO (glucose equivalents) Retained 5 min.	15 min.	30 min.
Peanuts	4.9mg	3.3 mg	2.6 mg
Dentyne Gum	5.0	3.9	3.1
7 UP	6.3	2.4	2.1
Chocolate Milk	7.4	3.8	1.9
Potato Chips	12.3	4.9	2.5
White Bread	16.1	10.0	3.6
Raisins	16.8	5.7	3.0
Sponge Cake	18.8	6.0	4.2
Caramel	19.0	4.2	2.5
Milk Chocolate	19.0	6.8	3.0
Cracker (Oil Sprayed)	23.8	8.5	3.7
Hard Mint	31.9	9.4	2.5
Cracker (Plain)	33.6	10.4	3.3
Sandwich Cookie	35.0	8.4	4.9

f. Measurements of pH of plaques Because acid formation on the tooth surfaces is the acknowledged cause of caries, it is logical to assume that comparisons of the amount of acid formed in the deposits or plaques on the teeth would be a good index of their cariogenicity. Thus, it happens that measurements of plaque acidity are highly favored as indicators of the strength of the caries attack produced by foods. However, as with the other measurements we have considered, plaque pH cannot be accepted as a reliable measurement of cariogenicity until it has been demonstrated that they do, in fact, give results that parallel caries production in man. To date this has not been done.

There are other reasons why it is premature to attach too much weight to plaque pH. One that we have already discussed is that acid production by oral bacteria does not parallel the amount of enamel destroyed. Therefore there are theoretical grounds for questioning the significance of plaque pH measurements as indicators of caries activity. The other, more practical one, is that there are questions relating to the methodologies of measuring plaque pH. The most favored methods do not give the same results.

The method developed in Zurich[28] for measuring plaque pH fits an electrode between the teeth in a dental prosthetic device. This has some theoretical advantages over other methods, but its technical difficulties and special requirement for adult test patients reduce its practical value. So far, investigators outside Zurich have had limited success with it.

The most used pH testing method collects samples of plaque from the tooth surfaces after eating and measures the pH on the laboratory bench. Several investigators,[29–31] including ourselves have measured the plaque pH produced by a number of foods. The depressions of pH were smaller than those given by the Zurich method but placed foods in the same positions relative to one another.

Both pH methods showed quite wide pH differences between foods, but it must be emphasized that the pH figures obtained by both are relative rather than absolute values. Figures 5 and 6 show examples of the types of results given by the two types of tests.

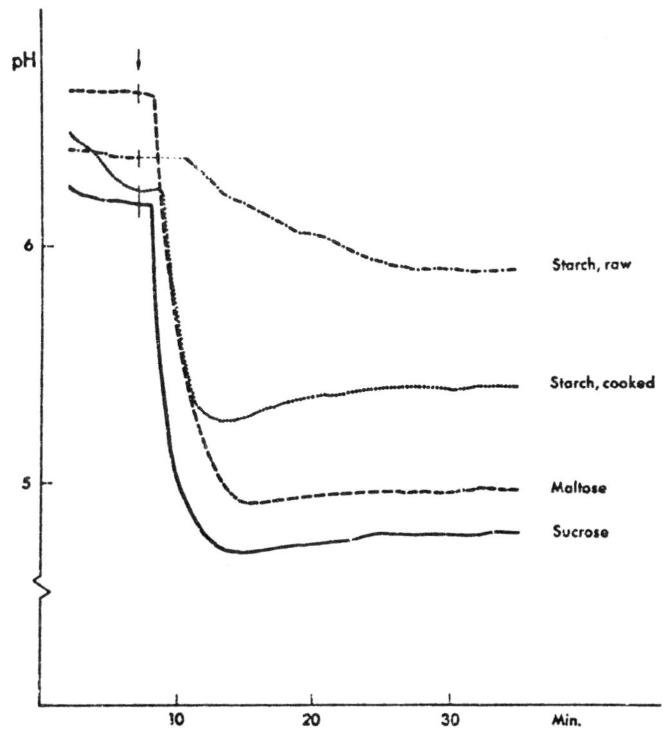

FIGURE 5. pH of dental plaque after exposure to sugars and starches measured by *in situ* electrode. (From Neff[31])

Evaluation of Tests on Characteristics of Foods

Having reviewed measurements that can be made of the characteristics of foods which are believed to determine their cariogenicity, and shown that each type of measurement varies widely among different foods, it is time to ask how such findings can be put to practical use. The answer is that if one or more of these characteristics can be proven to give a reliable index of the cariogenicity of foods it will offer a tool that could become important in caries prevention. It could be used by the dental profession to distinguish between caries-dangerous and safer foods, or by manufacturers to help them develop foods of lowered cariogenicity. Unfortunately, we are not at that stage yet.

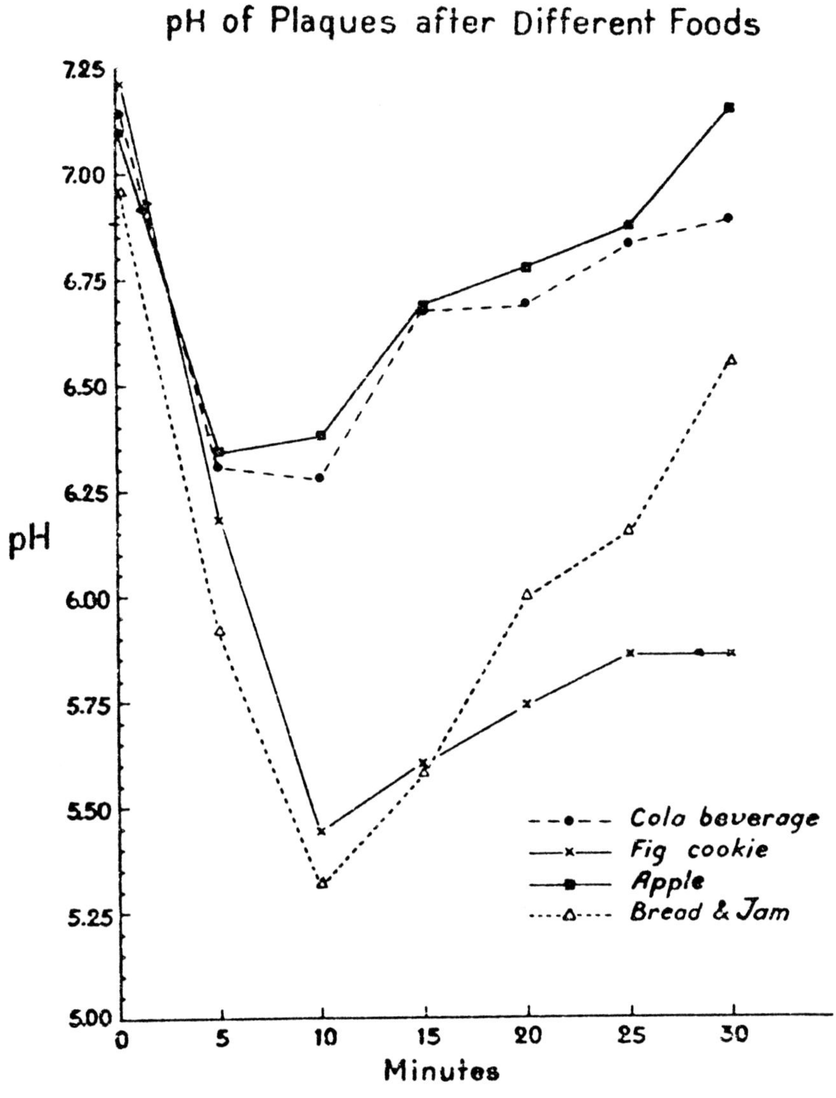

FIGURE 6. pH of dental plaque after exposure to foods—measured extraorally on removed plaque sample. (Ludwig and Bibby) •All Figures Mean of 5 Subjects.

It still has to be shown that the types of measurements we can make on foods are true indications of caries causation in man. Stated differently, it means that in order to have a laboratory measurement of a food characteristic accepted as a reliable index of cariogenicity, the indications it gives must be confirmed by tests on caries development in the human mouth. Ethics and regulations dealing with experimentation on human subjects make this almost impossible. Therefore, another way of correlating laboratory tests on foods with the caries they cause in human teeth has to be found. It is our opinion that a practical approach would be to subject a number of foods to all available types of laboratory animal and "semi-clinical" tests and determine by statistical methods which of them gives the best correlations with the other tests. Thereafter the most practical of the highly correlated tests could be used for rating the cariogenicity of foods.

Animal and "semi-clinical" tests are more difficult to run, and more time consuming and expensive than the previously discussed laboratory tests that have already been run on a number of foods. They are procedures that produce caries or caries-like changes in animal or human teeth. Most have been used with only one or two human foodstuffs, and then only in a preliminary way but their potential usefulness requires that they be given some mention. Those that will be discussed briefly are:

1. Caries tests in animals.
2. Production of in vitro "caries."
3. Demineralization of enamel blocks in the mouth.
4. Production of pre-carious lesions in vital human teeth.

Semi-clinical "Caries" Methods

Animal caries Rats and hamsters have been widely used for many types of caries experiments besides those dealing with food. The bulk of the feeding studies have been limited to comparisons of pure carbohydrates such as starch or sucrose but quite a number of breads, cookies, confections and fruits have been tested. Many of the findings are contradictory but the major conclusions seem to be that the sugars, particularly sucrose, are more cariogenic than starches, and that the cariogenicity of diets can be modified by the addition of mineral salts, fats or whole grain products. It appears that cooked starches are more destructive than their raw counterparts.

Unfortunately, most of the earlier work has little value because only recently it has been realized that achievement of meaningful results required regulation of the amount of the test foods offered and the frequency of eating. Special automatic feeding apparatus (Figs. 7 and 8) is now available to serve this purpose, but as yet has produced no significant body of information. The findings that have come from the four or five laboratories that are using the automatic feeding procedure have, as with *ad libitum* feeding, failed to show that the caries produced parallels the sugar content of the foods tested.

Monkeys have also been used for caries tests. Findings in them will be more applicable to the human mouth than those in rodents. Thus far, monkeys have not been used for making comparisons of caries production by different foods but it has been shown that glucose will produce caries, as does sucrose. In spite of the high cost of caries tests in monkeys they could be valuable for providing a standard against which other cariogenicity tests could be evaluated.

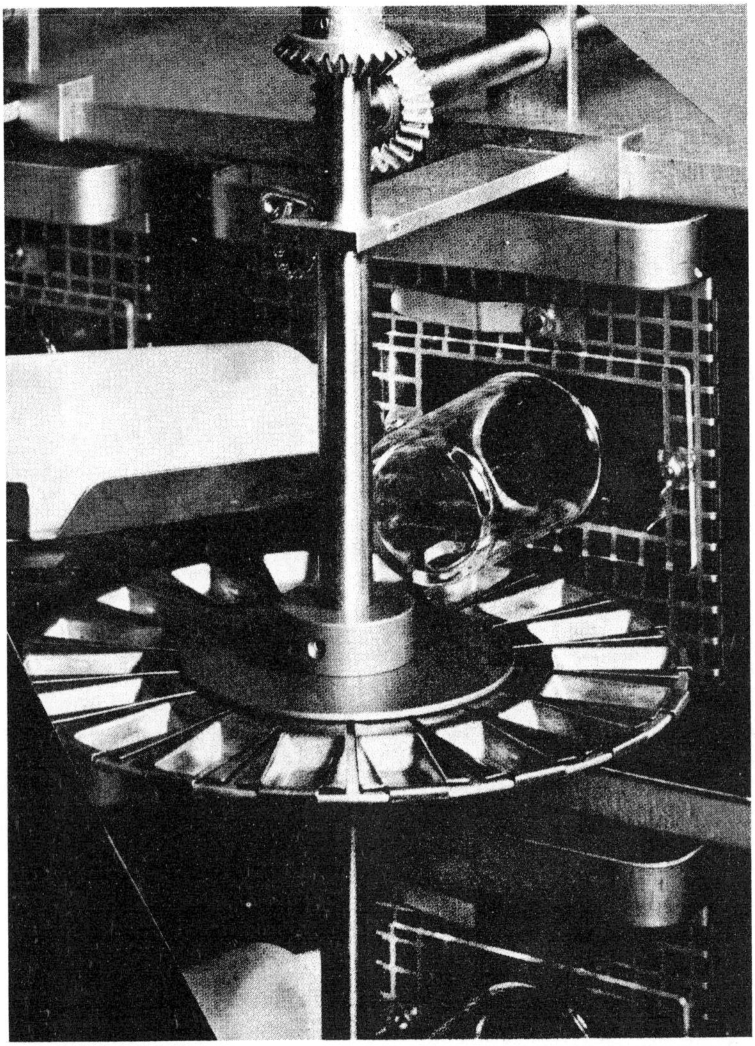

FIGURE 7. Automatic rat feeding apparatus showing food carrying disc that rotates under feeding tube from individual rat cage. (Hofer)

In vitro caries A number of laboratory systems have been devised for producing caries-like change in teeth. Of these we, naturally enough, favor the "Orofax" which we developed and use.[32] This produces "caries" in enamel sections held in a flow of human saliva (Figs. 9-11). Our tests on a number of foods show that they vary quite widely in the extent of "caries" produced. Parallelism to the sucrose content of the foods is not apparent.

Intraoral enamel demineralization In this procedure, blocks of enamel covered with gauze are fitted into a dental appliance which is worn in the human mouth except when it is exposed to test carbohydrates on the laboratory bench. Demineralization or "caries" is measured as changes of hardness

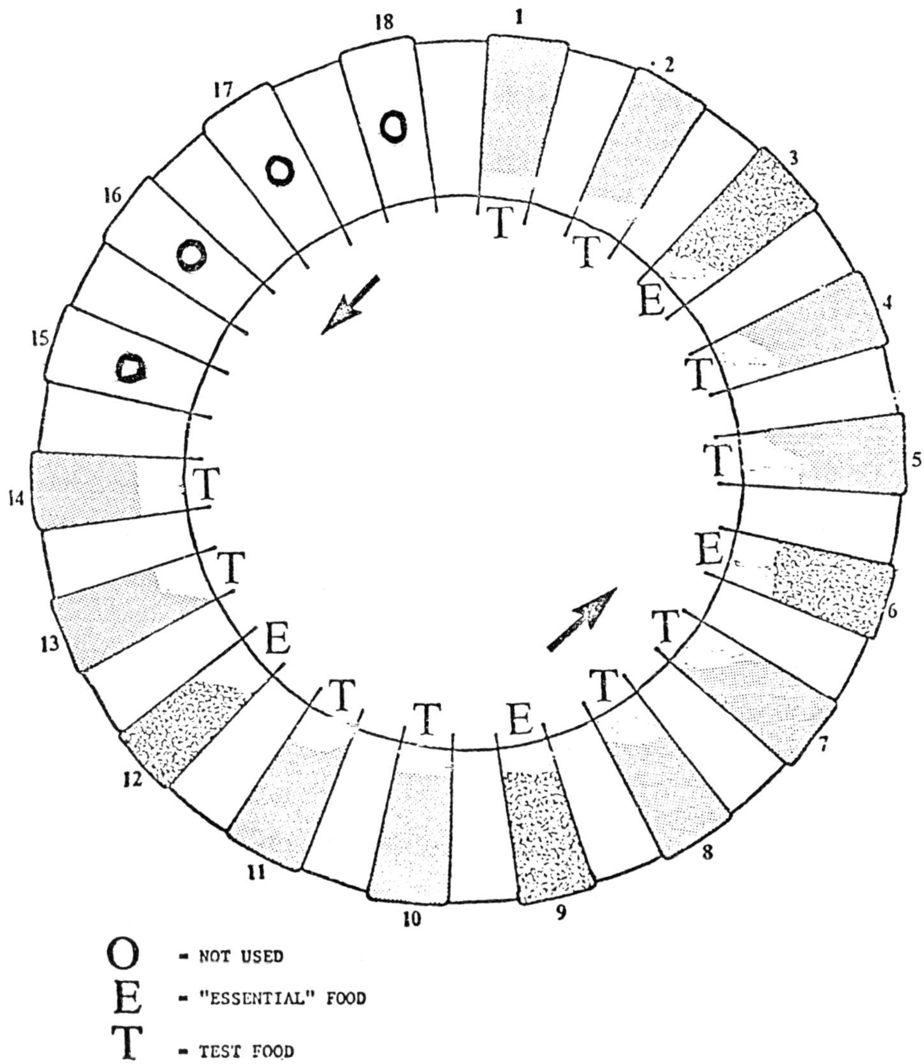

FIGURE 8. Schematic representation of food disc showing distribution of test and essential meals for one day.

in the test enamel. So far only differences in the cariogenicity of sugar solutions have been reported.[33] These showed no difference between sucrose and glucose which, however, were more destructive to enamel than some other sugars and sugar alcohols.

Caries in vital teeth We have made preliminary tests with a method that holds cells containing food against the enamel or vital teeth in the human mouth and uses special clinical examination methods to detect the first signs of caries.[34] We have found that a sucrose-starch mixture will produce pre-carious lesions in as little as three days (Figs. 12-14).

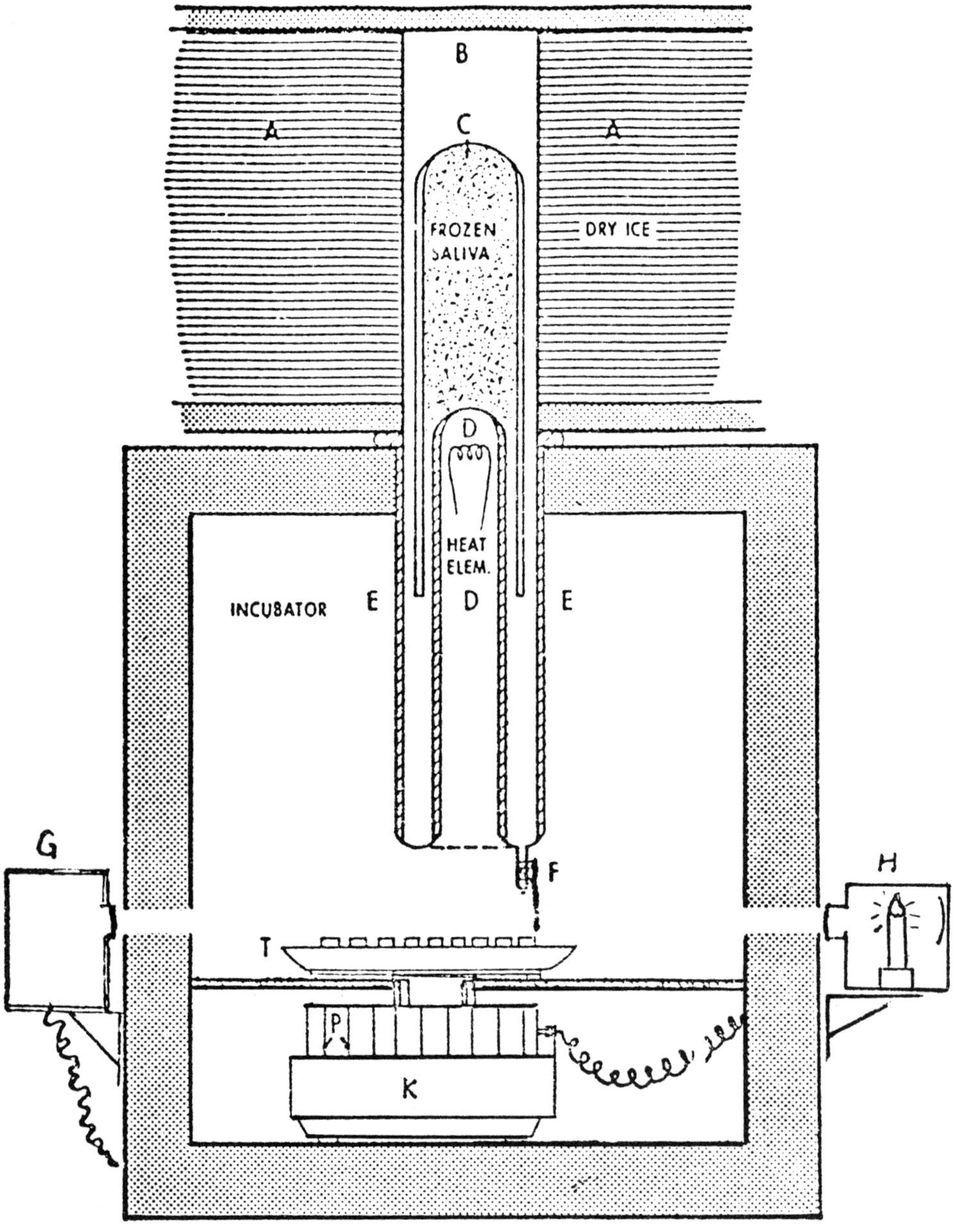

FIGURE 9. Schematic drawing of "Orofax" apparatus with frozen saliva reservoirs (C), thawing element (D), photo electric system (G,F,H,) and rotating specimen tray (T) impelled by carousel projector motor (K) activated from G.

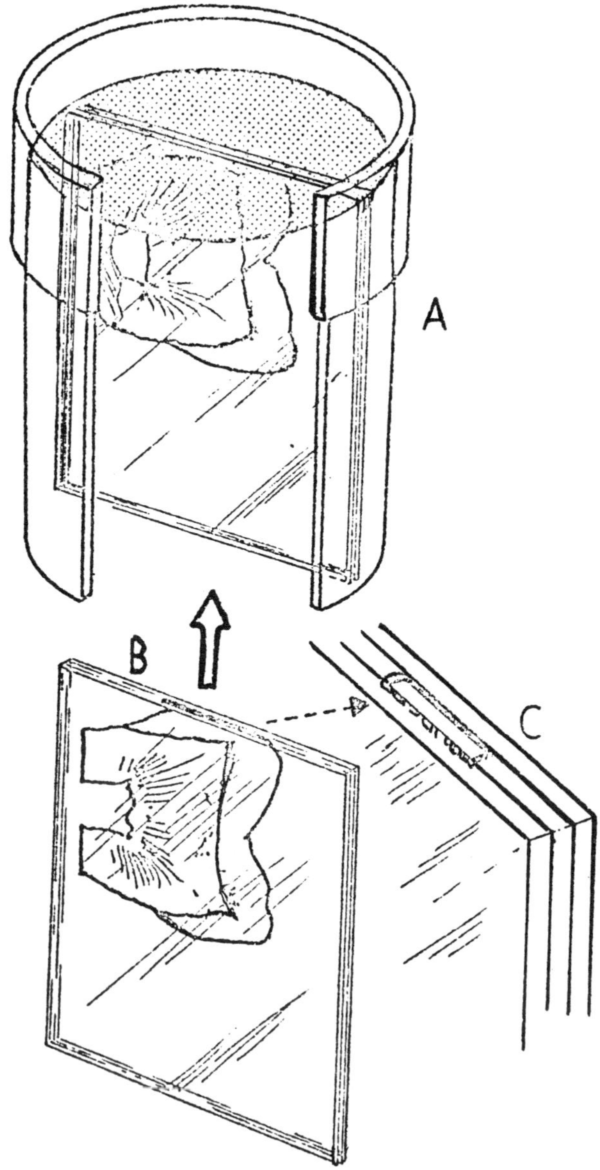

FIGURE 10. Method of mounting enamel sections between glass (B & C) and fitting in food holding capsule (A) for Orofax.

Concluding Comment

Having, at this point, touched upon most aspects of the relationships between food and dental caries, it is appropriate in the way of a conclusion to emphasize the following points.

Sucrose is the food constituent most closely associated with caries causation, but a proportionate relationship between caries and the sugar content of the diet, or that of individual food items, has not been established.

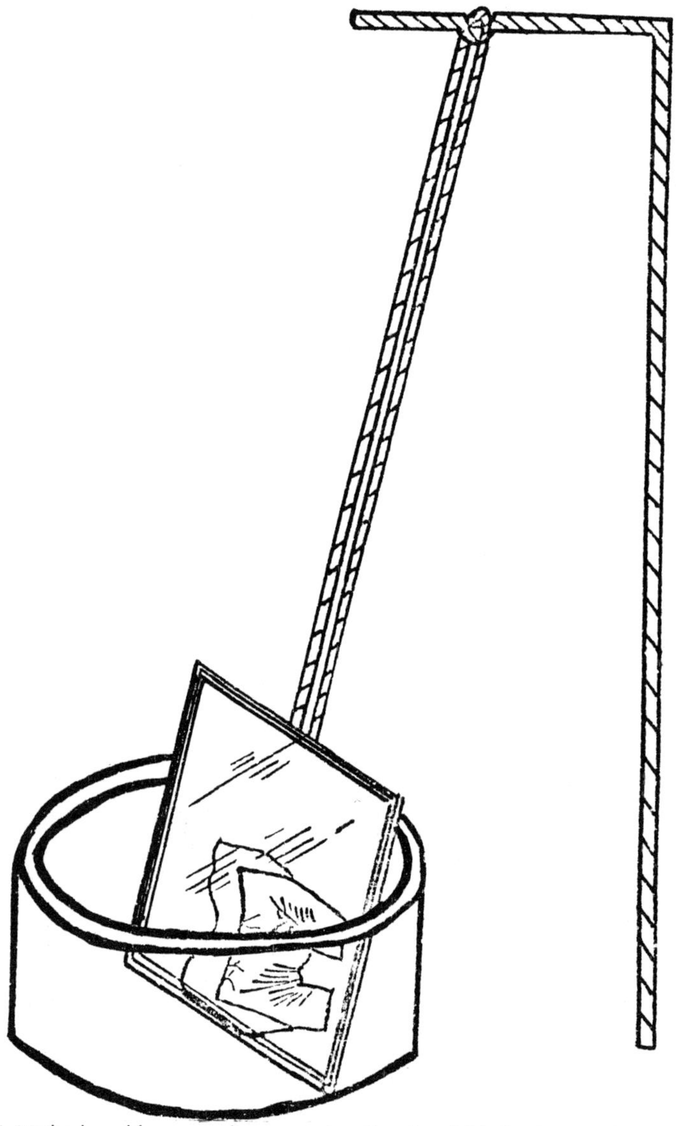

FIGURE 11. Method used for suspending enamel sections in soluble foods in Orofax.

Acid produced by bacterial fermentation of carbohydrates on the tooth surface is the activating cause of caries but clinical and laboratory evidence indicates that many foods provide factors that modify this effect.

The amount of caries produced by a foodstuff is determined largely by the frequency of use, the extent of retention on the teeth, its acid forming capacity in dental plaques, and its ability to dissolve enamel.

While measurements of these factors can provide some indications of the cariogenicity of individual foods, such evidence is open to question until it has been shown to correlate with caries production in man.

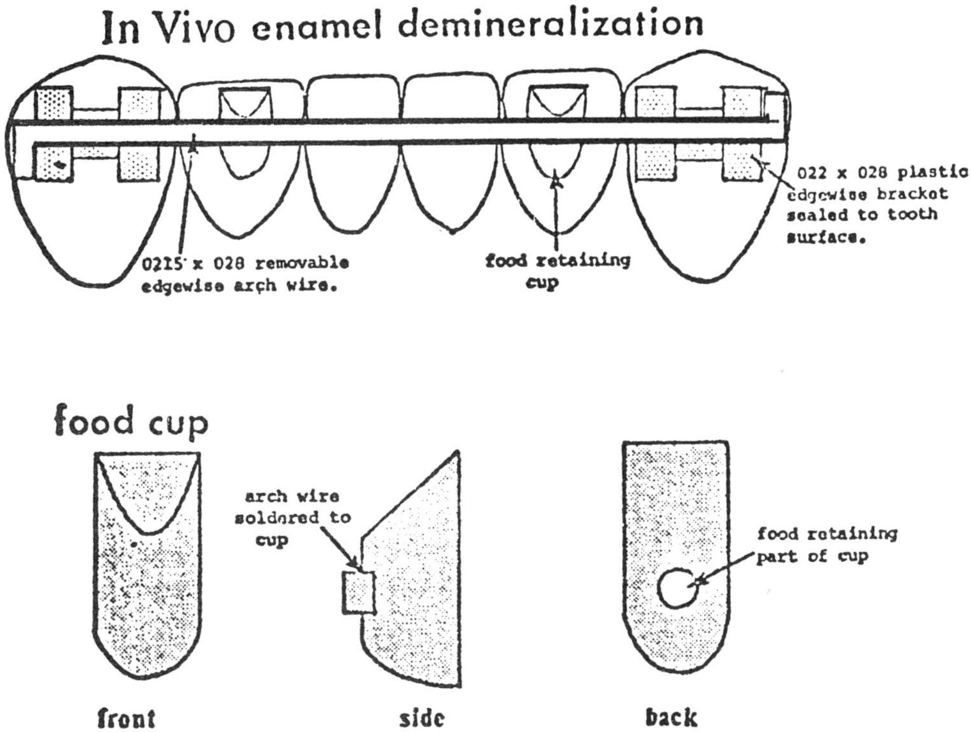

FIGURE 12. Schematic representation of food cups for *in vivo* "caries" test and apparatus for holding them in contact with the teeth.

Practical and reliable methods for measuring the cariogenicity of foods are needed, both as an aid to food selection by the public and as a guide to manufacturers interested in producing foodstuffs of lower cariogenicity.

It is probable that the reliability of tests for cariogenicity can be enhanced by evaluating them against test procedures that produce caries-like lesions in human or animal teeth.

REFERENCES

1. Aristotelis. Opera. Tomus IV (Problemata), Section 14, pp. 186-7
2. Black, G.V. *Operative Dentistry*. Vol. 1. Chicago, Med. Dent. Publishing Co., 1920
3. Fauchard, P. *Le Chirugien Dentiste*. Paris, Mariette, 1746.
4. Berdmore, T. *A Treatise on Disorders and Deformities of Teeth and Gums*. London, Private Printing, 1768.
5. Hardwick, J.L. The incidence and distribution of caries throughout the ages in relation to the Englishman's diet. *Brit. Dent. J.* 108, pp. 9-17, 1960.
6. Magitot, E. *Traite de la Caire Dentaire*. Paris, J.B. Baillure et Fils, 1867.
7. Robertson, W. *The Diseases of the Teeth in Which the Origin and Nature of Decay is Explained*. London, Hayward and Moore, 1845.
8. Miller, W.D. *The Microorganisms of the Human Mouth*. Philadelphia, S.S. White, 1898.

9. Bibby, B.G. Antibiotics and Dental Caries, in *Chemicals vs. Dental Caries*. Washington, American Chemical Society, 1970.
10. Orland, F.J. Use of the germ free animal technic in the study of experimental dental caries. *J. Dent. Res.* 33:147-74, 1954.
11. Kite, O.W., Shaw, J.H. and Sognnaes, R.F. The prevention of experimental tooth decay by tube feeding. *J. Nutrition* 42:89-94, 1950.
12. Kamrin, B.B. Local and systemic effects of refined dextrose solution fed to one animal in parabiosis. *J. Dent. Res.* 33:824-9, 1954.
13. Miller, B.F. Inhibition of experimental dental caries in the rat by fluoride and iodoacetic acid. *Proc. Soc. Exp. Biol. Med.* 39:389-95, 1938.
14. Dreizen, S. and Spies, T.D. Effectiveness of a chewing gum containing nitrofuran in the prevention of dental caries. *J. Amer. Dent. Assn* 43:147-53, 1951
15. Littleton, N.W., McCabe, R.M. and Carter, C.B. Studies in oral health in persons nourished by stomach tube. *Arch. Oral. Biol.* 12:601-9, 1967.
16. Marshall-Day, C.D. and Sedwick, H.J. Studies on the incidence of dental caries. *Dent. Cosmos* 77:442-52, 1935.
17. Osborn, T.W.B., Noriskin, J.H. and Staz, J. A comparison of crude and refined sugar and cereals in their ability to produce *in vitro* decalcification of the teeth. *J. Dent. Res.* 16:165-72, 1937.
18. Khanna, S.L. and Bibby, B.G. Enamel decalcification by cereals of different geographic origin. *J. Dent. Res.* 45:927-33, 1966.
19. Toverud, G. Decrease in caries frequency in Norwegian children during world War II. *J. Amer. Dent. Assn.* 39:127-136, 1949.
20. Gustafsson, B. The Vipeholm dental caries study. *Acta Odont. Scand.* 11:232-388, 1954.
21. Harris, R. Biology of the children of Hopewood House, Bowral, Australia. *J. Dent. Res.*42:1387-99, 1963.
22. Beck, D.J. and Bibby, B.G. Acid production during fermentation of starches by saliva. *J. Dent. Res.* 40:486-91, 1961.
23. Andlaw, R.J., Buonocore, M.G. and Bibby, B.G. Protective factors in wheat germ. *N.Y. State Dent. J.* 28:106-10, 1962.
24. Bibby, B.G. and Mundorff, S.A. Enamel demineralization by snack foods. *J. Dent. Res.* 54:461-70, 1975.
25. Lundquist, C. Oral sugar clearance. *Odont. Revy.* 3 Suppl 1, 1952.
26. Harris, M.R. and Stephan R.M. Effect of mixing water in the diet on the development of carious lesions. (Abstract) *J. Dent. Res.* 32:653, 1953.
27. Carlsson, J. and Egelberg, J. Effect of diet on early plaque formation in man. *Odont. Revy.* 16:112-25, 1965.
28. Graf, H. and Muhlemann, H.R. Telemetry of plaque from interdental area. *Helv. Odont. Acta* 10:94-101, 1966.
29. Frostell, G. Dental plaque pH in relation to intake of carbohydrate foods. *Acta Odont. Scand.* 27:3, 1969.
30. Edgar, W.M., Bibby, B.G., Mundorff, S.A. and Rowley, J. Acid production in plaque after eating: Modifying factors. *J. Amer. Dent. Assn* 90:418-25, 1975.
31. Neff, D. Acid production from different carbohydrate sources in human plaque *in situ* caries. *Caries Res.* 1:78-87, 1967.
32. Bibby, B.G. The Orofax. "Methods of Caries Prediction." *Microbiol. Abstracts,* Sp. Supp: 237-40, 1978.
33. Koulourides, T. Cariogenicity of nine sugars tested with an intra-oral device in man. *Caries Res.* 10:427-41, 1976.
34. Zero, D., Bibby, B.G. and Deeney, M. Experimental white spot development in vital teeth. (Abstract). *J. Dent. Res.* 57 (Spec. Issue A):1101, 1978.

EFFECT OF SEQUENCE IN FOOD INTAKE ON PLAQUE pH

W. Michael Edgar, B.D.S., Ph.D.

Ladies and gentlemen, last year[1] I had the privilege of talking to most of you on the subject of plaque pH changes. particularly referring to the two principal methods which have been applied in the study of these phenomena, and to which Dr. Bibby has referred . Today, I would like to tell you a bit more about our work in Newcastle on the subject, to amplify some of the points made earlier, and also to develop a few new points with you, particularly in relation to the study of plaque pH after eating foods in combination, looking at the way in which foods may or may not be eaten in normal use.

The study of plaque pH, of course, goes back to the classic work by Robert Stephan.[2]

The importance of plaque pH is that when the plaque pH falls after food consumption, it passes through zones of progressive hazard to the integrity of the tooth surface. The chemical basis of this is the pH dependence of hydroxyapatite solubility; the more acid, the greater the rate of dissolution. If you eat foods which don't provoke a large drop in pH, then the plaque pH remains in a safe zone throughout the period following food consumption and no caries should develop. If it passes some critical pH, then dissolution can occur. If we could keep the pH above the critical level all the time, we should expect no enamel dissolution. Current thinking may not be quite sure about the all or none nature of this so-called critical pH concept, but most theories of caries include the idea of a progressively larger hazard to the tooth as the pH on the tooth surface falls. Of course, many other modifying factors, protective factors, etc., may also play a part in controlling whether the tooth dissolves or not, as has been emphasized by Dr. Bibby. The idea has received some clinical confirmation from studying plaque pH changes in individuals with high and low caries experience following the same exposure to sugar, when high-caries subjects were found to have resting and minimum pH levels lower than those with low caries.[3,4]

We have chosen an extraoral pH measurement system because we feel more secure in the accuracy of the pH values that we record, although we realize that the pH values may refer to the pH of plaque which is growing in an area essentially not prone to caries.

The method is based on the use of a conventional pH meter and a slightly unconventional one-drop electrode, the pH-sensitive glass of which is in the form of a cup and contains a drop of water in which the plaque can be mixed. Samples of plaque are taken before and at timed intervals after eating a foodstuff. The plaque is removed from all accessible tooth surfaces with a nickel micro-spatula, placed in the cup-shaped electrode with a measured volume of water, and the plaque dispersed in the water with spatulation. The circuit is completed by lowering the reference electrode into the drop of plaque suspension.

Using this method we,[5-7] among other people,[8-11] have studied the pH in plaque following eating many individual items of foods in isolation, and have been able to rank snack food items in a hierarchy of acidogenicity, from low acidogenicity foods like peanuts, cheese and sugarless chewing gum, to those provoking a large pH drop (and thus potentially more cariogenic), including some hard candies, sugared tea or coffee, and certain biscuits.

Among the food characteristics we considered as contributing to the different effects on plaque pH are the quantity and concentration of fermentable carbohydrates, principally the soluble carbohydrates, especially sucrose. In addition, we considered the duration for which food is consumed and the time during which that food is retained in the mouth in contact with the plaque after food consumption; the nature of the food, its pH, its consistency; and the method of use — whether it is chewed, sucked, sipped, swallowed with gusto; and the all-important factor of the frequency with which the food is normally taken.

However, the factor which I would like to consider in greater detail today is the relationship between the food being consumed and other food; that is, is it a food which is characteristically eaten as part of a normal meal, or is it a snack food which is eaten in isolation and without relationship to other foods? Or is it both? Under which circumstances would it be more or less cariogenic? If the food is part of a meal, what is the effect of the order of the different courses of food items within a meal? Can we change the effect of a food by changing the order of eating, and can we find foods which, if eaten after a meal might tend to raise the pH of the plaque which had been lowered previously by an acidogenic foodstuff?

To illustrate the first point, I would like to describe some experiments[12] which were done a few years ago, but which may be unfamiliar in detail. We looked at a meal consisting of three experimental courses. They were not realistic courses of a meal, but the experiment serves to illustrate the kind of interactions which are possible.

The three courses were pears (half a tinned pear in syrup), a piece (15g) of cheese, and a cup of coffee with sugar and milk, and we studied the effect on plaque pH of eating these foods in various permutations.

The effects of the interactions were quite dramatic. If pears were eaten on their own, the plaque pH fell, but if pears were followed by eating a piece of cheese, the plaque pH rose immediately to exceed slightly the level at which it was under resting conditions, and remained high during the following 20 minutes. Cheese did not delay the pH drop, but appeared to abolish it. This effect of modifying the plaque pH response by sequences of foods, including an acidogenic food among other non-acidogenic items was explored in further experiments. If cheese was eaten before the pears, the cheese caused the resting plaque pH to go up, raising generally the drop in pH caused by the pears, but not so effectively as when cheese followed pears.

When a delay of 10 minutes was imposed between pear-eating and cheese-eating, the beneficial effect of cheese was reduced. And if a second acidogenic food, sugared coffee, was drunk after pears, the plaque pH fell further than with pears alone. Cheese after pears and sugared coffee was effective in restoring plaque pH toward resting values, but with the pattern: pears, cheese, coffee, the pH fall was delayed but reached levels equally as low as those occurring after cheese and coffee.

To study further this effect of food sequence, Fig. 1 shows some results[13] of an experimental breakfast which consisted of a soft-boiled egg, a piece of crisp bread with butter, and a cup of sugared coffee, the sugared coffee being consumed either before, or in the middle, or at the end of the meal, or sipped slowly throughout the meal. When sugared coffee was first, the pH dropped rapidly, but then quickly recovered when the egg was eaten, and there was very little pH drop in response to the crisp bread. When coffee was the central item, a similar rapid pH drop occurred, again followed by a rise after eating the crisp bread. But when coffee was at the end of the meal, it gave rise to a much more prolonged drop, although the minimum pH reached was higher than that when coffee was first or in the middle of the meal.

In order to analyze the different overall pH responses, we can calculate a parameter, pΣΔcH, which I have described previously, and which is calculated by estimating the area enclosed by the pH curve and an imaginary line drawn horizontal to the resting pH. Using this parameter, it was found to be just preferable to take coffee between courses rather than at the beginning or at the end of the meal. Apparently we can mitigate the effects of a highly acidogenic food by placing it between other foods. The taking of the coffee throughout the meal was preferable to taking it in the absence of other, nonacidogenic foods.

We have discussed the pH response to foods in combination and the effect of order, and these findings stimulated us to look again at the question of selecting foods which we might advise patients to eat at the end of meals to stimulate a rise in plaque pH. I have described the results of experiments to test the effects of apples and peanuts in stimulating such a rise. Here the previously eaten sugary food was represented by a sugar lump which was crunched up and eaten during a period of one minute. The pH fall resulting from the sugar lump alone was compared (in the same subjects) with the effects of apples eaten after the sugar lump, and we found the apple to have very little effect. This, we believe, is because apple itself is an acidogenic food, having high levels of malic acid, which in itself can directly influence the pH of the plaque, and with a reasonably high sugar content, which may also have a similar effect. However when peanuts were substituted for apples, a dramatically different response was seen. Taking a handful of peanuts after eating an experimental sugar lump caused a rise in pH of a similar form to that found with cheese. We have since done a number of experiments of this type, using various foodstuffs; for example, we have reinvestigated the effect of cheese, and have tried to titrate the pH drop against progressively smaller quantities of cheese. We can still find an effect with only 4 g, which is a cube 1.6 centimeters in each of its dimensions.

The mechanism of this response, we have reason to believe, is simply the effect of the pH and buffering power of the stimulated saliva, although as human physiologists, it is probably our training which leads us to think that it is a mammalian response rather than an effect of the foods on bacterial metabolism. It is well known, however, that increasing saliva flow from resting to maximum levels results in the pH of the saliva rising rapidly by a factor of almost 2 pH units. Thus, it is this flow of alkaline saliva that we believe is influencing the plaque pH, both the direct effect of the pH and the high buffering power of the bicarbonate in the stimulated saliva.

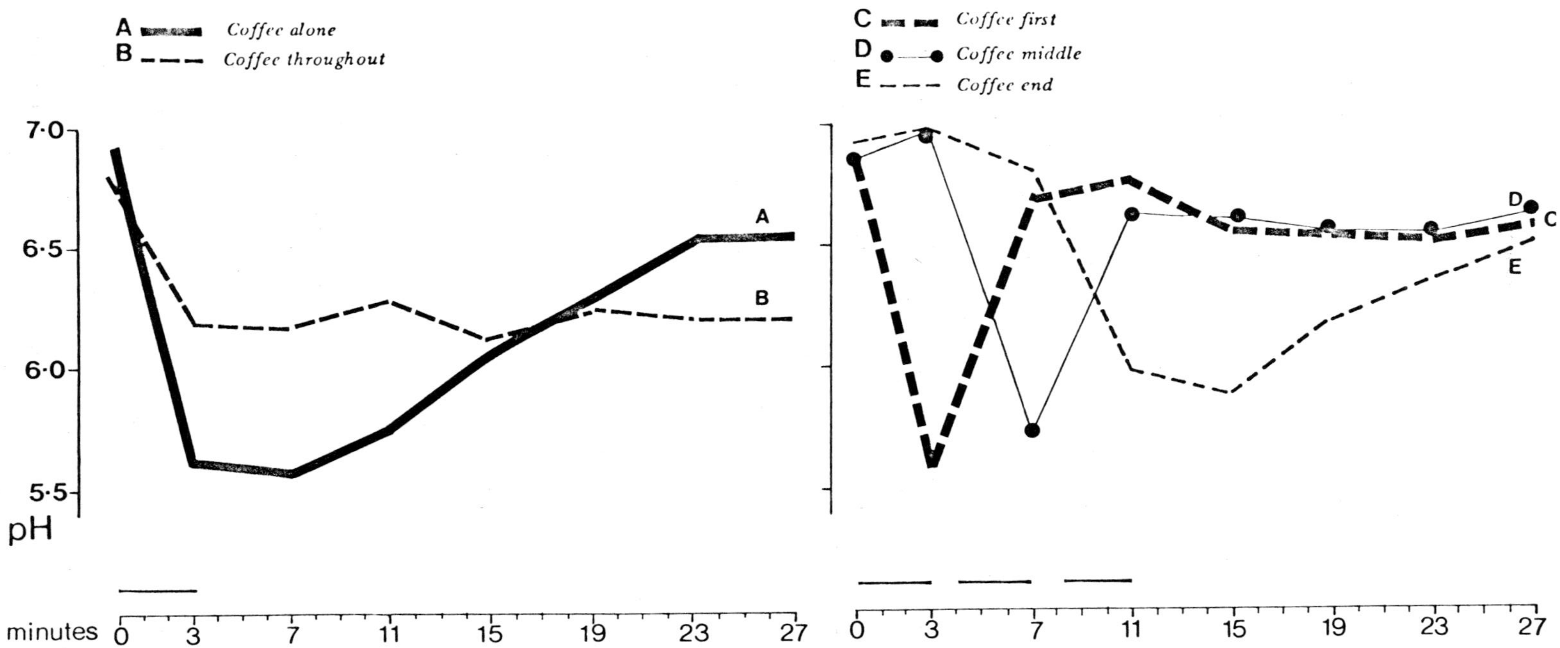

FIGURE 1. Effect of varying sequence upon the plaque pH response to an acidogenic stimulus (coffee with sugar). See text for details.

To test this point, we attempted to reproduce the effect of cheese on the response to a sugar lump by bathing the plaque *in situ* with bicarbonate solutions in the same concentration and at the same pH and the same volume as that stimulated by the cheese. The effect of the bicarbonate mouthrinses was similar to that of cheese; that is, solutions of salivary concentrations of bicarbonate are capable of buffering the acid of plaque (Fig. 2).

Some recent experiments we have done to evaluate some foods under realistic circumstances will illustrate some of my points. The foods concerned were four breakfast cereals, three of them pre-sweetened. The aim of the experiment was to assess the acidogenicity of the cereals as consumed, that is, with milk and, if not pre-sweetened, with sugar added because most people when they eat such cereals add sugar. Further, we wanted to assess effects of other breakfast constituents on their acidogenicity as part of a regular breakfast. The four cereals were Fruit Loops, Apple Jacks, Frosted Flakes, and Corn Flakes. Normal portions were eaten over a natural period (Fig. 3). The resulting plaque pH drop was not at all dramatic; in very few subjects did pH fall below 6.

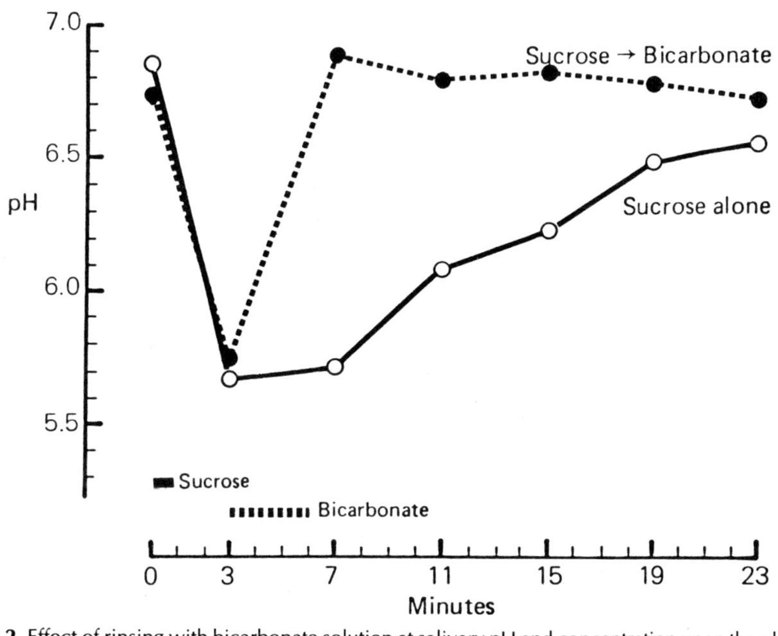

FIGURE 2. Effect of rinsing with bicarbonate solution at salivary pH and concentration upon the plaque pH response to sucrose.

As a control, to show that the plaque pH of these 16 subjects was capable of a drop in response to a fairly major stimulus, the subjects also rinsed for one minute with a 10% sucrose solution.

The differences between cereals were not significant, but the difference in minimum pH between the cereal giving the largest pH drop (Apple Jacks) and the sucrose rinse was significant ($p<0.025$).

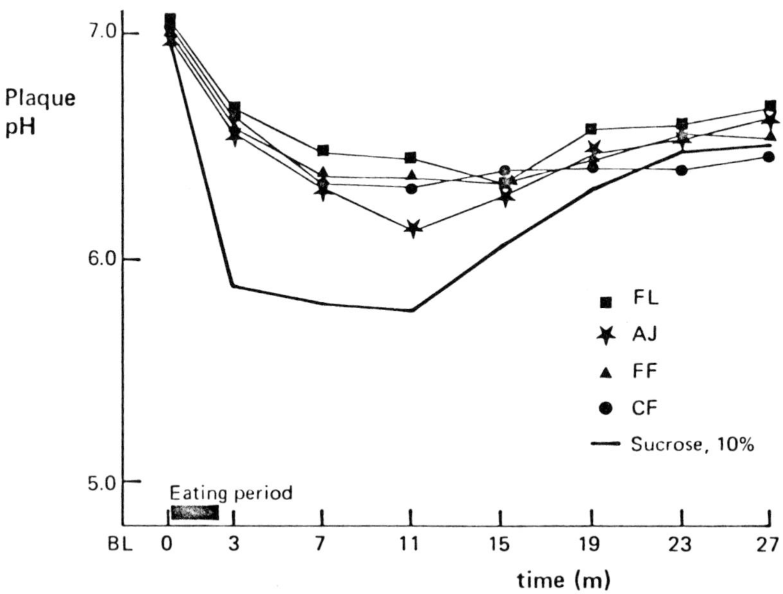

FIGURE 3. Effect of breakfast cereals upon plaque pH (mean of 16 subjects). (AJ=Apple Jacks; FL=Fruit Loops; FF=Frosted Flakes; CF=Corn Flakes)

However, for these 16 students, most of them highly motivated toward oral hygiene, the plaque pH fall in response to sucrose was, on average, rather small. Accordingly, the data were reexamined, selecting the 8 students showing the most acidogenic responses to the standard sucrose exposure. We call this group the "acid eight" for convenience. Results for the "acid eight" are shown in Fig. 4. These had a larger drop in pH with the sucrose exposure, but still the response to the cereals was small, the mean pH remaining above 6: there is no change in our interpretation that breakfast cereals as individual items of food are not markedly acidogenic when eaten normally with milk. Furthermore, Corn Flakes with added sugar give a similar response to that from presweetened cereals.

To look at the effect of other breakfast constituents on the acidogenicity of the cereals, we asked the subjects to eat their cereals preceded by a glass of freshly-pressed orange juice and followed by a slice of toast with strawberry jam. Only two cereals were tested — Corn Flakes, with added sugar and milk, and Frosted Flakes with milk.

Figure 5 shows the patterns for the two cereals as part of the experimental meal, and for the cereals on their own. Orange juice gave rise to a rapid drop in pH, but immediately upon eating the cereals, the plaque pH rose, and then after eating the toast and jam it rose once more, followed by a small pH fall in response to the toast and jam. This is rather reminiscent of the effect of the egg and crisp bread described previously, in that the cereal seems to be having a mitigating effect, reducing the acidogenicity of the orange juice.

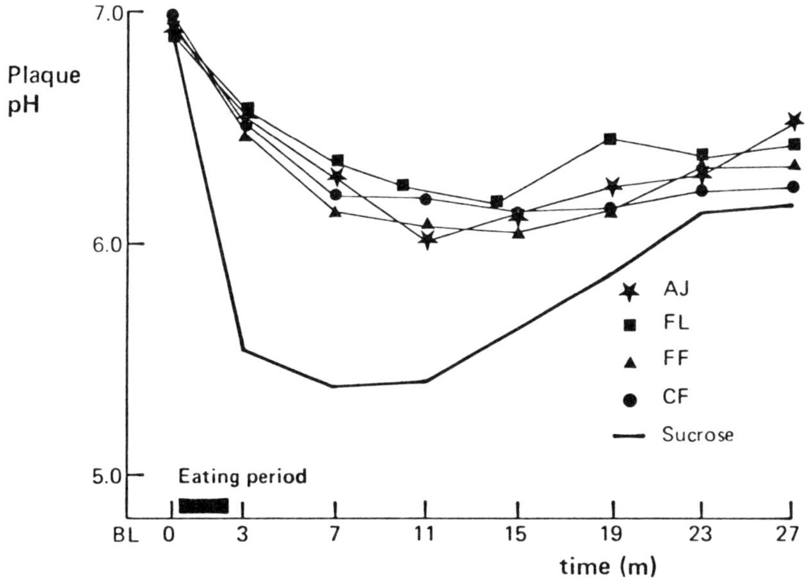

FIGURE 4. Effect of breakfast cereals upon plaque pH (mean of 8 subjects). For explanation of symbols see Fig. 3.

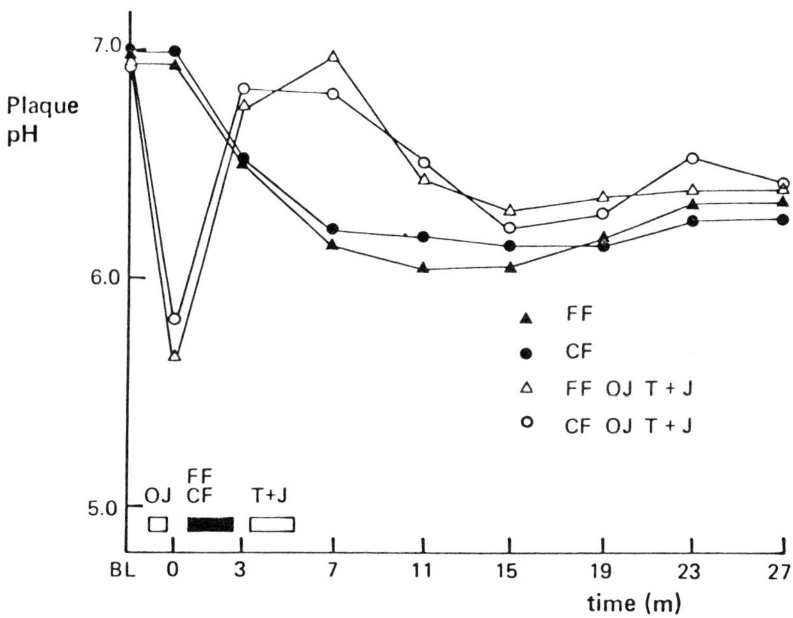

FIGURE 5. Effect of breakfast cereals with and without orange juice, toast and jam upon plaque pH (mean of 16 subjects).

Calculating the parameter pΣΔcH to estimate the overall severity of the pH responses after cereal consumption (i.e., ignoring the complication arising from the pH fall after orange juice) we find (Table 1) a greater response to the cereals on their own than when cereal was consumed as part of the overall breakfast, suggesting that sandwiching the cereal between orange juice and toast and jam had an overall beneficial effect.

TABLE 1. Mean pΣΔcH values, breakfast cereals eaten alone or as breakfast constituents (16 subjects)

	Mean pΣΔcH (±S.D.)
Corn Flakes, alone	5.61 (0.50)
Corn Flakes, orange juice, toast and jam	6.05 (0.75)*
Frosted Flakes, alone	5.71 (0.58)
Frosted Flakes, orange juice, toast and jam	6.11 (0.72)*

*Difference significant (p 0.01), dependent t-test.

CONCLUSION

The plaque pH response may be influenced, either by accident or by design, by changes in food sequence. And so, when we look at the relationship between food and caries, we should consider not only the foods in themselves, but also their relationship with other items of the diet with regard to their nature, timing, and order.

REFERENCES

1. Edgar, W. M. Plaque pH assessments related to food cariogenicity. Proceedings, Workshop on Cariogenicity of Food, Beverages, Confections and Chewing Gum. ADA Health Foundation, 1978.
2. Stephan, R. M. Changes in the hydrogen ion concentration on tooth surfaces and in carious lesions. *J. Amer. Dent. Ass.* 27:718-723, 1940.
3. Stephan, R. M. Intra-oral hydrogen-ion concentrations associated with dental caries activity. *J. Dent. Res.* 23:257-266, 1944.
4. Englander, H. R., Carter, W. J. and Fosdick, L. S. The formation of lactic acid in dental plaques. III. Caries-immune individuals. *J. Dent. Res.* 35:792-799, 1956
5. Edgar, W.M., Bibby, B. G., Mundorff, S. and Rowely, J. Acid production in plaque after eating snacks; modifying factors in foods. *J. Amer. Dent. Assn.* 90:418-425, 1975.
6. Edgar, W. M. The role of saliva in the control of pH changes in human dental plaque. *Caries Res.* 10:241-254, 1976.
7. Rugg-Gunn, A. J., Edgar, W. M. and Jenkins, G. N. The effect of eating some British snacks upon the pH of human dental plaque. *Brit. Dent. J.* 145:95-100, 1978.
8. Frostell, G. Dental plaque pH in relation to intake of carbohydrate products. *Acta Odont. Scand.* 27:3-29, 1969.
9. Frostell, G. A method for evaluation of acid potentialities of foods. *Acta Odont. Scand.* 28:599-608, 1970.
10. Frostell, G. Effects of milk, fruit juices and sweetened beverages on the pH of dental plaques. *Acta Odont. Scand.* 28:609-622, 1970.

11. Ludwig, T. G. and Bibby, B. G. Acid production from different carbohydrate foods in plaque and saliva. *J. Dent. Res.* 36:56-60, 1957.
12. Rugg-Gunn, A. J., Edgar, W. M., Geddes, D. A. M. and Jenkins, G. N. The effect of different meal patterns upon plaque pH in human subjects. *Brit. Dent. J.* 139:351-356, 1975.
13. Rugg-Gunn, A.J., Edgar, W. M. and Jenkins, G.N.. The effect upon plaque pH of altering the position of a sugar course in a meal, relative to two non-acidogenic courses. Abstracts, 26th Meeting, Brit. Division, I.A.D.R. Abst. No. 188, 1978.
14. Geddes, D. A. M., Edgar, W. M., Jenkins, G. N. and Rugg-Gunn, A. J. Apples, salted peanuts and plaque pH. *Brit. Dent. J.* 142:317-319, 1977.

LABORATORY STUDIES ON CARIES

James H. Shaw, Ph.D.

I. Evolution of Caries Assays in Experimental Rodents

The first known observations of dental caries in the molars of experimental animals were recorded in the pioneering nutrition laboratory of E. V. McCollum at John Hopkins University in 1922, which was relatively early in the modern era of systematic research on nutrition when the white rat was the most common subject.[1-4] The stock ration seems strange to us today, and consisted of 30% each of wheat, maize and rolled oats, finely ground together, plus 10% flaxseed oil, all of which was supplemented with whole milk *ad libitum* and fresh cabbage or carrots twice weekly. No caries-like lesions, pulp exposure, or osteodentin, or abnormalities in the "attaching tissues" were observed in rats maintained on this diet. However, when this diet was modified to produce protein, mineral or vitamin deficiencies, by gross switching among the major components, McCollum and co-workers observed such dental abnormalities relatively frequently, with the highest in rats fed diets deficient in protein, calcium and fat-soluble A.

They presented photographs of molar teeth and of the occasional histological section that strongly resembled carious lesions produced by today's procedures. Unfortunately these investigators tended to lump together all dental defects as if they had a common etiology so that the frequency of occurrence of carious lesions is obscured. In addition, because investigators of that era had little or no comprehension of the complex etiology of dental caries, they were biased toward finding nutritional relationships not only to dental caries but to other oral problems. As other investigators sought to repeat the observations reported by McCollum and co-workers, controversy arose either because carious lesions could not be produced under similar circumstances with similar diets or because deficiencies that resulted in one laboratory in increased caries did not in other laboratories.

At best, the overall situation with regard to knowledge about experimental caries was confused, but numerous investigators were convinced that the deficiency of certain nutrients such as calcium and phosphorus and of protein must produce carious lesions under the right conditions. This situation is not surprising in view of the facts that in this era the major nutritional deficiencies were being discovered and described, most dental studies were being done in nutritional research laboratories, and as yet there was no general recognition that fully developed teeth were unlike bone metabolism and remodelling.

Sugars obviously were not involved in the early study by the McCollum group, nor in many others conducted in this era. In one study reported in 1929 and 1930, Shibata reported that a diet of rice and greens mixed with 5-10% sucrose, glucose, lactose and maltose caused dental caries in 70-80% of his rats within 20 days.[5,6] Young rats were particularly susceptible to development of lesions, whereas adults were not: an observation that has often been repeated under various experimental conditions. American investigators who sought to repeat this experiment and were unable to do so ridiculed it on the basis that caries cannot be expected in less than 100 days of feeding. Despite all the writings in the dental literature about the probable role of sugars in human caries, investigators of that period did not rush to introduce sugars into their caries-producing diets.

The unpredictability of the occurrence of caries in laboratory rats continued to plague the field and confound interpretation of the data.[7] In the early '30s, investigators at Michigan State University pointed out one complicating factor, namely the particle size of the diet.[8,9] The diet (HWC) was composed of yellow maize meal, 60%; whole milk powder, 30% linseed meal, 6%; alfalfa meal, 3%; and sodium chloride, 1%. The only appreciable source of sugar in this diet is the whole milk powder, about 38% lactose, i.e., the overall sugar content of the diet was about 11%. Later the linseed meal was omitted and the corn proprotionately increased. When the components of this diet were finely ground, dental caries did not develop. However, when the corn was ground coarsely so that about half of the particles did not pass through a 20-mesh screen, substantial numbers of carious lesions developed. While the authors considered this to be an adequate diet, later studies, especially through the reproductive cycle, indicated it was not able to suport maximal growth in young rats, in which the capacity to grow is very rapid with adequate nourishment.

Thus the HWC diet drew attention to facets of the diet apart from its strict chemical composition that influenced caries development. The oral circumstances of the rats were such when the finely ground HWC diet containing about 11 percent lactose was fed that little or no caries occurred. However, when the coarse particle HWC diet was fed, particles of this particular size were apparently pressed into the sulci during mastication and were retained there to act as a nidus for bacterial action and dissolution of tooth substance. Investigators of that day speculated whether physical damage to the enamel of the sulci was caused by these particles establishing points where acid easily could begin the process of decay or whether simply the physical presence of the particles as bacterial substrates only was essential to establish the decay process.

The rat is the only species where such a particle size phenomenon has been shown to play a role, and in this species the phenomenon is only operative in this type of cereal that otherwise can be considered to have a low cariogenicity. Large particles did not appear to bear any significant relationship to caries in hamsters, presumably because the sulci were so broad in comparison to those of the rat that there was little or no likelihood of particles being wedged between the cusps. In the cotton rat, where the sulci are much narrower and more slit-like, large particles again were irrelevant because fine particles were readily able to enter the sulci and remain there to support bacterial activity. This anatomical situation probably predisposes animals of this species to be highly prone to dental caries when fed almost any carbohydrate-containing diet that is able to enter the sulci.

While one hopes that a diet having HWC nutritional characteristics would not be used today, experiments with it and numerous modifications of it tended to dominate the scene through the '30s and early '40s, largely because this diet was one of the few that would produce caries in rats with reasonable frequency. This category of diets and the results obtained with them tended to point up for the first time in a well-defined way that certain physical requirements of the diet were related to the oral environment and had to be fulfilled in order to develop carious lesions.

One serious problem about the use of natural diets such as HWC and its modifications related to the difficulty to modify them to change their chemical composition, even of gross components such as the source of carbohydrate or protein, and the almost total inability to modify them with regard to vitamin or mineral composition of the ingredients used in natural diets varies from season to season and from source to source.

Along in the late '30s and '40s, diets composed of chemically better defined ingredients than natural products began to be used extensively in nutrition laboratories. This change became possible as a result of general progress in nutritional research that had identified and characterized almost all of the essential nutrients. The latter became available in pure form at reasonable cost so that the investigator had the increasing ability to produce a chemically defined diet of predictable and reproducible composition. This development made possible many modifications of the complete maintenance diet to evaluate the role of the major nutrients carbohydrate, fat, and protein, and the minor nutrients, vitamins and minerals, in the initiation and progression of dental caries. Almost invariably, an adequate semi-purified diet supported better growth and reproduction than did diets composed of natural ingredients. Their use began to enter the dental field in the early '40s. They had the advantages of being easier to modify for evaluation of the roles of major and minor nutrients in dental caries, more predictable composition, and the ability to support more nearly maximal growth. Dental investigators should strive to approach optimal nutrition in all of their experimental animals unless a specific nutritional deficiency is being studied.

A continuing problem in laboratory caries research has been the relative unpredictability of the occurrence of lesions. Highly cariogenic diets in one laboratory with a given strain of rats did not cause caries in another laboratory under similar conditions. Not infrequently, rats of a different strain or rats of the same strain from a different commerical source did not develop a usable level of caries in a laboratory where carious lesions were readily produced with their own standard diets and strains. Keyes specified an essential component in the puzzle, one that was certainly not new but was not well understood and often disregarded.[10] While dental caries was known to result from bacterial action on the tooth surfaces, investigators assumed that the ordinary laboratory animal would have the oral microbiota necessary for initiation and progession of carious lesions. Frequently experiments, often large and elaborate, were conducted with a highly cariogenic diet with little or no attention to whether an appropriate oral flora was present. Keyes demonstrated for the hamster that this assumption of an adedquate flora was not necessarily correct. Oral inoculations of flora from "caries-active" hamsters resulted in the development of extensive lesions in "caries-inactive" hamsters fed a cariogenic diet. In other words, experimental animals could be susceptible to dental caries and be fed cariogenic diet but not develop caries until the appropriate oral flora was provided and was able to implant in cares-prone sites on the teeth. From these studies, the interlocking three factors of agent, host and environment came to typify the gross interrelationships essential for the production of experimental dental caries. When any one of these three factors was not present, the other two were incapable of causing caries. Similarly, when all three were present, the rate of development of carious lesions was little or much, depending on the composite effect provided by the three.

König reviewed the relationship of frequency of eating by experimental animals to the extent of dental caries that would develop.[11] He concluded that under highly cariogenic circumstances of diet, microbial flora, and inherent proneness to caries, about 60 minutes per day seemed to be the minimum time that food had to be in the mouth to initiate caries. Under less cariogenic conditions he considered that a minimum of 100 minutes per day would be necessary. He pointed out the value of programmed feeding machines that would offer food at repeated intervals for short periods throughout the day to insure that the experimental animals did feed long enough each day to exceed these minimum values. He noted that anything in the diet or a food that was being evaluated for its cariogenicity that altered either the amount or frequency of consumption probably would alter the amount of caries produced and thereby the investigator's perception of that item's cariogenicity.

While various individual investigators or pairs of investigators have often tried to explain why strikingly different results were observed in similar experiments, the first major attempt to standardize experimental conditions in the attempt to have thoroughly reproducible results from different laboratories was quite recent.[12] In six laboratories, a simple two-group experiment was conducted simultaneously with rats of the same strain from the same source, fed MIT diet 200 prepared and distributed from a central point, and provided with deionized drinking water from a common supplier. The 12 rats in each of the six Groups A served as controls with no oral infection beyond that endemically carried by rats from that source; the 12 rats in the Groups B were inoculated early in the experiment with *Streptococcus mutans* 6715-5, again from a common source. At the end of the 56-day trial, all caries evaluations were made by a single investigator using the method of Keyes.[13] The authors indicate: "The similarity of results for the six geographically separated groups in this study is of more interest than the variations. The differences in caries development between the various laboratories was one of magnitude only; the pattern of caries development was the same for all groups. That is, the highest number of carious areas was always found in the sulci, the lowest on the buccal-lingual surfaces, and the animals infected with *mutans* showed increases largely on the proximal surfaces."

It is interesting to look more specifically at the variations than the generalization to indicate something of the range that occurred despite the fairly rigorous attempts to standardize procedures. The purpose for the following comparison is to point out not just the range of values but, importantly, pitfalls in excessively minute comparisons of data. The mean values and standard errors for lesions in the sulcal regions of the molars for rats in Group A varied from 10.1 ± 2.0 to 18.3 ± 1.8 and for Groups B from 11.6 ± 1.9 to 21.6 ± 2.2, with the lowest means for both A and B in the same laboratory and the highest means for both A and B in another laboratory. The comparable values for smooth surface lesions on the buccal and lingual surfaces in Group A varied from 0.2 ± 0.2 to 2.6 ± 0.7 and in Group B from 0.1 ± 0.1 and 2.5 ± 1.3. In the case of this carious lesion site, the lowest values were from two laboratories, each different from the laboratory that had the lowest values for Groups A and B sulcal lesions; the highest values came from the same laboratory, but a different laboratory had the high values for sulcal lesions. The values for the lesions of the approximal surfaces of the molars from Group A were 0.5 ± 0.4 to 5.6 ± 0.9 and 5.6 ± 1.2, with two laboratories reporting the same highest scores with different standard errors; and for Group B these scores varied from 3.9 ± 1.7 to 11.6 ± 0.9. The low value for Group A came from a laboratory that had no other low value; one of the two high values for Group A came from a laboratory that had other high values. The low values for approximal lesions in Group B came from a laboratory that had no other low values while the high value for Group B came from a laboratory that had other high values. Despite these variations, it is important to note with the authors that "while some data differ from each other, the results of each investigator are not unlike those of at least two others."

This type of consideration of low and high values for individual lesions in specific groups selected out of the total statistical evaluation for the entire experiment tends to be dangerous because the lowest two or three or the highest two or three were not statistically different from each other. Yet this type of minute comparison is what tends to occur frequently when people unjustifiably compare data between laboratories or even from one procedure to another in the hope of getting absolute agreement between data comparing several products. If such group for group or one laboratory versus another comparison in a tightly controlled trial such as that by Larson, *et al.* is not justified, certainly broader comparisons of various experimental conditions are not justified.

A second experiment was conducted by the same researchers with replication of a three-group experiment in each laboratory, with animals, diet and drinking water provided from common sources (unpublished data). Again, good correlations were observed among the results from the laboratories even though a different strain of rat, a different cariogenic diet, and the caries-preventing ability of fluoride were evaluated.

In addition to rodents such as the hamster, white rat and cotton rat, sub-human primates have been used in limited fashion for caries assays of etiologic parameters. The monkey has the advantages of larger teeth that are much more similar anatomically to man than those of rodents, permitting the collection of plaque as well as more careful oral examinations than are possible with rodents. However, the use of the monkey probably will always be limited because of the expense of maintenance, the small number that can be included in a group, and the increasing scarcity of some species for experimental purposes.

Much of what we know about the complex etiology of dental caries has come from animal studies, if for no other reason than many of these studies could not have been conducted in comparable fashion in man. From the large number of studies of dental caries that have been conducted with experimental animals with a cariogenic diet and a caries-producing oral flora, the following generalizations can be made about food components and experimental caries. Using the terminology that Dr. Newbrun has spelled out so precisely, these generalizations could be called consensus views that most knowledgeable investigators in experimental dental caries would accept. A minority of experiments and probably of investigators might not be in full agreement about some points.

1. Food introduced into the body without passage through the mouth is not capable of producing carious lesions.

2. Food must be available and consumed for periods of at least 60 to 100 minutes per day for carious lesions to occur. Caloric restriction causes reduction in dental caries activity because of reduced eating time rather than reduced availability of calories.

3. Carious lesions do not occur in the absence of carbohydrate in the diet, even when such penalties as surgical removal of the salivary glands are imposed.

4. Carbohydrates have differing abilities to produce carious lesions. Raw starch under most circumstances has a low ability to produce caries; dextrin and partially cooked starch have slightly higher caries-producing abilities; the mono- and disaccharides have the highest caries-producing abilities of all carbohydrates that have been studied.

5. The type of cariogenic flora, the species of experimental subject, and possibly the site of the carious lesion influence the relative caries-producing ability of the mono- and disaccharides. In the hamster, sucrose tends to be more cariogenic than other mono- and disaccharides, probably because *mutans* may be of greater importance than in the white rat and the cotton rat because of the different cuspal configurations; in the rat, superinfection with *mutans* also appears to increase the caries-producing ability of sucrose beyond that of other mono- and disaccharides, especially on buccal and lingual surfaces.

6. The composition of the rest of the diet is tremendously important in determining how cariogenic a given amount of sugar will be. For example, in high fat diets with relatively low carbohydrate, more sugar is required to reach the minimal threshold for producing caries than in a low fat, high carbohydrate diet. As little as 2-5% sugar is adequate to reach the threshold for caries production in the presence of 50-70% starch; five or more times as much is necessary when only sugar is present in a high fat diet with just adequate protein, vitamins and minerals. The same kind of elevation in the threshold of sugars may be necessary to produce minimal caries activity with increased protein or phosphates or other minerals. To my knowledge these influences have not been investigated.

7. Introduction of water into a cariogenic diet reduces its cariogenicity. On a gram-for-gram basis, sugars in solution are less cariogenic than sugar by itself or in a powdered diet.

8. The sugar alcohols, xylitol, sorbitol and mannitol, tend to have no ability to initiate or support the caries process in most experiments; an exception to the generalization may have been found by Navia,[19] for whom the sugar alcohols at low levels appear to be cariogenic. The circumstances in his laboratory seem to be more conducive to higher caries activity under standardized conditions than in many other laboratories, including my own.

9. The addition postdevelopmentally of many phosphates to cariogenic diets at levels well beyond those required nutritionally results in major reductions in dental caries. If the high levels of phosphates necessary to reduce caries in rodents are equally necessary for comparable benefits in man, the daily level of phosphate ingestion may well be in excess of physiologically appropriate intake. Possibly this objection may be overcome by the use of calcium phosphate instead of the comparable sodium or potassium salt. Another possibility may be to add the phosphate only to the most cariogenic of foods and confections.

10. The addition of adequate amounts of fluorides to the diet or drinking water, either during tooth development or postdevelopmentally, results in major reductions in proneness to dental caries.

11. The effects of a variety of trace elements provided during and after tooth development on dental caries have led to equivocal and controversial results.

II. Estimations of Caries-producing Ability of Foods and Confections

In comparison to the very large number of studies summarized very briefly in the foregoing section, only a limited amount of time and energy has been expended on efforts to estimate the cariogenicity or cariogenic potential of human foods and confectionary items in an animal model system. Here and throughout the rest of this paper, I use the terms cariogenicity and cariogenic potential, carefully and advisedly. Like Dr. Bowen, I urge that we be careful to use these terms only when we are indeed producing and measuring carious lesions, not some parameter such as pH or demineralization that we believe may be involved in caries production. Even in animal model systems, we must use cariogenicity or cariogenic potential of a food or confection in a limited sense with specific reference only to its caries-producing properties in that species under the conditions of that model system. At the moment, any wider generalization is not justified to other model systems, to other species, and least of all to man. I also should point out the parallel situation; we are probably not justified yet in drawing generalizations from any one *in vitro* test to any other unless perchance the two tests are variants of one another. In every case, as in the animal model system, we are in the situation of an individual investigator who has developed animal or laboratory procedures that in his or her wisdom have the potential to estimate some parameter that is sincerely believed to be intimately related to the causation of caries in man. How we put all the parts together to get the right answer is not yet within our grasp, as far as I can discern. We are here to describe the available information and seek to determine the most constructive ways to go forward. The missing link now, and possibly always, will be the ability to test as adequately as we would like the cariogenicity of specific products and combinations of chemical components in human populations for a variety of reasons: adequacy of control and frequency of intake, expense, and ethical considerations.

The amount of time and energy devoted to attempts to evaluate cariogenicity in animal model systems has been minimal in relation to the need. Many investigators of experimental dental caries have emphasized the collection of basic science information about the etiology of dental caries and neglected to think about or collect the kinds of applied science information that we need today. The latter is harder and more time-consuming; for many, the applied studies are not as interesting or challenging; and applied trials have been found difficult to support financially in the past. In any case, the paucity of studies is unfortunate in view of the potential for human benefit.

I cannot predict that a better or less expensive estimation of cariogenicity of foods can be obtained with an ideal animal assay than with a single test or a battery of *in vitro* tests. However, I am impressed by the high number of the generalizations from animal studies appearing to be entirely consistent with the knowledge that we have about caries in humans. In addition, on the basis of the vast amounts of information applicable to man's well-being that has been contributed by animal studies over the past 50 years in many areas, I believe that more time and effort need to be put into the development and evaluation of possible ways to estimate cariogenicity of foods in experimental animals. Future evaluations obviously will involve attempts to correlate laboratory trials and clinical investigations. I expect that the extrapolation of data from *in vivo* careful evaluations in animals to man are likely to be much less hazardous than attempts to extrapolate from *in vitro* tests directly to man. Yet we must realize that some products are going to be well nigh impossible in their original form to evaluate with animals. Such parameters as excessive hardness, chewiness and stickiness as well as unusual flavors can pose insurmountable difficulties in having rodents consume enough by weight and frequency for a meaningful test. However, the rodent is not a particularly fastidious or discerning subject, so that literally hundreds of products can be evaluated carefully if the motivation is there to do so.

Rodent studies to estimate the cariogenicity of human foods fall into four general categories. In the first of these, several investigators have sought to determine whether human diets as a whole were cariogenic. Instead of using one of the formulated cariogenic diets typical of the basic science studies described here in Section I, they have mixed together human foods in an approximation of the combination that an average person might eat, based on human surveys. One such study was that of Zepplin *et al.* with cotton rats, where a natural diet containing 17.3% sucrose was found to be as cariogenic as their laboratory's high sucrose caries-producing diet.[14] Doubling the amount of sugar in the human diet did not further increase its cariogenicity. Deletion of the sugar resulted in a diet with very little potential to cause caries. Addition of as little as 2% sugar to the diet caused an appreciable increase in caries. Diets [19,20] prepared by other investigators to resemble human diets also proved to be cariogenic. This does not particularly resemble the human's use of the same foods for these investigations were conducted with foods that had been thoroughly mixed together and fed in dry particulate or pureed form. The same mixture was consumed *ad libitum* by the rodents throughout the experimental period instead of the variable food consumption by humans at meals and snacks.

In the second category, individual foods are fed as the sole source of nutrients throughout the experimental period. This procedure has the advantage of making single items the only material in the mouth of the experimental animals; therefore, in combination with saliva and oral flora it has the ability to express itself as the only food in the oral cavity during a given period. This procedure, too, is unlike any human dietary habit except in underdeveloped areas where food resources are limited. This procedure has the great disadvantage that very few foods are able to sustain life alone for the length of a caries assay. As soon as animals are depleted of one or more nutrients during this kind of deficient regimen, systemical and oral complicating factors enter to confuse any interpretation of the relation of this food item to caries production. A good example of the problems in this approach is in the comparison of Corn Flakes, Cap'n Crunch, and Life, in which 46% of the rats fed Corn Flakes and 33% of those fed Cap'n Crunch died during a 28-day experiment (Table 1). One possible approach to correct this problem might be fortification of a single food item to remove deficiencies. However, this procedure immediately brings in the complicating problem that the food itself is no longer being evaluated.

TABLE 1. Food and sugar consumption, weight gain, and caries occurrence in rats given different cereal diets

Diet Group	Sugar Content (%)	Weight Gain/ Day (gm)	Diet Consumption Daily (gm)	Daily Sugar (gm)	Rats Examined	Carious Teeth	Total Lesions
Corn Flakes (100%)	8.0	-0.3	3.0	0.24	10	12.0±0.0	26.5
Corn Flakes (100%)	8.0	-0.3	3.6	0.29	8	11.3±1.2	22.7
Cap'n Crunch (100%)	43.0	-0.2	4.1	1.76	10	10.0±1.2	23.6
Life (100%)	19.0	2.2	6.3	1.20	15	5.4±4.6	9.9
Life (100%)	19.0	1.9	6.5	1.23	12	4.4±3.9	6.8
Life (100%)	19.0	2.9	8.0	1.52	11	5.7±3.9	12.1
Laboratory Chow	....	5.6	14.2	....	14	0.0±0.0	0.0
Corn Flakes (64.8%)	5.2	5.0	11.2	0.58	17	10.1±3.0	16.7
Cap'n Crunch (64.8%)	27.9	5.1	10.4	2.90	18	9.6±3.3	16.3
Life (64.8%)	12.3	4.9	10.7	1.32	15	7.5±4.8	11.7
CD-30 (100%)	64.8	4.5	10.2	6.61	9	10.3±2.1	20.2

Chuong, U.B., Bibby, B.G. and Losee, F.L.[15]

In the third category are the trials in which a food is mixed in known proportions with a cariogenic diet. As the conditions in most caries assays have been designed to produce the maximum amount of caries in the minimum time feasible, the typical cariogenic diet has a very high capability to produce caries in a model system in which the oral flora and the experimental subjects are favorable to the development of caries. Thus the cariogenic diet may, and probably does, have the potential to obscure the true cariogenicity of any food incorporated into it, even in relatively large amounts. For example, from many past studies with rats (summarized in Section I), the expectation is high that the chemical composition of Shredded Wheat is such that it seems highly likely that in ground form, Shredded Wheat will not be cariogenic for rats. However, when a mixture of as much as 1 g of Shredded Wheat per g of cariogenic diet was fed to rats, the mixture was not less cariogenic than the cariogenic diet itself[16] (Table 2). Here what is theoretically non-cariogenic for the rat gives the appearance of being cariogenic under this experimental condition. Probably, the addition of foods that are theoretically highly cariogenic to one of our standard cariogenic diets is not likely to increase its cariogenicity. This procedure has the ability to nourish the subjects adequately in that the cariogenic diet can be made sufficiently nutritious that even very deficient foods can be incorporated into it in relatively large amounts without seriously compromising its nutritional quality. If a diet of borderline cariogenicity were to be used instead of one of today's cariogenic laboratory diets, the incorporation of items of low cariogenicity into it might reduce the composite cariogenicity to the point where caries would not be produced. Similarly, the incorporation of a

TABLE 2. Influence of cereal supplements to a highly cariogenic diet on caries activity in white rats

Experiment No.	Group No.	Diet	No. of Rats	Gain in Body Weight (gm) M	F	Carious Lesions in the Occlusal Sulci: No. of Carious Molars	No. of Carious Lesions	Extent of Carious Lesions
1	1	2700	22	160.5	115.5	6.8	10.8	37.4+
				(5.1)	(3.2)	(0.4)	(1.0)	(4.1+)
	2	2700 + 25% Shredded Wheat	21	167.9	117.8	5.8	8.8	31.6+
				(7.3)	(4.7)	(0.4)	(0.9)	(3.7+)
	3	2700 + 50% Shredded Wheat	21	157.3	111.4	5.6	8.9	30.1+
				(7.5)	(5.1)	(0.5)	(0.8)	(2.9+)
3	1	2700	17	196.6	125.5	7.2	11.0	40.1+
				(10.3)	(8.2)	(0.5)	(1.1)	(4.1+)
	2	2700 + 35% Special K	19	182.1	123.5	6.6	10.4	38.2+
				(9.4)	(5.1)	(0.4)	(0.9)	(2.5+)
	3	2700 + 35% Product 19	20	170.3*	115.5	6.9	12.2	44.6+
				(7.6)	(4.6)	(0.5)	(1.0)	(3.9+)

Note: Values in parentheses are standard errors of means. Statistical comparisons were made by Student's t test for groups 2 and 3 with group 1 in each experiment. *$P<0.05$.
From König, K.G.[12]

highly cariogenic item into such a borderline cariogenic diet might cause measurable increase in the caries activity produced by the composite diet.

The fourth category probably has received the least attention, and yet by my reasoning may have the greatest potential. Possibly the first investigator to propose this procedure was König, although he does not seem to have followed up intensively.[17] In addition to using his programmed feeder to demonstrate so clearly that the frequency of eating a cariogenic diet was directly related to the dental caries experience of experimental rodents, he also alternated feedings of a cariogenic diet with feeding of a food such as bread. The ideal modification of his early procedures appears to be the feeding of a highly nutritous, low cariogenic diet for part of the day and the test food for part of the day.

In this experimental situation, the nutritious diet is provided for a sufficient length of time each day and has a sufficient amount of protein, vitamins, and minerals that the test object supplied at other times need only provide additional calories. This procedure has the real advantage of certain times in the 24-hour day in which the test substance is the only nutritive substance in the mouth. This procedure may be used in the programmed feeder where "meals" of the nutritious diet and the test substance are provided at the desired frequency. The same procedure may be conducted in suspended cages, in which an appropriate amount of the nutritious diet is provided for an appropriate interval once each day and an appropriate amount of the test substance is provided for the rest of the day. The programmed feeder has the advantage of greater control of the amount and the specific frequency at which both the nutritious diet and the test substance are consumed. The amounts of care and labor involved with the programmed feeder are sufficiently high that its use will probably need to be limited to the estimation of cariogenicity for those products that the rat needs to be coerced into eating. For many products that are desirable to the rat, the combination of appropriate amount and length of time for the two different materials make possible the use of regular suspended cages.

We have explored this alternating procedure with about 30 foods and confections commonly used in the human diet. We use a high and a low caries control group. The low caries control group is fed continuously the highly nutritious diet that has a low caries-producing ability by reason of its low sugar concentration. The high caries control is fed the low caries-producing diet part-time and sugar the rest of each day. The increase in caries caused by the sucrose in the high caries control group is given a value of unity; the ability of the remaining substances to increase caries above the low caries baseline is calculated as a ratio relative to the increase caused by sugar. Products such as Shredded Wheat, soda crackers, Cheerios, oatmeal, Cream of Wheat, and bread, white or whole wheat, do not increase the caries activity appreciably above the low caries control; in other words, they have cariogenicity ratios of 0.1 to 0.2 in comparison to 1.0 for sucrose. Various cookies, candy, and breakfast cereals such as Corn Flakes and Frosted Flakes, have ratios of 0.4 to even in excess of 1.0 in some trials (unpublished data).

Much remains to be done to standardize caries assays in order to make the most use out of the potential that experiments offer for this kind of testing of foods and confections. Hand in hand should go suitable non-animal laboratory tests and detailed chemical analyses not just of carbohydrate and sugars, but fat, protein and major, possibly even minor, minerals.

III. Laboratory Evaluations other than Animal Trials

Space does not permit a detailed description of the numerous laboratory studies that have been conducted to simulate caries production or some parameter thereof in a simplified situation in contrast to the complex milieu in animals and in man. Indeed, my expertise concerns animal assays rather than the evaluations that tend to be grouped under the heading *in vitro*. Dr. Bibby has given examples of data from such experiments; I will only list available procedures and comment briefly about them.

The principal laboratory tests that have been used can be grouped into the following categories, each of which has numerous modifications devised to provide the kind of situation considered ideal by its investigator-proponent:

1. **Acid production from foods incubated in saliva or in a bacterial medium** In this type of study a known amount of the food to be tested is incubated in human saliva or in a bacterial medium with a bacterial inoculation for a given period after which the change in pH or the amount of titratable acid is determined. This test is a measure of the potential that the test foods have under this static situation to produce acid and—presumably—to demineralize tooth substance. Why should anyone be surprised that bread fermented under this type of situation should produce as high an amount of titratable acidity and as low a pH as the same weight of sugar?

2. **Demineralization of enamel blocks when incubated in saliva or a bacterial medium with foods** After a suitable period of incubation, pH changes and calcium increases in the medium or demineralization of the enamel block are measured as indications of the extent to which foods alter the characteristics of the enamel block under this type of stagnant circumstance.

3. **Artificial mouth** In attempts to remove some of the static features of the above procedures, investigators have established systems in which teeth or enamel blocks are bathed in a slowly changed, inoculated bacterial medium or saliva in the presence of various compounds or foodstuffs.

These three groups of methods are strictly *in vitro* in that they are conducted in the laboratory detached from any animal or human relationships other than the investigator. In addition, the measurements are on very limited parameters that are presumed to be involved in the etiology of dental caries.

4. **Adherence of foods and confections in the oral cavity** Various studies along this line have been conducted to evaluate the amount of food or confection retained in the mouth or on tooth surfaces to act as caries substrates after a standard chewing or rinsing procedure. Here one evaluates the amount of a food that may be retained in the oral cavity without any judgment that it may be cariogenic. The latter estimation would be more appropriately attempted in one of the first three categories.

5. **Measurement of pH in plaque** In this procedure the change in pH is measured from the resting status, during and after the consumption of a food or beverage until the pH has returned to a resting point. This procedure involves human subjects, with the presumption that the pH at the interface between plaque and tooth substance is pivotal in caries production.

6. **Demineralization or hardness changes of enamel blocks in vivo** Standard blocks of enamel are placed in appliances that are worn by subjects under standardized conditions. The enamel may be protected by various agents or be bathed periodically with test substances. The influence on the enamel block is normally measured by changes in hardness as an indication of the extent of demineralizing or remineralizing.

Many variations in these general categories have been described and still others are no doubt possible. Such studies in general are relatively straightforward and require less time and money than caries assays in animals, and far less than the typical clinical trial. Many reasons exist for continued use of laboratory trials as long as their limitations are recognized and care is taken in the generalization without adequate testing to human situations.

In general, laboratory trials tend to be simplistic, measuring a single parameter or a set of parameters among the very complex series of interrelated parameters in the etiology of dental caries. Some of these laboratory trials tend to be very static in contrast to the dynamic situation in the mouth with the constant exchange of saliva, the periodic addition and depletion of substrates and the metabolic influences of the pulp and exchange through the enamel and dentin. In addition, in numerous laboratory trials there is no guarantee that the inoculum of microorganisms from saliva or from a bacterial medium is the same as the actively metabolizing microorganisms on the interface between plaque and tooth substance or at the depth of an enamel lesion with dentin adjacent to it.

In summary, animal assays under carefully standardized conditions offer the potential for estimation of the cariogenicity of many human foods and confections when the latter are fed in adequate amounts with sufficient frequency in circumstances where their differences in cariogenicity can be expressed. These studies need to be combined with a small battery of carefully selected *in vitro* tests and both correlated with detailed knowledge of the compositon of the food items.

REFERENCES

1. McCollum, E.V., Simmonds, N., Kinney, E.M. and Grieves, C.J. The relation of nutrition to tooth development and tooth preservation. I. A preliminary study of gross maxillary and dental defects in two hundred and twenty rats on defective and deficient diets. *Johns Hopkins Hospital Bul.* 33:202, 1922.
2. Grieves, C.J. A preliminary study of gross maxillary and dental defects in three hundred rats on defective and deficient diets. *J. Amer. Dent. Assn.* 9:467, 1922.
3. Grieves, C.J. The effect of defective diets on teeth. The relation of calcium, phosphorus and organic factors to caries-like and attaching tissue defects. *J. Amer. Med. Assn.* 79:1567, 1922.
4. Grieves, C.J. The effect of defective diets on teeth. The relation of calcium, phosphorus and organic factors to caries-like and attaching tissue defects. *J. Amer. Dent. Assn.* 10:573, 1923.

5. Shibata, M. On the experimental dental caries of molars of the white rat. *Shikwa Shimpo* 32:1, 1929. Japan. J. Expt. Med. 7:247, 1929.
6. Shibata, M. Sugar and teeth. *J. Nippon Dent. Assn.* 23:214, 1930.
7. Cox. G.J. Experimental dental caries in animals. Chapter in Survey of the Literature on Dental Caries, ed. by Toverud, G., et al. Publication #225, National Academy of Sciences, National Research Council, Washington, D.C., 1952.
8. Hoppert, C.A., Webber, P.A., and Cannitt, P.L. The production of dental caries in rats fed an adequate diet. *Science* 74:77, 1931.
9. Hoppert, C.A., Webber, P.A., and Canniff, P.L. The production of dental caries in rats fed an adequate diet. *J. Dent. Res.* 12:161, 1932.
10. Keyes, P.H. Dental caries in the molar teeth of rats. II. A method for diagnosing and scoring several types of lesions simultaneously. *J. Dent. Res.* 37:1088, 1958.
11. König, K.G. Feeding regimes and caries. J. Dent. Res. 49:1327, 1970.
12. Larson, R.H., Amsbaugh, S.M., Navia, J.M., Rosen, S., Schuster, G.S. and Shaw, J.H. Collaborative evaluation of a rat caries model in six laboratories. *J. Dent. Res.* 56:1007, 1977.
13. Keyes, P.H. Dental caries in the molar teeth of rats. II. A method for diagnosing and scoring several types of lesions simultaneously. *J. Dent. Res.* 37:1088-1099, 1968.
14. Zepplin, M., Smith, J.K., Parsons, H.T., Phillips, P.H. and Elvehjem, C.A. Dental caries in the cotton rat. XI. The effect of feeding a natural diet comparable to a human diet. J. Nutrition 40:203, 1950.
15. Chuong, U.B., Bibby, B.G. and Losee, F.L. Some effects of breakfast cereals on caries in rats. *J. Dent. Res.* 52:504, 1973.
16. Shaw, J.H. Influence of cereal incorporation in a caries-producing diet on caries activity in rats. *J. Dent. Res.* 53:397, 1974.
17. König, K.G. Caries activity induced by frequency-controlled feedings of diets containing sucrose or bread to Osborne-Mendel rats. *Arch. Oral Biol.* 14:991, 1969.
18. Navia
19. Stephen
20. Steinman

INFLUENCE OF DIETARY IRON ON THE DENTAL CARIES EXPERIENCE AND GROWTH OF RATS FED AN EXPERIMENTAL DIET

Jorge L. Sintes, D.M.D., Ph.D.

The development of teeth and salivary glands is intimately associated with the nutrient supply. Teeth and oral tissues exhibit the same formative changes that are the hallmarks of development of all tissues and organs. Critical periods indeed exist in the development of teeth and salivary glands during which imposed stress (nutritional imbalance) will lead to irreversible changes in these oral tissues.[1]

Menaker and Navia[2-4] demonstrated that the offspring of female rats fed a low protein diet grew slowly, were smaller in size and had significantly increased susceptibility to caries relative to control animals. Shaw[5,6] and Menaker and Navia showed that changes in the form, morphology and eruption patterns of teeth, as well as alterations in salivary gland morphology and function are attributable to deficiency of protein during critical developmental periods.

The effect of diets low in mineral salts have been studied on rat's teeth. It was found that the weights of the incisors were lower than in control animals and that the percentages of ash were reduced and of water increased. Another important difference between the behavior of bone and teeth was that when a diet with normal salt content was fed to animals which were mineral-deficient, the ash content of the bone returned to normal, but that of the teeth formed during the deprivation period remained unchanged.[7]

Although iron is a major mineral element and is important to hemoglobin formation, normally it is not considered part of the apatite molecule and bone structure. However, iron appears essential for the formation of the orange-brown pigment that is characteristic of the enamel of the rodent incisors.[8,9] The pigmentation of the enamel is characteristic of the rat incisor and does not occur in the rat molars; it does offer another method of evaluating experimental effects upon teeth. Smith[10] for example, observed an absence or diminution of pigment in the incisors of anemic rats.

Implicit in the use of the standard caries-promoting diets, MIT 200 and NIH 2000, is their nutritional adequacy for growth and development of the young animal and maintenance of the mature rat. Little is known, however, concerning these parameters, particularly in terms of long periods of exposure, as caries studies are generally restricted to fifty days of feeding or less.

Materials and Methods

Animal husbandry Sprague Dawley rats of the CD strain obtained from Charles River Breeding Laboratories were used. Animals were housed under controlled humidity (50-55%) and temperature (72±2°F) with equal hours of light and darkness.

Experimental design The influence of caries promoting diets on the growth and development of Sprague Dawley rats was examined in 3 stages of life:

(1) during pregnancy, on growth and development in the offspring;
(2) during lactation, on growth and development in the offspring;
(3) after weaning, on growth and development of the animal.

Each experimental period involved the following study groups:

Group A 25% protein diet, without inoculation (control)
Group B 25% protein, with inoculation
Group C MIT 200 diet, without inoculation
Group D MIT 200 diet, with inoculation
Group E NIH 2000 diet, without inoculation
Group F NIH 2000 diet, with inoculation

The principal purpose of this work was to determine whether two frequently used caries promoting diets (i.e., MIT 200 and NIH 2000) were nutritionally adequate to support growth in the young rat and maintenance in the adult rat, in comparison to a diet that satisfies the requirements established by the National Research Council. By analysis, it was determined that the caloric density of diet MIT 200 was lower than that recommended by NRC standards because of its lower fat content. In addition to being hypocaloric, NIH 2000 also was deficient in other essential nutrients. Measuring growth by weight gain of the animal revealed that both caries-promoting diets, under the experimental conditions, did not sustain growth at a rate comparable to animal fed control diets (Table 1).

TABLE 1. Composition of experimental diets

Nutrient	Control	MIT 200	NIH 2000	NRC
Protein	25.0	20.0	14.0	12.0%
CHO	51.9	67.0	78.4	%
Fat	15.0	3.0	0.8	5.0%
Ca	4.7	3.42	4.4	0.5%
Cu	24.0	10.5	5.8	5.0 mg/kg
I	0.12	0.87	---	0.15 mg/kg
Fe	45.6	33.0	16.0	35.0 mg/kg
Mg	0.39	0.35	0.09	0.04%
Mn	38.0	51.0	54.0	50.0 mg/kg
P	3.12	2.65	3.93	0.4%
K	0.393	0.223	0.568	0.18%
Na	0.377	0.260	0.956	0.05%
Zn	36.0	41.7	17.2	12.0 mg/kg
Biotin	0.5	0.1	0.13	mg/kg
Choline	4000.0	3000.0	449.0	750.0 mg/kg
Folate	2.0	2.0	1.24	mg/kg
Niacin	50.0	20.0	29.9	15.0 mg/kg
Pantothenic acid	50.0	30.0	14.1	8.0 mg/kg
Pro-Vit A	1.0	3.6	3.13	0.6 mg/ret/kg
Piridoxine	10.0	3.0	2.46	7.0 mg/kg
Riboflavin	2.0	6.0	8.37	2.5 mg/kg
Thiamine	1.0	0.8	1.6	1.25 mg/kg
B_{12}	5.0	3.0	1.79	0.005 mg/kg
Vit E	40.0	50.0	27.0	35.0 mg/kg
Vit K	0.5	0.3	---	0.05 mg/kg
Vit D	1000.0	4000.0	1080.0	1000.0 I.U./kg
Vit C	20.0	100.0	20.0	mg/kg

All animals were weaned at 19 days of age. At the same time, the animals to be challenged were infected with a pure culture of *Streptococcus mutans* I.B. 1600 for three consecutive days. The inoculum also was added to the water for the three days. At the end of the inoculation period animals were placed on suspended stainless steel cages, two per cage. The implantation of *mutans* was checked by swabbing animals at the end of the first week, after four weeks and the day before they were killed.

Enumeration of organisms obtained by oral swab in different growth media revealed a difference among various diets in the counts of bacteria on M.S.A. (Fig. 1). The effect was due probably to the increase in the number of streptococci associated with increased carbohydrate in the diet. A similar difference was also observed on M.S.B. a medium favoring the growth of *mutans* with increased carbohydrate availability.

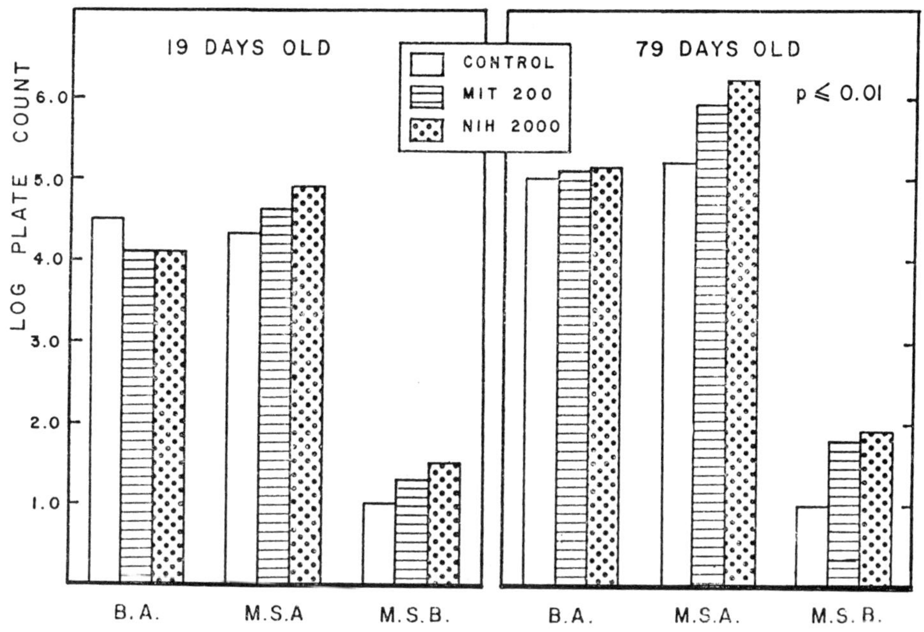

FIGURE 1. Relative counts of bacterial sampling from male albino rats on B.A.[a], M.S.A.[b] and M.S.B.[c] at 19 and 79 days of age. ([a] Blood agar;[b] mitis salivarius agar;[c] mitis salivarius agar + bacitracin)

The inoculation of animals at day 19 with labeled *mutans* did not affect the nutritional status of the animal. This was confirmed by the fact that no difference between inoculated and non-inoculated animals in final weights and weight of organs was observed at autopsy. The only observed difference was in the caries scores (Table 2).

TABLE 2. Average caries scores for all surfaces of right mandibles for 60 days post-weaning rats[a]

Lesion[b]	Control	MIT 200	NIH 2000
	Buccal		
E	0 (0.4)	0 (0.5)	3.3 (5.6)
D_s	0 (0.1)	0 (0.3)	2.6 (3.9)
D_m	0 (0)	0 (0.3)	1.5 (3.3)
	Sulcal		
E	0.1 (3.5)	6.7 (9.4)	7.7 (9.9)
D_s	0 (1.3)	2.7 (4.9)	4.2 (6.9)
D_m	0 (0)	0.3 (1.0)	1.3 (4.1)
	Proximal		
E	0 (0)	0 (0.1)	0.7 (1.1)
D_s	0 (0)	0 (0)	0 (0)
D_m	0 (0)	0 (0)	0 (0)

[a] The numbers in parentheses are scores for inoculated animals.
[b] E=enamel only; D_s =slight dentinal and D_m =moderate dentinal

Animals were weighed and measured[11] from the day of arrival, twice a week to 35 days, and weekly thereafter. Animals were observed daily for condition of skin, hair, tail, etc. Eight and twelve weeks after birth, eight animals in each group were guillotined.

Weight as a measure of growth of the animal revealed that caries promoting diet MIT 200 supports growth comparable to that of the control until approximately 5-6 weeks of feeding, when growth of animals fed this diet levels off in contrast to that of the control in which growth continues throughout the experiment (60 days post weaning). This is a critical period, for it is the time when the animal is reaching maturity. Results suggest that the higher caloric need of this age is not met by the diet. Diet NIH 2000 did not support growth when compared to the control at any period of the experiment. This was not unexpected, in view of the various nutrient deficits of the diet. No differences in food intake were observed among the various groups until the sixth week after birth, when the animals fed the NIH 2000 started to lose their appetites (Figs. 2-4).

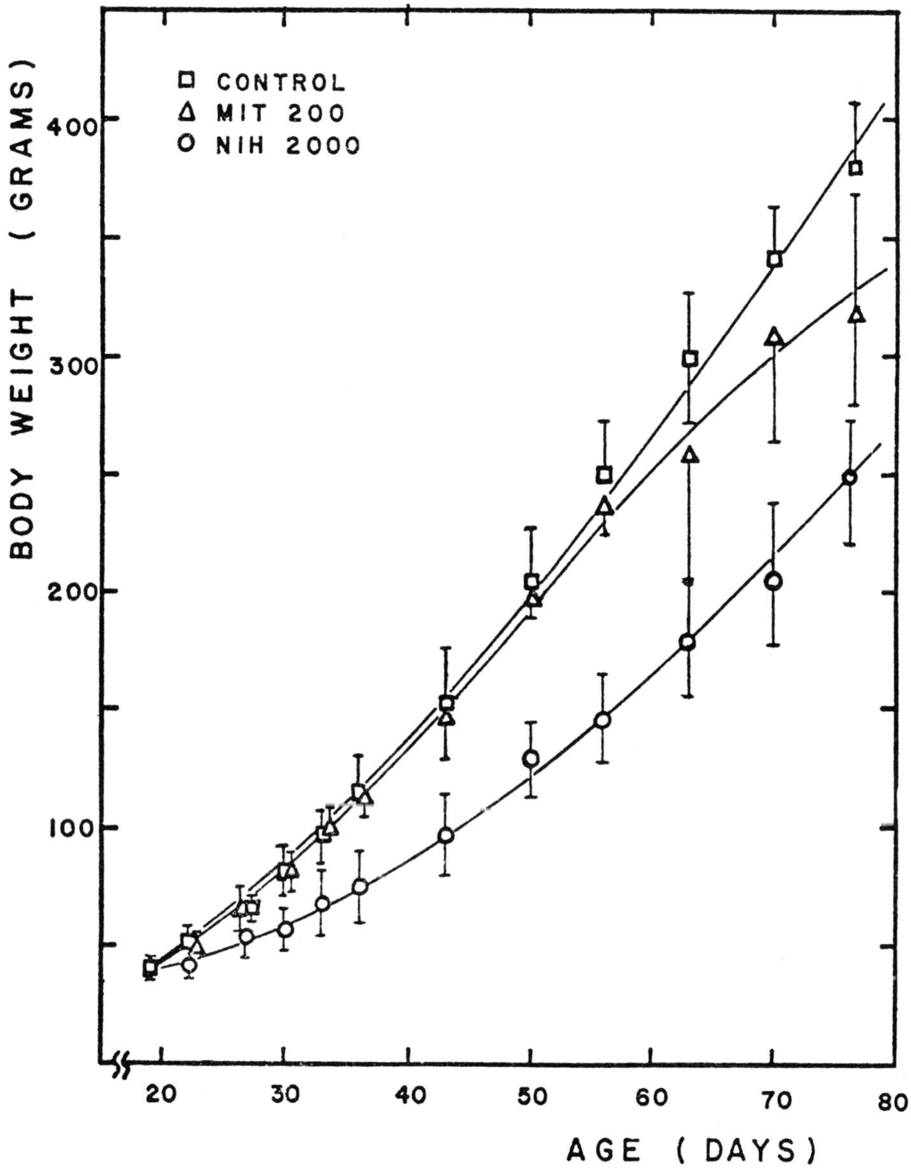

FIGURE 2. Growth curves of male albino rats fed a caries promoting diet post-weaning.

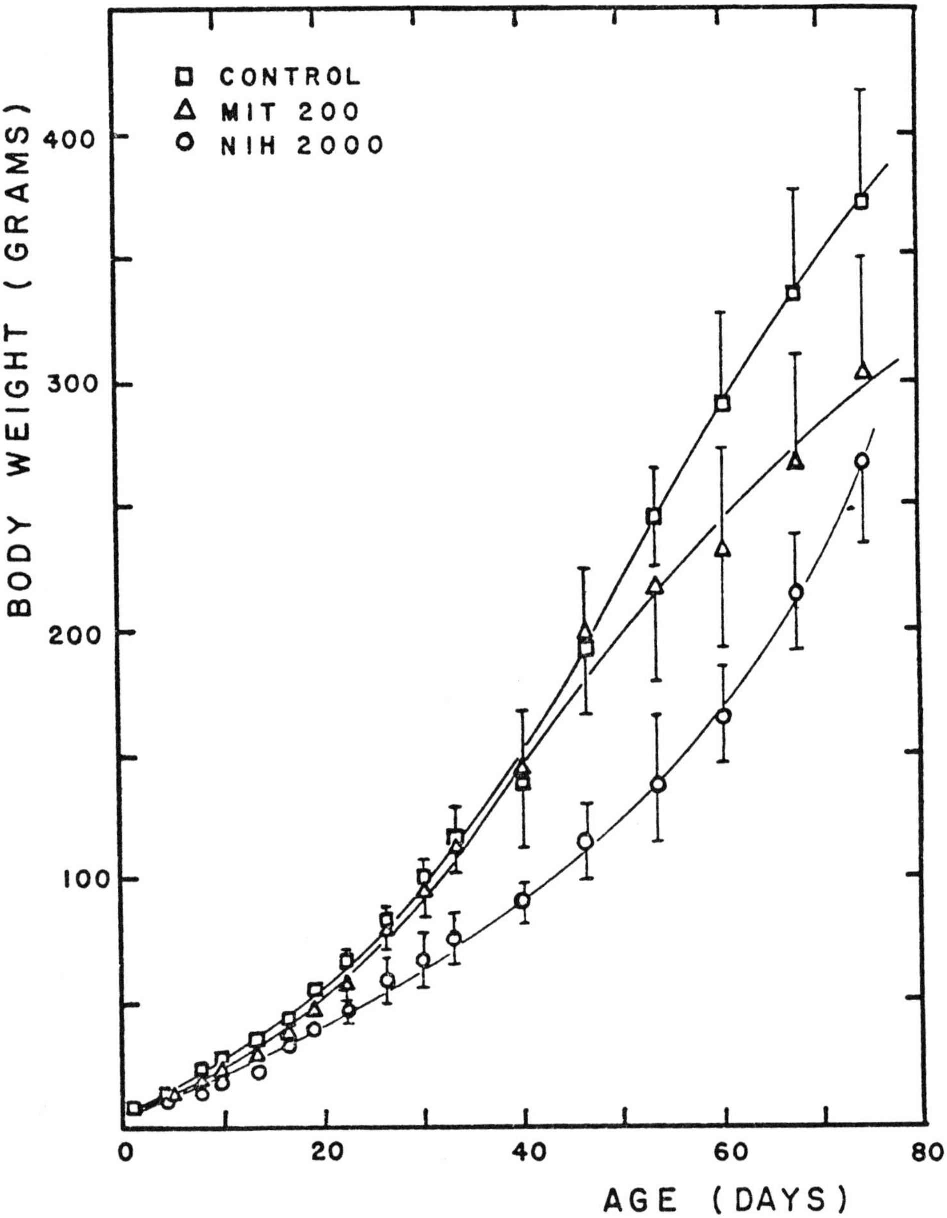

FIGURE 3. Growth curves of male albino rats fed a caries promoting diet during lactation and weaning.

The right half of the mandible was radiographed and the exposed radiographed mandible was used to measure anatomical landmarks. The mandibular films were examined and measured for anatomical landmarks. Differences

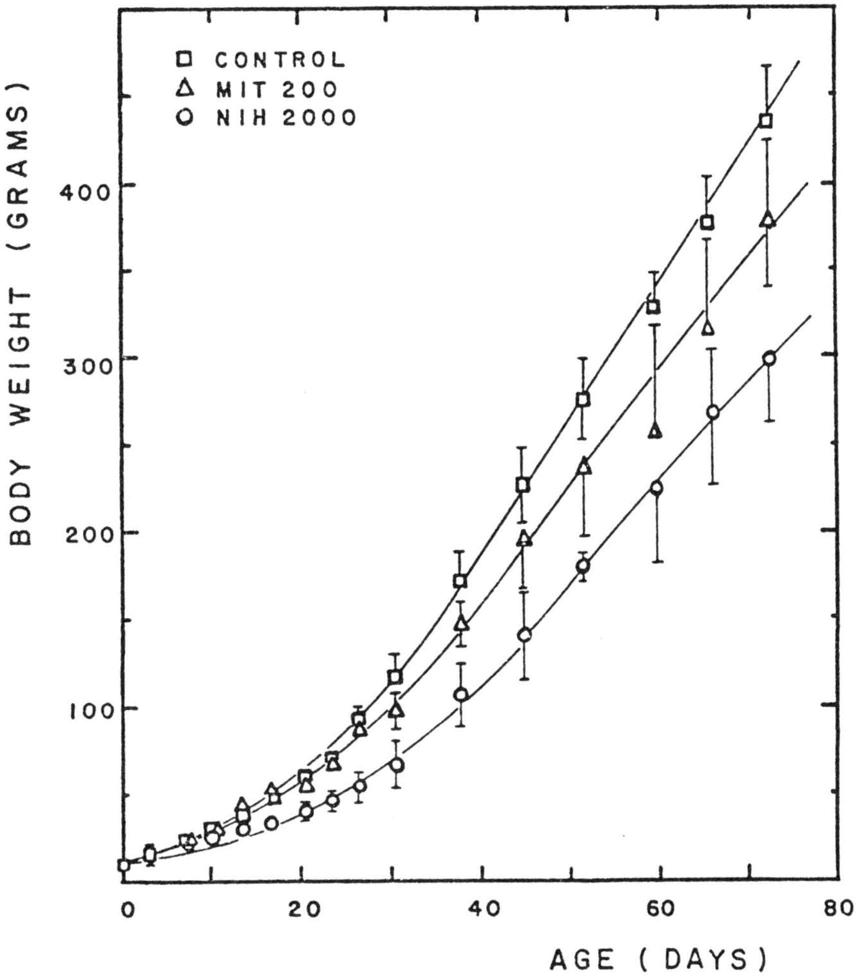

FIGURE 4. Growth curves of male albino rats fed a caries promoting prenatally, in lactation and weaning.

were observed in all parameters between control and the NIH 2000 groups except for the combined mesiodistal length of first and second molars (Fig. 5, Table 3).

The technique used for removal of intact teeth from jaws was described by Navia *et al.*[12]; a ficin solution was prepared.

Upper right first molars were measured directly with an INOX Dial Caliper accurate to 0.1 mm. Both mesiodistal and buccolingual diameters were determined and the length from tip of mesial cusp to the end of the root. The size of the first upper molar of the animals fed NIH 2000 in the post weaning group was not different from that of controls. This was expected, for these teeth were already formed when the animals were exposed to the diets (Table 4).

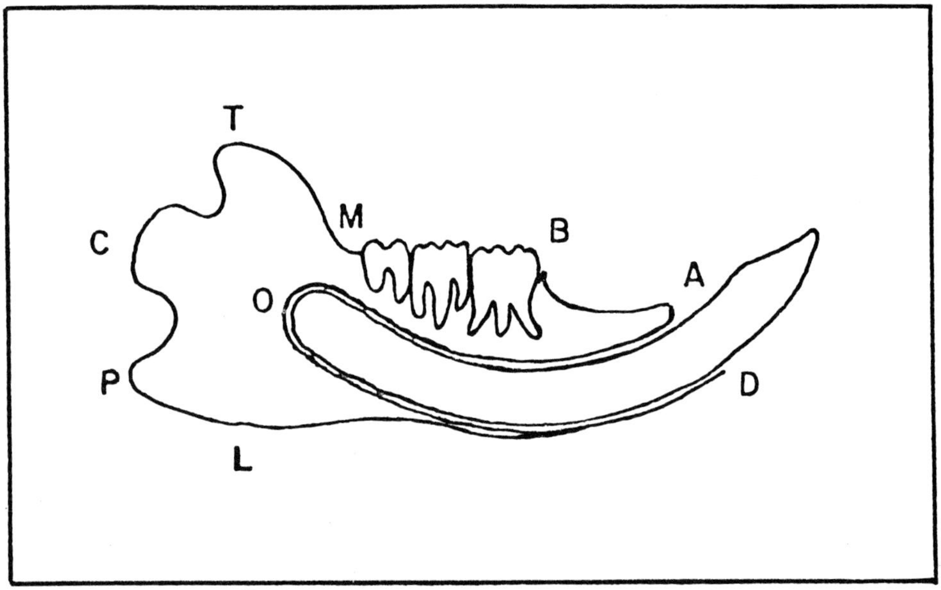

FIGURE 5. Measurement of landmarks on radiographs of rat mandible. (Bunyard[18])

T-L Perpendicular height from upper point of coronoid process to lower border.

D-P Base length from bony crest on labial side of incisor to most posterior part of body.

A-C Condylar length from bony crest on lingual side of incisor to greatest convexity of condyle.

B-M Combined mesio-distal length of first and second molars.

A-B Length of diastema, from bony crest on lingual side of incisor to bony crest next to medial surface of the first molar.

A-O Length of unerupted portion of incisor, from tip of enamel organ space to lingual bony crest.

Mandibles with teeth, teeth alone, upper incisor teeth, upper first molars and upper second molars were weighed. There was no difference in weight of mandible, the extracted teeth of the mandible, the upper incisors, upper first molars and upper second molars at 40 days in the post weaning group, but there was a significant difference at 60 days for all parameters measured (Table 5).

Mandibular caries were scored by the Keyes method.[13] To have a better delineation of the extent of involvement of the carious process, mandibles were stained with murexide. The caries scores were lower in animals fed the control diet than in those fed NIH 2000. It is interesting to note that there were more smooth caries lesions in animals fed the NIH 2000 diet than in other groups. The affected area was still immature when the molars erupted and when the animals were stressed not only with weaning but also with super inoculation as well as exposure to the caries-promoting diets. There was also a difference between the caries scores of the non-inoculated and the inoculated groups (Table 6).

Pigmentation of the incisor teeth was assessed as the normal orange color, partly depigmented or completely white. The normal orange pigmentation of

TABLE 3. Averages of mandibular anatomical landmarks for 40-60 days post-weaning rats[1]

Landmark[2]	Days	Control (mm)	MIT 200 (mm)	NIH 2000 (mm)	p
T.L.	40	11.4	10.9	9.9	<0.1
	60	12.5	12.0	11.2	<0.1
D.P.	40	22.9	22.1	20.4	<.01
	60	24.6	23.9	22.8	<.01
A.C.	40	24.2	23.7	22.3	<.01
	60	25.9	25.7	24.2	<.01
B.M.	40	5.1	5.1	4.9	<.05
	60	5.0	4.9	4.9	n.s.
A.B.	40	6.3	6.3	5.7	<.01
	60	6.6	6.8	6.3	<.01
A.O.	40	17.5	17.5	16.5	<.01
	60	17.7	17.7	17.1	<.01

[1]The lines joining pairs denote that these treatments have not been shown to be significant ($p<.05$)
[2]T.L.=perpendicular height from upper point of coronoid process to lower border; D.P.=base length from bony crest on labial side of incisor to most posterior part of body; A.C.=condylar length from bony crest on lingual side of incisor to greatest convexity of condyle; B.M.=combined mesio-distal length of first and second molars; A.B.=length of diastema, from bony crest on lingual side of incisor to bony crest next to medial surface of the first molar and A.O.=length of unerupted portion of incisor, from tip of enamel organ space to lingual bony crest.

the incisors was present at the end of both periods in all developmental stages and in all experimental groups with the exception of teeth from animals fed NIH 2000. In these animals, the pigment was absent; thus the teeth were totally white or partially white.

The appearance of the fur was good for the control group and those fed the MIT 200, but the NIH 2000 group started to show skin lesions with specific areas of alopecia on the dorsal side of the neck; the skin of the tail was slightly to moderately scaled. Dental caries, obviously, is the least of these animals' problems.

Because of the low content of iron in the NIH 2000 diet (16 mg/kg of diet), hemoglobins and hematocrits were assayed. Hemoglobin and the hematocrit of the NIH 2000 group was lower than the control group in all experimental periods (Table 7).

Saliva was collected by the Menaker and Navia technique[14] and protein was determined by the modified method of Lowry *et al.*[15] Pooled saliva samples were analyzed by disc gel electrophoresis.

TABLE 4. Average for size of upper first molars for 40 and 60 days post-weaning rats

Distance[1]	Control (mm)	MIT 200 (mm)	NIH 2000 (mm)
	40 Days		
MD	3.6	3.7	3.3
BL	2.1	2.1	2.1
L	3.8	3.9	3.7[2]
	60 Days		
MD	3.5	3.3	2.9
BL	2.1	2.1	1.9[2]
L	4.1	4.1	3.9[2]

The lines joining pairs denote that these treatments have not been shown to be significant ($p<.05$).

[1]MD=mesio-distal; BL=buccolingual; L=Length of mesial cusp to tip of root.

[2]$p<.05$

Analysis of stimulated salivary volume during a fixed period of time revealed a significant statistical difference ($p< .01$) between controls and NIH 2000 in post-weaning animals at both ages. If diets were introduced during the suckling period, there was no significant difference at both ages. The salivary protein content differed in both experimental groups fed either MIT 200 or NIH 2000 when compared to controls, especially when diets were introduced during the suckling period (Table 8).

Disc gel electrophoresis of whole saliva revealed a protein pattern different in all experimental groups. This was assumed to represent evidence of the effect of the different protein compositions of the diets. If we compare an electrophoretogram from human saliva with that of the rat, and assume that the lower band (which include the acidic proline-rich proteins) is present in the rat as well, it is seen that this band is missing in saliva from animals fed the NIH 2000 diet (Plate 1).

Autopsies were performed immediately after sacrifice. Vital organs such as brain, lungs, heart, kidneys, liver, adrenals, thymus, spleen, parotid and submandibular glands were dissected and weighed. At autopsy, the weights of several organs were compared to those of the control group. In the animals fed the NIH 2000 diet, the weight of the heart, expressed as percent body weight, increased. Examination of the heart revealed hypertrophy of the left ventricle and dilation, chiefly of the right side. This pathology was present in animals as young as age 59 days (post-weaning group). Examination under the light microscope revealed no morphological differences between the control diet and experimental diet NIH 2000 in the bone, muscle, liver, heart or spleen.

TABLE 5. Average weight of mandible; teeth only; upper incisors; upper first molars and upper second molars of post-weaning rats

	Control (g)	MIT 200 (g)	NIH 2000 (g)	p
		40 Days		
1[1]	0.5472	0.4739	0.5139	n.s.
2[2]	0.1829	0.1704	0.1696	n.s.
3[3]	0.1046	0.1028	0.0954	n.s.
4[4]	0.0360	0.0325	0.0369	n.s.
5[5]	0.0184	0.182	0.0217	n.s.
		60 Days		
1[1]	0.8000	0.6330	0.6433	<.01
2[2]	0.2641	0.2441	0.2237	<.01
3[3]	0.1734	0.1568	0.1401	<.01
4[4]	0.0450	0.0422	0.0351	<.05
5[5]	0.0301	0.0277	0.0220	<.05

The lines joining pairs denotes that these treatments have not been shown to tbe significant ($p<.05$).

[1]Mandible

[2]Teeth only

[3]Upper incisors

[4]Upper first molars

[5]Upper second molars

TABLE 6. Combined average caries scores for all lesions (buccal + sulcal + proximal)[1]

Lesion[2]	Control	MIT 200	NIH 2000
	Weaning		
E	0.1	6.7[3]	11.7[3]
	(3.9)	(10.0)	(16.6)
D_s	0	2.7	6.8[3]
	1.4	5.2[4]	10.8[3]
D_m	0	0.3	1.5[5]
	(0)	(0.3)	(7.4)
	Lactation		
E	1.3	5.4[4]	15.2[3]
D_s	0	1.9	8.6[3]
D_m	0	0	6.7[3]

The lines joining pairs denote that these treatments have not been shown to be significant ($p<.05$).
[1]The numbers in parentheses are scores for inoculated animals.
[2]E=enamel only; D_s=slight dentinal and D_m=moderate dentinal.
[3]$p<.01$
[4]$p<.05$

Supplementation of Diet MIT 200 and NIH 2000

After determining the nutrient deficiencies of these diets, a supplementation experiment was designed.

Supplementation of NIH 2000 diet produced a better growth pattern than that of the non-supplemented group but one still significantly lower than that of the controls. Supplementation also improved hemoglobin and hematocrit. The pigmentation of the incisor teeth did not disappear when supplemented diets were fed. Finally, there was a 50% reduction in buccal caries lesions in the supplemented NIH 2000 diet when compared to the nonsupplemented basal diet (Fig. 6, Table 9).

Supplementation of MIT 200 diet with or without 1% fat revealed a growth pattern similar to that of the controls. Body weight and organ weights at autopsy revealed no significant statistical differences from controls.

Finally, a supplementation study was conducted to rule out the effects of iron on diet NIH 2000; basal diet 2000 was supplemented with 35 mg of $FeSO_4$, 3% fat or both. Caries scores in the iron supplemented groups were reduced from approximately 14 buccal lesions (NIH 2000 basal) to 3 (NIH 2000 + iron). There was a significant reduction of caries when iron was introduced into diet NIH 2000 (Table 10).

TABLE 7. Hemoglobins and hematocrits of male albino rats exposed to diets during different developmental periods[1, 2]

		Control	MIT 200	NIH 2000
		40 Days		
Hematocrit	W	45.5 ± 2.9	42.7 ± 4.0	39.8 ±2.9[3]
(%)	L	44.0 ±2.6	42.2 ±2.6	39.5 ±1.7[3]
	P	51.7 ± 2.9	48.2 ± 0.8	36.9 ± 2.2[4]
Hemoglobin	W	14.3 ±2.1	13.5 ±0.5	10.8 ±1.4[3]
(g%)	L	14.4 ±1.4	13.4 ±2.1	11.9 ± 0.6[3]
	P	15.9 ± 1.0	14.6 ± 1.0	10.7 ± 0.4[4]
		60 Days		
Hematocrit	W	48.2 ± 1.0	48.0 ± 0.0	40.0 ± 3.0[4]
(%)	L	50.1 ± 1.9	47.0 ± 0.6	41.2 ± 1.7[4]
	P	51.8 ± 1.7	50.0 ± 1.9	40.5 ± 3.0[4]
Hemoglobin	W	14.4 ± 1.0	14.3 ± 0.6	11.0 ± 2.9[4]
(g%)	L	15.6 ± 1.0	14.5 ± 0.6	12.4 ± 0.6[4]
	P	16.5 ± 0.8	15.8 ± 1.0	12.5 ± 0.4[4]

[1]W=post-weaning L=lactation; P=pre-natally
[2]The lines joining pairs denote that these treatments have not been shown to be significant (p<.05)
[3]p<.05
[4]p<.01

TABLE 8. Salivary protein content in a fifteen minute period

Age (Days)	Control (mg%)	MIT 200 (mg%)	NIH 2000 (mg%)
	Weaning		
59	426.0 ± 6.1	445.0 ± 5.6[1]	522.0 ± 3.7[2]
79	490.0 ± 9.4	449.0 ± 9.2	491.0 ± 4.5
	Lactation and Weaning		
59	599.0 ±7.9	445.0 ± 5.4[2]	481.0 ± 8.0[2]
79	551.0 ± 4.2	477.0 ± 2.2[2]	472.0 ± 3.2[2]

The lines joining pairs denote that these treatments have not been shown to be significant (p<.05)
[1]p<.05
[2]p<.01

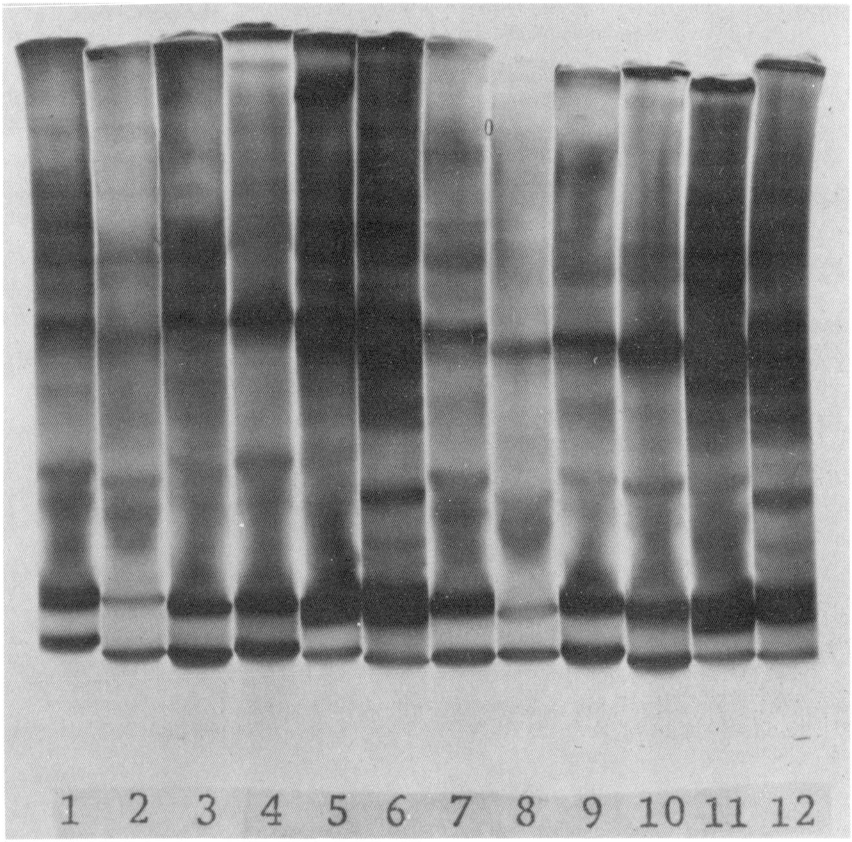

PLATE 1. Whole saliva electrophoretogram for the rat. (Gels 1, 3 and 5, Control; 2, NIH 2000 and 4, 6, MIT 200. Gels 7-12 same but diluted 1:2)

Final body weights and organ weights at autopsy revealed a statistical difference between those obtained from controls and those fed the supplemented NIH 2000 diet.

Depigmentation of incisor teeth was not recovered when animals were placed on a diet supplemented with iron after two weeks on the basal diet or the supplemented diet with fat.

Skin lesions were abolished with iron supplementation; scaliness of the tail was abolished with fat supplementation. This was interpreted to mean that iron is necessary for the maintenance of the appearance of the fur and that essential fatty acids are necessary to maintain a healthy tail.

Purvis[16] points out that 90% of American children less than one year of age do not satisfy the recommended dietary allowance of iron.

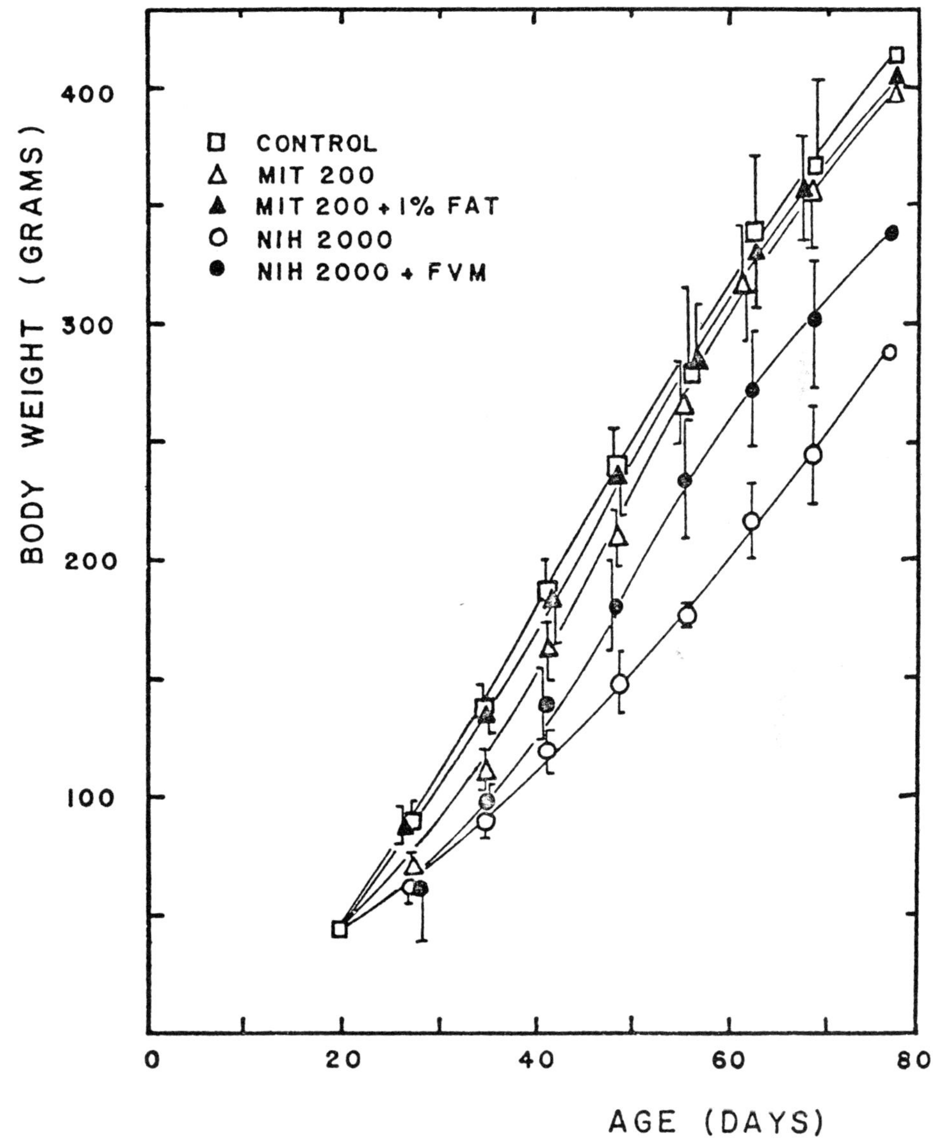

FIGURE 6. Growth curves of male albino rats fed a caries promoting diet supplemented with essential nutrients.

Summary

A multifactorial explanation must be suggested to describe the mechanism by which the NIH 2000 produces increased caries susceptibility. This must include marginal iron deficiency and would explain:

1. The constituents of the diet; for example, whole wheat flour has been suggested as a possible metal-binding agent.

2. The amount of iron in the diet, 16 parts per million versus 45 parts per million in the RDA, is marginal for the rat.
3. Collagen biosynthesis is dependent upon essential co-factors such as vitamin C and iron. It is inhibited under conditions of limitation of iron, a necessary co-factor for protocollagen-proline-hydroxylase. If this limitation occurs early in development, a permanent reduction occurs in the ability of some tissues to synthesize this protein, even after iron rehabilitation. The host is left vulnerable to disease under appropriate stress. For example, poor oral hygiene would result in gingival and periodontal irritation.
4. A proline-rich salivary protein has been identified as present in normal humans. Its amino acid composition is similar to collagen, and it is cleaved readily by clostridial collagenase A.
5. Reduced salivary volume and the amount of protein produced is one reflection of the decreased functional capacity of the salivary gland when stressed with a marginal deficiency such as protein or iron.
6. Pigmentation of rat incisor teeth is dependent on iron and disappears in anemic rats.

Therefore, we can hypothesize that one of the marginal deficiencies demonstrated with caries-promoting diet NIH 2000 is caused by iron. This diet produces high caries scores, especially in the buccal surfaces of molars,

TABLE 9. Average caries scores for all surfaces of right mandibles for 60 days post-weaning rats[1,2]

Lesion[3]		MIT 200		NIH 2000	
		Basal	Suppl.[1]	Basal	Suppl.[2]
		Buccal			
E	0	1.3	2.8	6.3	3.4
D_s	0	0.3	0	3.5	1.1
D_m	0	0	0	3.3	0.3
		Sulcal			
E	2.4	12.9	11.4	12.8	12.3
D_s	0.4	1.6	9.3	12.5	8.6
D_m	o	0.8	3.8	6.0	2.6
		Proximal			
E	0	0	0.1	1.1	0.6
D_s	0	0	0.1	0.8	0
D_m	0	0	0.1	0.8	0

[1]Supplemented with 1% fat.
[2]Supplemented with 3% fat, 3% mineral mix and 1% vitamin mix
[3]E=enamel only; D_s =slight dentinal and D_m =moderate dentinal.

TABLE 10. Average caries scores for all surfaces of right mandibles for 40 days post-weaning rats[1,2,3]

			NIH 2000			
Lesion[4]	Basal	Basal[5]	+Iron[1]	+Fat[2]	+Fat[6]	+Iron, Fat[3]
			Buccal			
E	6.8	6.5	2.4	7.0	3.0	2.3
D_s	3.5	3.0	0.9	4.0	1.0	0.8
D_m	3.5	2.5	0	2.5	0	0.3
			Sulcal			
E	13.3	12.8	8.1	12.8	11.5	7.1
D_s	12.3	10.5	0.8	12.0	4.5	2.1
D_m	6.0	5.5	0	4.5	0.5	0
			Prosimal			
E	1.8	1.5	0	2.0	1.0	0
D_s	1.3	1.0	0	1.3	0	0
D_m	0.5	0.3	0	0.3	0	0

[1]Supplemented with 35 ppm of $FeSO_4$;
[2]Supplemented with 1% fat;
[3]Supplemented with 35 ppm of $FeSO_4$ and 1% fat;
[4]E=enamel only; D_s=slight dentinal and D_m=moderate dentinal;
[5]basal recovered and
[6]fat recovered.

because it reduces the salivary volume and content of proteins. It also interferes with the biosynthesis of salivary proteins dependent on iron, such as the proline-rich proteins identified by Oppenheim *et al.*[17] It also may be true that these proteins are those associated with the remineralization processes, which are well known to occur on enamel surfaces *in vivo* as well as *in vitro*.

It is clear from the preceding that a significant portion of the effects of this diet NIH 2000 is due to iron deficiency and possibly to a lack of several other nutrients. This work not only raises the issue of the role of dietary iron in the caries process, but also brings into doubt the value of NIH 2000 as a model diet for the study of the cariogenic process, particularly when it is used in a sucrose model. Such models, by definition, must be adequate diets in all respects if they are to be useful in the study of diet and caries formation.

REFERENCES

1. DePaola, D.P. and Kuftinec, M. M. Nutrition in growth and development of oral tissues. *Dent. Clin. N. Amer.* 20:441, 1976.
2. Menaker, L. and Navia, J. M. Effect of undernutrition during the perinatal period on caries development in the rat. II. Caries susceptibility in underfed rats supplemented with protein or calories during the suckling period. *J. Dent. Res.* 52:680-687, 1973.
3. —III. Effect of undernutrition on biochemical parameters in the developing rat. *Ibid.*688-91.

4. —IV. Effects of differential tooth eruption and exposure to a cariogenic diet on subsequent dental caries development in the rat. *Ibid.* 692-697.
5. Shaw, J.H. and Sweeney, E. A., in "Nutrition in relation to dental medicine" in *Modern Nutrition in Health and Disease*, R.S. Goodhart and M. E. Shills, eds. Philadelphia: Lea and Febiger, 1973, pp. 733-769.
6. Shaw, J. H. Protein deficiency and tooth and salivary gland develoment. *Nutr. Rev.* 32:24, 1974.
7. Jenkins, G.N. The influence of diet on the oral structures, in *The Physiology of the Mouth*. Oxford; Blackwell Scientific Publications, 1960, pp. 164-217.
8. Navia, J. M. Effects of minerals on dental caries, in *Dietary Chemicals vs Dental Caries*, R. Gould, ed. Washington; American Chemical Society, 1970.
9. Schour, I. and Massler, M. The teeth, in *The Rat in Laboratory Investigation*. J. Q. Griffith and E. J. Farris, eds. Philadelphia; J.B. Lippincott Co., 1942.
10. Smith, M. C. and Lantz, E. M. Changes in the incisors of albino rats accompanying a deficiency of vitamin A. *J. Home Econ.* 25:5, 1933.
11. Hughes, P. C. R. and Tanner, J. M. A longitudinal study of the growth of the black-hooded rat: Methods of measurement and rates of growth for skull, limbs, pelvis, nose-rump and tail lengths. *J. Anat.* 2:349-370, 1970.
12. Navia, J. M. Harris, R. S., Nizel, A. E. and Moor, J. R. Technique for removal of intact teeth from jaws of experimental animals. *J. Dent. Res.* 42:1251, 1963.
13. Keyes, P. H. Dental caries in the molar teeth of rats. II. A method for diagnosing and scoring several types of lesions simultaneously. *J. Dent. Res.* 37:1088, 1958.
14. Menaker, L. and Navia, J. M. Effect of undernutrition during the perinatal period on caries development in the rat. V. Changes in whole saliva volume and protein content. *J. Dent. Res.* 53:592-597, 1974.
15. Lowry, O. H., Rosenbrough, N. J., Farr, A. L. and Randall, R. J. Protein measurement with folin phenol reagent. *J. Biol. Chem.* 193:265-275, 1951.
16. Purvis, G. A., Wallace, R. D., Skeberdis, G. H. and Stewart, R. A. The role of diet in the nutrition of U. S. infants. XI Internat. Cong. Nutrition, Rio de Janeiro, Brazil, 1978.
17. Oppenheim, F., Hay, D. J. and Franzblau, C. Proline-rich proteins from human parotid saliva. I. Isolation and partial characterization. *Biochem.* 10:4223-4238, 1971.
18. Bunyard, M. W. Effects of high sucrose cariogenic diets with varied protein caloric levels on the bones and teeth of the rat. *Calc. Tiss. Res.* 8:217-277, 1971.

DISCUSSION

Dr. Schiff: Dr. Edgar, when you take plaque samples every two or three minutes, do you take samples from different parts of the mouth to make comparisons? Do you always take plaque samples from the same area when you compare one specific food? And if you do so, how do you manage to have so much plaque?

The second question that I have is, what is the age of the plaque? Is this fresh plaque, two-day plaque, three-week plaque, etc.?

Dr. Edgar: The plaques were grown by volunteers for 24 hours, not following a prophylaxis, but following their normal, pretty good, oral hygiene practices. The sampling is done by removing small bits of plaque from all surfaces on each occasion at each time, so that one is returning repeatedly to the same areas, but all areas are covered in the sampling procedure. The sampling is done all around the mouth each time and pooled together, of course.

Dr. Ciancio: In Zurich your paper about cheese created quite a furor because the results were different from the work of Mühlemann and co-workers. Some of the controversy seems to revolve around the method you use and the characteristics of the cheese used—for example, the pH of the cheese, and the taste of the cheese, and how the cheese stimulates taste, etc.

Dr. Edgar: Professor Mühlemann has published experiments which repeated our work fairly closely, but using his technique. In fact, he eventually selected the same kind of cheese that we were using, so that he was doing the same thing as closely as possible. The results of his experiments were good and bad from our point of view and from the general academic point of view, too; good in the sense that we agreed essentially in the direction which the pH changes took. The pH tended to go up after eating cheese in his experiments, as in ours. But in our experiments the pH went right up to the resting level or even beyond, whereas in his experiments the pH did not rise dramatically, it it rose at all. The pH sometimes just stayed the same instead of going further down. So there is a difference in interpretation.

The reason for this difference lies in the design. Our plaque samples are removed from essentially non-cariogenic areas. If the acid theory of caries is right, then you wouldn't expect the pH to drop very much anyway. And, perhaps because of some of the geometry of the indwelling glass electrode, there is created a slightly anomalous situation; in fact, in a sense the electrode is being pushed into a cavity within a tooth surface.

Your point about the cheese is very important. We should try to determine just what the effects of the various foods which can do this trick are, and the properties of that food. The cheese we were using happened to be on the acidic side. I would imagine that there is a spectrum of pH in cheese which we haven't begun to investigate. Various other properties, particularly the sharp flavor of the cheese, must be important parameters as well.

Dr. Ciancio: One of the problems is the complete disagreement, or differences between different groups in their methodology. Therefore we can't really compare many of the results—pH values of the foods being used, taste factors, etc.

Most of Dr. Edgar's measurements are made in 30 minutes, after which the pH returns about back to normal. Dr. Bibby showed us the effect of some different foods on pH. There was relatively no difference in the drop in pH of the foods but there was a difference in enamel solubility, occurring over a six-hour period. How does that relate to the 30-minute time change that was pointed out by Dr. Edgar and Dr. Mühlemann? Did the maximum drop in pH occur at 30 minutes?

Dr. Bibby: We have made no correlations at the same site of the same food at the same time. I don't see technically quite how we can combine that. The point is that our results seem to show that acid production is not proportionate to enamel dissolution. If enamel dissolution is of some value as an indicator of the cariogenicity of foods, then the two measurements ought to be combined in some way. If I want to evaluate a food I would want both the pH measurement and a test of the food to make sure that the amount of acid formed meant greater or less enamel solubility for that particular food. I can see two foods forming the same pH but leading to quite wide differences in caries or enamel solubility. In fact, one series exists on this point. I had 16 breakfast cereals and modifications of them tested in Zurich by Dr. Mühlemann. There was no parallel between the pH and the amount of dissolution or, in the three cereals we tested, the amount of rat caries. These are the results just of several experiments, not from a unified experiment. Nevertheless, it supports my concept that the pH measurement should be treated with suspicion until it is more firmly established. Some of these other measurements should, of course, be related to human caries.

Dr. Mackay: I think it is clear that pH is part of the story, that the nature of the anion is the other part of the story. The acids have been rated according to cariogenicity. It is the food acid and clearly not just pH. It is partly the chelation ability of the acid formed.

Dr. DePaola: The students that you used for these studies, were they all high caries students, or where they low caries? What is their potential? Initial observations of Stephan and many other people have indicated that the real difference in terms of the plaque pH between groups was in the initial pH and not really in the precipitous drop that occurs. As all the pH's of your students started somewhere above 6.5, does your sample reflect a low caries potential? Would you think the curves would be the same if you had a different caries potential group, a more highly susceptible group?

Dr. Edgar: The students were a mixture. I suppose that there were one or two with very low caries experience. In general, it is our observation that on the average, people with a low caries experience tend to have a very shallow pH drop from a high initial value—not going down very far. The contrary isn't necessarily true—that subjects with very high caries experience have a very deep, profound plaque pH drop.

This raises the question of current caries activity versus previous caries experience, a question that will complicate matters somewhat. When we looked at the more acidogenic—the "acid eight" as I referred to them—we did this to see if we could increase the discriminatory capacity of the test by trying to increase the spread of results. Those "acid eight" subjects probably exclude some of the less susceptible subjects, although they do not necessarily include all of the highly susceptible subjects.

We do tend to find, like Stephan, that the inital pH rather than the change in pH is affected. The pH drop from 7.5 to 6.5 is as large as from 6.5 to 5.5. Of course, this reflects an enormously different amount of acid being produced by the bacteria.

Dr. Chichester: We really don't have a consensus on how to measure the caries-causing properties of food. As we cannot determine the cause or the sequence of events, it is difficult to combat them. But aside from that, I think from a nutritional point of view there are a number of points to be made, and also from a food technological standpoint. We have heard a passing reference by two speakers to the fact that the rats and the animals used in the experiments don't always eat the foods supplied to them. Man, the human animal, is unique among mammals. He is one of the few animals that responds to sweetness. Sweetness is a built-in genetic factor and not an acquired taste. This is not the case in most other animals, including those that are used to test for caries-causing properties of foods. You are giving animals a diet they don't particularly like and to which they don't respond, while the human is very responsive to it.

This also makes it difficult to change the diet—the dietary properties of the diet that the human consumes—because he has an inherent drive for sweetness that other animals do not have.

Equivalently sweet foods, in general, do more than sweeten the human diet. They produce flavors and they produce colors, all of which contribute to the various attributes of food that make it pleasant to eat. This is a problem of cost-benefit, if you are proposing a major modification of the human diet. From a nutritional standpoint, most of the sweeter foods also contain some of the very essential elements of the diet in the form of vitamins and minerals, so their elimination or modification must be considered very carefully. We saw from the work at MIT that diets developed for caries and other testing may be nutritionally inadequate, and modifications to human requirements may cause the same thing.

Finally, sweet foods in general also supply calories to the diet at a comparatively low cost, so modifications here also must be considered carefully.

Dr. Shaw: I wouldn't underestimate the ability of the white rat to adapt to a fantastic number of diets, sweet and sour and starchy and otherwise. That is the least of our problems; my strain of caries-susceptible animals, for example, has been on a 67% sucrose diet for 30 generations, and I don't know of any strain of animal obtained from an animal dealer that doesn't—within hours—start consuming the high-sugar, caries-producing diets with no hesitation whatever.

That concept is something of a red herring. It may be that the rat, under given circumstances, would not take a sweet diet if he had something else to choose. When the rat is offered such a diet, he eats very, very well.

Dr. Sintes: The rat model is a suitable model for caries. However, the animal diets that have been used most commonly in this country are nutritionally inadequate. Therefore, the possible role of other nutrients in the caries process must be raised.

Dr. Zoumas: I am struck by the very low threshold for maximum cariogenic potential of the animal diet, a threshold for sugar at 2, 3, or 5% of the diet. If you extrapolate that to humans, someone eating between 2,000 and 3,000 calories daily would need only between 15 and 18 g of sugar to get maximum caries exposure. This is about the amount of sugar in one glass of orange juice or a banana. In fact, you could eliminate totally all sugars added to the diet and you would still be above that level because of the sugar present in natural foods.

Dr. Shaw: In a very high carbohydrate diet, in other words, up to 60 to 70%, as little as 2 or 3% sugar will be the threshold value, not the maximum value. Furthermore, the data today in the United States indicates something like 40% fat in the average human diet. Under those circumstances, the threshold value for sugar to produce caries in rats was something like 5-15%, depending on the amount of fat and other characteristics of the diet.

It really is not correct to say that I was talking about the maximum threshold for rat caries being 2-5% sugar in the diet. Certainly that is far from the truth in the experimental situation.

Dr. Chilton: As I understand, they were 16 students from the general population, of whom 8, the "acid eight," produced more acid more rapidly.

Your data showed mean values for all 16 or all 8, but there was no indication of the dispersion around these means. Was there more variation in the 8 who were non-acid than in the acid-formers? Would the higher acid-formers all have mean values which had less variation around them, or those in the general population greater disperson? There was no indication of this, and mean values can have a rather large spread.

Dr. Edgar: I think it would be true that the "acid eight" would have a smaller standard deviation arising from intrasubject variation than the rest of the group, certainly than the group as a whole. But I think they would have been selected to have a smaller standard deviation. This was reflected by sharpening up the level of statistical significance that went from 2.5 down to 1, even though the number of subjects was reduced.

Dr. Chilton: Do those people who tend to form acid have less variation in repetitive readings than other populations? Is this a characteristic of certain types of people, rather than the general population at large?

Dr. Edgar: We did not replicate studies because we had 16 subjects and a lot of work to do on them. We have done them in the past, but I can't say whether they showed more or less intra-subject variability than the general population. My hunch would be that this was not the case.

Mr. Cornell: We have done some work in that area, and just as a cue, we found generally the changes from day to day in a person were fairly small compared with the changes between people. As that was not the major difference, I suspect you will find that the other would be very difficult to measure. Within a person, you generally get fairly good reproduction.

Dr. Edgar: I think that would have been my hunch, although I do not have the figures at hand.

Dr. Bowen: It has been well known for a decade or more that the diet 2000 that is used in NIH is less than nutritionally optimum. This has been described to my knowledge by at least two people, Weatherell in England and Kanopka in NIH itself.

As to the depigmentation of the incisors, we certainly don't see it in our rats on the diet 2000, and iron deficiency is not the only thing that will give rise to depigmentation. Vitamin E deficiency produces the same effect; here the pigmentation can be restored by feeding the animal selenium. Even if the diets are nutritionally deficient—and I would accept that they are—I don't think it in any way invalidates either the animal or the system as a model to study the main factors in the disease, and certainly does not invalidate the model as a means of investigating methods to prevent dental caries.

If you look at the diet as a whole, you will find it is deficient in fluoride. If you add sufficient fluoride to any diet, you prevent dental caries. I am not saying that dental caries is a fluoride deficiency disease, but nevertheless, fluoride is an essential nutrient and you can prevent dental caries by adding it to the diet.

I might also add in passing that Graf, by the way, many years ago described the addition of ferrosulfate to the diet of hamsters to prevent dental caries. Possibly, he suggested, the animals didn't eat the diet.

I must have seen between 1,000 and 2,000 rats in NIH, being fed diet

2000. I have never, never seen rats in the condition shown in the pictures today.

Dr. Sintes: Some reports about depigmentation (Bunyard) of incisor teeth attribute it to a deficiency of protein and the biosynthesis of a nutrient such as vitamin A_2. I have not said that the model used was an incorrect model. I accept that, according to what had been published, it was adequate. My study, done on at least 1,000 animals covering three developmental periods: pregnancy, lactation and weaning, followed the exact techniques published by other researchers, and I encountered the lesions in all animals at all developmental periods. I have not reproduced this information, but I look forward to reproducing the same information just presented.

Dr. Shaw: I must have at least six papers in the literature where I compared the growth on diet 2000 with our 2700, and invariably got better growth with 2700 than 2000. When I supplemented diet 2000 with protein—a growth improvement; with a mineral mixture—a growth improvement; with corn oil—a growth improvement; and with all three simultaneously, an even larger growth improvement. I do not think there is any way to avoid the fact that diet 2000 is less than desirable for growing animals, and I have never yet been able to get it to support reproduction decently. Yes, there are some pregnancies and some offspring, but compared to a stock colony diet such as lab chow or diet 2700, diet 2000 falls far short in supporting good reproduction.

Dr. Daniels: You referred to the "acid eight" vs. the normal individuals. Are children different from normal adults? Have we ever been allowed to do the research? Are they similar to the "acid eight"?

Dr. Edgar: I am not aware of any experiments of this type on children. I could see that it might just be possible to do such an experiment in England. I do not suppose that it would be possible in the United States.

Dr. Shory: We always compare foods and speak of the soft drinks, being in solution, as not being as detrimental as sticky foods, candy, etc. Have we ever measured the techniques of eating these foods? One big bar can be eaten in two bites and about five minutes. For a 12 ounce soft drink, you have about 30 minutes of sugar exposure. In the film, "Food That Stays," a very straightforward comment was made by children that the soft drink was not as detrimental as a piece of candy. Can we really support that, when we know that a child takes a great deal longer time to consume a soft drink than a small piece of candy or cake or cookie?

Dr. Bibby: We are fully aware that one can't duplicate in the laboratory what goes on in the human mouth. Experiments, by their very nature, are approximations of what goes on in the natural condition. As to soft drinks, we are on a completely different subject. Soft drinks, obviously, won't ferment; to pH 4 there is no fermentation because it is inhibited. There you have direct demineralization.

Now, clinical dentistry, to its shame, has not yet come up with a clear differentiation between direct demineralization, i.e. etching, and caries. Where does one merge into the other, or does one lead into the other? Is it not appropriate to ask us in the laboratory to be intelligent about putting these things together when we don't have the basic question yet offered from the clinic? One of our greatest lacks in caries research is good, critical, clinical observation. That is what we need.

There are technical problems. We have used all sorts of mixtures. But if you have a dry cookie, you can put anything with it and nothing is going to happen. To make contact, you have to have some moisture. We are aware of these problems, but we need better suggestions and we need better definition of the problem before we can make the progress desired.

Dr. Edgar: On the plaque pH front, you are right, of course. The way of handling drinks can vary enormously. We have evidence that changes in the way the drinks are handled can influence dramatically the effect of plaque pH, which may or may not be related to their cariogenicity. It would be a generalization, but a reasonable one, to say that, for instance, equal volumes of a soft drink might not be so harmful perhaps as a similar volume of coffee to which sugar has been added, perhaps because a soft drink of its nature is drunk rather rapidly, whereas a cup of coffee is sipped over a long period of time. I think that is an indication of the sort of variation that one can get.

Dr. Ross: This is really not a question, but Dr. Bibby said we needed some clinical observations, and it is related to the question that was asked. In the good old days before we had the soft drinks available in cans and other non-direct flow containers, and before there were so many competing brands, when I was in clinical practice I used to see many patients come in with a ring of caries in the anterior teeth that circled in almost a complete and full circle, covering the upper and lower anteriors. I used to be considered very much an ESP person because I would say to a new individual who came in with this appearance, "You drink coke from the bottle, don't you?" And variably, the correlation was 100 percent.

Now, I don't know if this relates to your clinical observation of what the continuous consumption of soft drinks does to teeth.

Mr. Jorgensen: I would like to direct this question to Dr. Edgar and also to Dr. Shaw. Not being a dental scientist, maybe you will forgive me for over-simplifying. But the question occurred to me, how far are we from the point of predicting by chemical and physical analysis what is necessary to design foods which would be low in cariogenicity? I have heard it said that a food that has minerals such as calcium, phosphorous, iron, and so forth helps, and that you need a strong buffering agent, bacteriostats would help, physical cleansing agents like liquids or nuts, peanuts, and an anti-sticking agent like fats, lipids, silicones, and what have you. Maybe if you had a product designed like that, a little sucrose in there wouldn't hurt anything.

It seems to me that—and again, I guess I am going to have to plug cheese—I have heard it done several times. But to me it looks like processed cheese and cheese spreads almost meet these requirements. They are high in calcium and phosphorous. They have sodium phosphates added, which would be good buffering agents. They have sorbates which would be good bacteriostats, and lactates. I don't know that they have a physical cleaning agent at all, but they do have anti-sticking agents which are fats and lipids and so forth.

If you design—and I won't hold you fellows to this question; maybe this is one that should be answered by Mr. Snyder—but if you did design such a product, I wonder what the regulatory people would say if you wanted to say you designed it for this purpose.

Dr. Hoerman: Dr. Sintes, the proline-rich salivary protein to which you referred is, I believe, considerably higher in molecular weight than collagen. It is a bit dangerous to suggest that there is a relation in biosynthesis between the two without further evidence.

What reference to human caries did you intend when you made reference to Purvis' work studying United States infants and iron deficiency?

Dr. Sintes: As to the salivary protein: this was a combined effort with Dr. Oppenheim *et al.* from Boston University, who have been working with the identification of salivary proline-rich protein. The amino acid profile is similar in its composition to collagen. So I am speculating that collagen is dependent upon iron for its biosynthesis.

If we have populations with a problem such as early iron deficiency, then we might encounter similar conditions in underprivileged populations such as in Guatemala, where dentition is totally lost by age 2 1/2 years. This may result from malnourishment—protein deficiencies and perhaps some mineral deficiencies during pregnancy and early lactation.Thus, a nutrient so essential as iron could be playing a role, a very important role, in the control of dental caries.

Dr. Purvis: I agree with the comment. The intent of the presentation is descriptive and points up the most frequent dietary problem for infants in the United States. The usual index used to measure the iron deficiency clinically would be the blood picture. This brings another focal point to iron nutrition. I think the point is well taken and deserves consideration.

Dr. Clydesdale: If we could eliminate between-meal snacks and beverages and after-meal desserts, including ice cream, all of which contain sugar plus other things, in an adolescent male this would probably amount to between 1,500 and 1,800 calories per day. If we were then to replace these things with fresh fruit and juices totally, 1,500 to 1,800 calories per day, which would be 15 to 18 apples or oranges, chewing all day, on the basis of either Dr. Bibby's studies or Dr. Edgar's, would this reduce dental caries?

Dr. Bibby: As a fruit lover, I would like to think it would, but I don't know.

Dr. Edgar: There is much documented evidence of potential danger to the dentition from excessive eating of citrus fruits and of apples. This has been reviewed recently in the British literature. That much fruit consumption would be regarded as excessive.

Dr. Shaw: It seems to me the wealth of cereal products, vegetables, etc., would be much more valuable nutritionally, and for oral health, than that kind of intake of fruits and fruit juices.

Dr. Clydesdale: Nonetheless, many dentists in our area make that recommendation very blithely by saying that all snacks, desserts, and ice cream should be replaced by fruits. These dentists forget that these foods add up to around 1,500 calories in the adolescent male.

Dr. Chilton: Most of the emphasis and the discussions so far have been on enamel-dentinal caries. Epidemiological studies have shown that about half of the population, between the ages of 40 to 49, have root caries. I have seen patients who were caries-immune until their late '30s and '40s, who then became subject to root caries. Breakfast cereals with a great deal of sugar, that are believed in some quarters to be cariogenic, are eaten also by older people. Older people, particularly those who are trying to break the smoking habit, and these people are usually very oral, will chew a lot of confections and other things. There is no enamel at the roots, so demineralization goes through the very thin layer of cementum and into dentin.

Because the American population is getting older, root caries is becoming a more important problem. Many of us have seen patients who have had full mouth rehabilitation and then develop root caries, because the gingiva has been displaced either physiologically or through disease, exposing root surfaces. These patients, who are still eating highly cariogenic diets, actually experienced even more rapid caries than they did as children.

Dr. Newbrun: Dr. Bibby made the point that *in vitro* methods are not related to caries in man. And I want to reemphasize that. The idea of doing *in vitro* testing in nothing new. Willoughby Miller, in 1890, tested meats and bread and other carbohydrates, and Dr. Bibby and his associates and graduate students over the years have done many different variations of *in vitro* tests.

We all recognize that the *in vitro* model is rather remote from the real life situation. One of the problems which must be emphasized in the sort of assay that Dr. Bibby uses with his Orofax, whether it is a static model or the dripping model, is that he uses saliva. The salivary flora is well-known by microbiologists. It is known that for at least 15 and possibly 20 years—that salivary flora is not representative of the plaque flora. It represents far more than that of the tongue. The tongue has a much larger surface area, and you get many more bacteria off the tongue by chewing paraffin. There are very serious drawbacks to these *in vitro* models.

It is not surprising that in those *in vitro* models, Bibby and his associates have found that a parallel did not exist between the amount of enamel dissolved and the amount of acid produced, or between cariogenicity as determined by his test method and the sugar content of food.

What do we know from clinical and epidemiological experience with humans? Consider, for example, the hereditary fructose intolerance (HFI) studies to which we have already alluded. Certainly not all carbohydrates, especially starches, are cariogenic as they are consumed by HFI patients with relative impunity. They eat bread, potatoes, noodles, rice and similar types of starch. Yet, according to the *in vitro* tests that Dr. Bibby has described, starchy foods like various breads and bagels and even potato chips cause more enamel demineralization than chocolate, cookies, cakes and pastries.

When such *in vitro* tests run counter to extensive clinical and epidemiological experience, one must conclude that the test model does not really measure cariogenicity and should be discarded as irrelevant.

Dr. Bibby: I expect that deserves a reply. I don't think anybody has claimed that the test represents cariogenicity. It is an index we can qualitate. But while I must admit that I am very surprised at some of the findings we get, I am aware of the fact that the important thing is to find out, and then interpret subsequently.

We think we have tried to open up some fields, because they need to be opened up. We need more people to come and improve them. And maybe, Dr. Newbrun, you know more about my Orofax machine than I do, about the bacterial composition, but we have looked at it and we have no reason to think it is associated with the tongue flora.

We are not trying to disprove anything. We believe that carbohydrates are the major cause of caries. We want to know which carbohydrates, and which modifications of those carbohydrates make them more or less cariogenic. We have the same objective. We want to make foods available which will have lower cariogenicity, which will have shelf life, be available, and be taste and cost-competitive with more cariogenic foods, and the only way they are going to be obtained is by finding something about the principles which make foods more or less cariogenic. When we know those principles — and we have made a start — then those who want to make foods, the manufacturers or whoever wants to get into it, have at least a starting point.

We can criticize manufacturers for not getting to work at it, but we in academia haven't given them the tools with which to work. We should be providing the basic information about relationships of various carbohydrates under various conditions to demineralization, and to anything else.

XI. ADVERTISING

Walter Wolman, Ph.D., Chairman

ISSUES IN ADVERTISING TO CHILDREN

Wallace S. Snyder, J.D.

The topic under consideration here, the role of sugar in the producing of dental caries, certainly is very timely. Indeed, the nondisclosure of dental health risks in television commercials for sugared products is one of the central issues in the *Childrens Advertising Rule* now under way at the Federal Trade Commission (FTC).

The dual issues — the role that foods containing sugar play in the production of dental caries and other health and nutrition problems, and the role that advertising directed to children plays in conveying possibly misleading information about sugared products — have been under active consideration by industry and government groups at least throughout the past decade. As you are aware, the Federal Trade Commission, whose responsibilities include the regulation of the advertising of foods and other products directed to children, has determined that these significant issues, as well as broader issues relating to the fairness of advertising at all to very young children who do not understand its selling purpose, should be addressed now in a public rulemaking forum. This proceeding will provide the opportunity for many diverse public and private groups to present their viewpoints on these important issues. It is expected that relevant information and opinions will be offered by industry and consumer groups, by the academic community, by the dental, medical and nutrition community, by expert government organizations, and very importantly by the general public. It is anticipated that the hearings will include the views of dental and medical researchers and practitioners, developmental child psychologists, and nutritionists. Experts in children's advertising and marketing research will explain their respective positions on the effects of advertising directed to children. In addition to the expert testimony, I expect that advertising and marketing research studies as well as animal studies and clinical trials relating to the role of sugar in producing dental caries will be placed in the record. I am confident that the same spirit of cooperation shown by the participants of this conference will be present during the Commission's rulemaking proceeding.

Factual and legal issues will be addressed in the Children's Advertising Rulemaking proceeding in a certain setting. I will provide a description of that setting. This will include background about the manner in which the Federal Trade Commission regulates food advertising, including how it resolves underlying scientific issues relating to the performance and safety of food products.

Finally, I would like to provide my response to one of the central questions raised in the agenda of this conference: "What can industry do?"

Before going further, I must state that the views that I express are my own, and not necessarily those of the Commission or of any one Commissioner.

First, I would like to deal with the legal and public policy framework within which the issues of food advertising is addressed by the federal government in general, and the Federal Trade Commission in particular. The health consequences resulting from consumers' food choices, as well as the relatively high percentage of their income that consumers pay for food, dictate from a policy viewpoint that the federal government play a significant role in this vital area. The Food and Drug Administration (FDA), the United States Department of Agriculture (USDA) and the FTC play the principal federal roles in the regulation of food advertising and marketing. For example, the FDA regulates the ingredients which may be added to food, specifies the ingredients a product must contain to be sold under a specified name, and requires certain nutritional information to appear in a standardized format on some food labels: USDA requires the disclosure of ingredients on meat and poultry products and operates a voluntary program under which agricultural products are graded for quality and appearance. At present, USDA permits (but does not require) certain nutrition information to appear on meat and poultry product labels.

The Federal Trade Commission has jurisdiction over unfair and deceptive practices in food advertising and marketing, and over anticompetitive practices in the food industry. With respect to the health implications of food choices, the Commission plays a significant role by regulating the claims made and the information presented in food advertising. It is in this capacity, of course, that the Commission initiated its investigation into advertising directed to children for sugared products.

Because of this shared jurisdiction over food and nutrition matters, and the fact that many of the issues with which the Commission must grapple in this area are also issues which other agencies must address, there is a need for cooperation and coordination with other agencies.* For example, in regulating food advertising, the Commission must decide which statements are likely to be misleading, what information is necessary to prevent deception from claims about food, and how this information can best be conveyed — issues similar to those that FDA or USDA must consider in regulating food labeling. Other issues present similar opportunities to share expertise or conduct joint research with other agencies.

In determinimg whether an advertisement for a food is false and misleading, the Commission considers both the expressed and implied representations contained in an advertisement. It is important to note that the Commission looks to the "net impact" of the ad. In television advertising, filming techniques, such as movement and graphics, background sounds and music, and nuances, as well as the verbal content, are important in conveying a message to consumers; this may be particularly important when the audience is composed of children.

*Since 1971 the FTC and the FDA have had a formal liaison agreement, which specifies that the FTC shall have primary responsibility with respect to the truth or falsity of all advertising of foods, and the FDA shall have primary responsibility for preventing the mislabeling of foods.

An advertisement also can be found to be false and misleading if it fails to disclose important information needed to qualify the advertising claims, or fails to disclose important information with respect to the consequences which may result from use of the product under the customary manner in which it is consumed. As I shall describe below, one of the issues in this proceeding is whether ads directed to children for sugared products are false because they fail to disclose any adverse dental health and nutritional consequences that may follow from overconsumption of these products or from "snacking" on sugared products.

In determining whether food advertising, or advertising for other products, is false and misleading the Commission may use a case by case approach or an industry-wide trade regulation rule. An example of the individual case approach involved the *Wonder Bread* case where the Commission, after reviewing all of the evidence, determined that the "Builds strong bodies twelve ways" campaign falsely represented that Wonder Bread was an extraordinary source of nutrition. The Commission ordered the company to cease disseminating this false advertising campaign.

Rulemaking proceedings are initiated by the Commission where, as in the case of advertising of sugared products to children, the issues presented involve an entire industry or are at least extremely wide-spread. The Commission has been authorized by law to prescribe industry-wide rules which define unfair or deceptive practices and to require remedies to prevent the unfairness of deception. When the Commission initiates a rulemaking proceeding it does so without preconceived notions of whether there have been law violations or whether certain remedies are appropriate; rather, only after the entire proceeding has been completed and the entire record reviewed can the Commission reach final determinations.

There are several advantages to a rulemaking proceeding. First is economy of action. The Commission is able to set standards for advertising for an entire industry in one proceeding, rather than by suing individually the companies comprising an industry. More importantly, it is fairer and more equitable when a standard is set which is applicable to an entire industry rather than only those companies which the Commission has sued. A further advantage of a rulemaking proceeding — which is a public proceeding — is that the Commission is afforded valuable input from as many members of the industry as wish to comment (and not just from a single company under the case by case approach) *and* from associations, consumer groups, the academic and research community, and the rest of the public. This additional input should allow the Commission to make a judgment as informed as is possible in relation to the factual, legal and policy underpinnings of the matters under consideration.

I think it would be of interest to you to turn now to a description of the type of evidence that the Commission finds probative in rulemaking proceedings. It is important to note that the views and opinions of qualified experts, such as the scientific members of this conference, are accorded much evidentiary weight in our proceedings. In past Commission cases and rules, experts who have been qualified to testify by their education, training and experience have been relied upon by the Commission for major medical, as well as communication, findings. Oftentimes these experts are able to refer to scientific studies on point, which they have either conducted or with which they are familiar. Courts have upheld Commission findings concerning health issues based solely on properly qualified expert opinions. For example, in the recent *Listerine* case, the Commission relied on the testimony of virologists, infectious disease specialists, clinical pharmacologists and microbiologists for the conclusion that Listerine mouthwash could not have a therapeutic effect on colds and sore throats. No laboratory or clinical studies were introduced for this proposition. As you can see, expert opinion testimony is very, very important.

Scientific studies relevant to the issues under consideration also are highly probative in Commission cases and rulemaking proceedings. Of course, the purpose for which the study was conducted must be relevant to the specific scientific issues being considered. Further, parties to the rulemaking proceeding may well "cross-examine" the manner in which the study was designed, conducted and analyzed to determine that there are no major defects that would adversely affect the reliability of the findings. In a recent case, the Commission concluded from the testimony of expert clinical researchers that a study offered on behalf of the effectiveness of an over-the-counter drug contained potentially biased results because of a defect in the manner in which the study had been conducted.

Expert opinion evidence and consumer and marketing research often are introduced into Commission proceedings to assist the Commission in determining what the advertisement under challenge "meant" to consumers. These studies also must be designed, conducted and analyzed in an appropriate manner that will insure the reliability of the proffered results.

I must also note that the Federal Trade Commission as an independent regulatory agency that has regulated advertising for more than sixty years, has been afforded an "expertise" to determine the messages of an advertisement without resorting to expert opinion or empirical data. Nevertheless, the Commission has found copy tests and other consumer research to be helpful in assisting it in ascertaining the meanings that flow from advertising campaigns.

Having presented the framework within which the children's advertising rule will be considered, I would like to turn now to a statement of the broad issues presented in this important proceeding. As already noted, the Commission determined that the controversial issues presented in the advertising of sugared and other products to children should be investigated and resolved through the rulemaking process. That decision was based upon recommendation, from such prestigious organizations as the American Dental Association, that the advertising of sugar-rich products to children should be prohibited. The Commission's decision to investigate children's advertising of sugared products has been supported by health and nutrition organizations such as the American Academy of Pediatrics and the Society for Nutrition Education, as well as by one of the most important federal officials dealing with health and nutritional issues, Dr. Donald Kennedy, the Commissioner of the Food and Drug Administration. Further, the Commission's action in proposing a trade regulation proceeding on children's advertising was predicated by petitions filed with the Commission by the following respected consumer organizations: Action for Children's Television, Center for Science in the Public Interest, Consumer's Union, and Commitee on Children's Television.

I believe that both the extensive amount of television directed to children, and the themes contained in that advertising justify that the Commission consider the issues raised by the prestigious organizations. Children are exposed to more than 20,000 television advertisements directed to them each year. The majority of these advertisements are for sugared products such as candy, cookies and pre-sweetened cereals. Our monitoring of the three commercial networks on Saturday morning, April 22, 1978 revealed that 58% of the children's commercials were for sugared products.

A large proportion of the foods advertised to children on Saturday (or Sunday) day-time television are ready-to-eat cereals. Many of these are between 40 and 60% sugar. In the most extreme case, the sugar content exceeds 70%. Further, these sugared products are advertised to children almost to the exclusion of any other foods — the principal *apparent* exception being fast-food restaurants whose products include such sugared items as desserts, "thick shakes," and carbonated soft drinks. In fact, of the food ads directed to children on that Saturday morning in April, 81% were foods containing sugar.

I would like to read a consecutive list of food commercials observed on a random Saturday this past summer (July 29, 1978, 8:30 - 11:00 am, CBS): Nestle $100,000 Candy Bar, Kool-Aid, Cap'n Crunch pre-sweetened cereal, Honeycomb pre-sweetened cereal, Kool-Aid, Cap'n Crunch pre-sweetened cereal, McDonald's Shake, Cap'n Crunch pre-sweetened cereal, McDonald's Hamburger and Shake, Kool-Aid, Nestle's Crunch Candy Bar, Coco Krispies pre-sweetened cereal, Sugar Crisp pre-sweetened cereal, Kool-Aid, Eggo Waffles, Cap'n Crunch pre-sweetened cereal, McDonald's Shake, Post Alphabits pre-sweetened cereal, McDonalds Shake, Bubble Yum Bubble Gum, Cheerios Cereal, Nestle's Quick, Cookie Crisp pre-sweetened cereal, Burger King Hamburgers, Snickers Candy Bar, Cracker Jack, Cookie Crisp pre-sweetened cereal, and Honey Comb pre-sweetened cereal.

Millions of dollars are spent annually in designing and disseminating advertisements that are effective in creating a demand for sugared products in ways that may be deceptive or unfair to children. Communication experts relying on sophisticated marketing research measuring the effectiveness of different advertising techniques on children are able to design enormously persuasive advertisements. One expert, who has studied the effects of advertising on children for several years, concludes that the 30-second television commercial is the most effective device ever invented to implant an idea in a child's mind.

The advertising themes one finds in commercials for sugared products directed to children often are that eating sugar is desirable and fun; that this is the normal, accepted way to satisfy hunger, either at breakfast or between meals; and that boys and girls who do this are healthy and happy, with no signs of tooth decay, obesity or any other problem.

Very importantly, these ads contain no warnings about the threat of dental caries that can result from over-consumption of sugared products of from between meal snacking of these products. In this context the ads may be deceptive.

In general, the advertisements make no reference to the nutritional qualities of foods. Therefore it is not surprising that only 3% of the children in one study cited nutrition as a reason for requesting cereal.

As part of our efforts to determine whether material facts about dental health risks have been omitted from advertising, one of the underlying issues in this proceeding will be whether the consumption of sugared products by children produces dental caries. In a report prepared for the FDA by the Federation of American Societies for Experimental Biology, sucrose, which is one substance found in most sugared products advertised to children, was found to be one of the most cariogenic substances. The report listed among the characteristrics which could influence the cariogenicity of products the frequency of their consumption, the duration of the exposure of the sugar in the mouth, and the form of the sucrose. It has been suggested that between meal snacking of sugared products is a particularly harmful pattern of consumption likely to contribute to tooth decay.

Another major issue in the proceeding will turn on the effects of advertising of sugared products on children. Does this advertising present a misleading picture resulting in over-consumption of sugared products, which in turn leads to dental decay in children? Does certain of the advertising affirmatively urge children to consume candy and other sugared products between meals while failing to disclose to children the dental risks associated with over-consumption and snacking of sugared products? Remember, I stated earlier that the Commission is required to find that advertising is deceptive if it fails to disclose to the intended audience any health risks associated with the customary use of the product. Collateral issues under this question include whether certain sugared products are consumed between meals, whether this consumption results in the formation of dental caries, and whether children are aware of the risk of consuming the product in this manner.

Another major issue in this proceeding is whether the advertising for sugar products conveys to children an inaccurate perception of the role of sugar in a well-balanced diet. Does such advertising shape the nutritional beliefs of children? Consumer research suggests the effectiveness of advertising in shaping the beliefs about the value of sugar. For example, in a survey of children 4 to 12 years old, one question asked whether the child thought that "sugar is good for you." Among heavy viewers of Saturday morning television (2 or more hours), 23% said that sugar was beneficial.

Aside from the dental health and nutritional issues raised by the advertising of sugared products to children, this proceeding is investigating the fairness of advertising any product to young children aged seven and under. Research seems to indicate that these young children may not comprehend the sales purpose of an advertisement. Unlike adults, they may not understand that they are being advertised to, and because of this lack of understanding tend to place indiscriminate trust in the advertising. Yet these children can play back names of products that are advertised and are motivated to want the product and to demand it of their parents. Assuming it is proven that young children fail to understand the selling purpose of advertising, is it fair to direct advertising to them as is currently done?

There is also evidence indicating that young children have not developed the cognitive skills necessary to perceive correctly the advertising directed at them. Child psychologists have demonstrated that children's sensory-motor intelligence processes are limited at young ages and mature only in slow stages, that their apprehension of space and time and causality are confused, that their mental images are concrete and not abstract, and that they lack adult notions of judgment. Assuming this lack of cognitive development in a young child, will that child inherently be deceived by television advertising?

I have taken some time to explain both the major issues that will be considered in the Children's Advertising Rulemaking proceeding and the legal and policy framework within which these issues will be addressed. In doing so my intent has been to provide information that you might find helpful in deciding whether to make a formal comment in these proceedings. While I am a staff member at the Commission, I want to assure you that in a rulemaking proceeding it is my job to insure that the Commission receives a full range of comments on the many issues presented. That includes views on the themes contained in advertising and its capacity to deceive children through omission of information relating to dental health and nutritional issues. It would be particularly appropriate to receive comments from the various participants of this conference as to the role that sugared products play in the production of dental caries. More specifically, it would be helpful to have your views about what the characteristics of sugared products are that determine whether that product will produce dental caries. Research about the relative cariogenicity of food products, of course, would be very relevant to this proceeding. At this point, what reasonable judgments can be made about those products that are and are not cariogenic? What preventive measures including dietary modification are likely to be feasible and particularly effective in preventing caries?

The Commission also would welcome your views on what, if any, appropriate remedies you believe would be effective in dealing with the advertising of sugared and other products to children. The remedies that might be appropriate include prohibiting certain techniques in children's advertising, such as host selling and certain themes, such as that "snacking" of sugared products is desirable; require affirmative disclosures within the context of ads concerning dental and other health warnings and nutritional messages; require affirmative disclosures outside the ads, perhaps in separate 30-second public service announcements;** and prohibit advertising to children too young to understand its selling purpose, and advertising of the most cariogenic products.

The remedies involve difficult questions about their effectiveness and their feasibility. The Commission will choose the remedy least onerous to the industry which will be effective in dealing with any problems found to flow from advertising directed to children. We hope that we will receive comments about these remedies from many different facets of the public, including children's advertisers and the manufacturers of sugared products.

**I note that the American Dental Association has participated in the development of television spots intended to inform children of the dental harms associated with the consumption of sugar. Other organizations have developed spots on nutrition themes. Unfortunately, very few of these spot messages appear on television, especially in relation to the 7,000 advertisements that appear annually on television urging the consumption of sugared products.

My answer as to what industry can do regarding the question of the role sugar plays in the production of dental caries is the same answer I would propose to the rest of the public. I would urge all of you to bring your expertise and your opinions to the Children's Advertising Rulemaking proceeding and assist in building a complete record upon which the Commission can base its conclusions regarding an issue that is important to all of us.

I can assure you that the Commission is engaging in an open and impartial review of these important issues. In announcing this rulemaking proceeding, the Commision emphasized that it needed input from the public before an informed decision could be reached as to whether there was a need to take action and, if so, what the appropriate action should be. I urge you to assist the Commission in its search for truth.

The remarks of this statement represent only the views of a member of the Federal Trade Commission staff. They are not intended to be, and should not be construed as, representative of offical Commission policy.

DISCUSSION

Mr. Choate: How and when people can comment to the FTC on this issue?

Mr. Snyder: The written comments are due on November 24. They can be filed by individuals or by groups, and they simply have to be sent to the Federal Trade Commision, and those comments will be put on the public record, will be put in the rulemaking record, and will be considered. People may testify orally in hearings that will start in January in San Francisco, and then will continue in Washington.

Dr. Ayer: There is question as to whether the child understands or even carries away after that point of exposure any understanding of what it is you have done to try to educate him, stemming from Piagetian concepts about the cognitive development of the child. He can parrot back facts, but be doesn't understand those facts. Do you really believe that controlling advertising at this level will have any impact? At this level of cognitive development of the child, it is only an instantaneous kind of thing, a here-and-now kind of thing that he doesn't take away later on.

Mr. Synder: As to the effects of advertising on a young child, we have seen some studies indicating that it is effective in the sense that the child wants to have the product, is able to take that much away from the commercial, is able to recall what the product was, and wants the product.

Yet, it may be, and some studies may demonstrate, that the child is deceived as to what the product can do and what it cannot do. The ultimate result of that, I suppose, is that the child was not happy with the product. That, to me, is an injury that needs to be managed. It can result in an economic injury.

Turning the question around, if there are problems of cognitive development of children, one might ask why the ads for those products are not directed to adults rather than to children, thereby avoiding the issue altogether.

Dr. Schiff: My problem with the whole issue is really one of timing. I have been involved in this program of the American Dental Association for some 2 1/2 years. We listened for two major conferences to well-known scientists, leaders in their field, who cannot yet agree about what is carciogenic, how to measure cariogenicity, the extent of which sugar is causative or noncausative, etc. Now I hear that you are going to make decisions within the next four to six months, when we scientists are trying to plan a very concentrated program to assess the truth of the statements you are trying to investigate.

Wouldn't that become very harmful to the industry which is now trying to solve the problem — to try to prejudge that they are wrong before scientists make a decision? Nobody really can prove these things to be harmful to children when we really don't know.

Mr. Synder: The answer to that question will come at the conclusion of the hearings, when all of the evidence of the clinical studies now in existence is reviewed and a decision is made as to whether there is enough evidence now at least to make certain judgments about certain foods.

The Commission certainly could not go beyond what that evidence demonstrates at the time. We are going to have to wait to see the record. Some people may be of the opinion that there is sufficient evidence, at least in regard to certain products, to form conclusions. That is why we need comments in the record.

Dr. Geiselman: This can go to the extremes. For example, would you consider hearings on the fact one may die of metal poisoning by the collision of a truck with a passenger car? I think the principle applies all the way down the line to advertising of any type. And it may end up that we don't have any television advertising at all.

Mr. Synder: The question has been raised, why pick children's advertising? Why not pick other types of advertising? We have a program at the Agency which is not focused just on children's advertising, and we try to make selections based upon the public interest and whether there is injury.

Mr. Geiselman: I can't believe that any child has ever died of tooth decay, to be absolutely honest with you. And I would like to see the American Dental Association or anyone else decide that sugar cannot be used as a table-top sweetener or even in food manufacture.

Mr. Synder: Well, I don't think you would urge that the Commission be stopped from proceeding against false advertising unless there was a chance of death occurring. There is a lot of economic injury in advertising, and I don't think that we should really take lightly dental decay and the cost of that to the public in health and medical bills each year.

Dr. DePaola: Do you perceive that the Federal Trade Commission is going to engage in a parenting job?

Mr. Synder: No.

Dr. DePaola: Isn't that part of the issue?

Mr. Synder: That is not the issue at all. The issue is one of deception in advertising. For years, the Commission has brought actions in the area of children's advertising so that children would not be deceived by advertising. I don't think that you would want to create a free fire zone for deceptive advertising to children, and we don't either. There is just no reason why advertising directed to children should be deceptive, and our mandate from Congress is to prohibit that sort of thing.

Nor do I want to try to interject myself into the role between the child and the parent. My concern is to make sure that the advertising is non-deceptive.

Dr. Alfano: You indicated that your primary goal was to obtain as fair a hearing as possible. And I am sure you are aware that the FTC issued a number of contracts or grants to a variety of agencies to assist in developing an additional data base for these hearings. Are you aware of some of the grants that have been given?

Mr. Synder: Yes.

Dr. Alfano: One was awarded to the Society for Nutrition Education (SNE), and as a member of that Society, I received a letter not too long ago in which the first paragraph indicated that, "As you know, advertising about food on children's television programs has drawn a great deal of professional and popular discussion. The Society for Nutrition Education is conducting a survey to ascertain SNE members' views on this issue. The study is being conducted under contract with the Federal Trade Commission." Are you familiar with this survey?

Mr. Synder: Yes.

Dr. Alfano: Well, I would have to make the comment that it is probably the most biased survey I have ever seen, with one exception, and that was a survey that was printed in Prevention Magazine about the use of calcium. For the benefit of the people in the audience who haven't seen some of the questions, I would like to read some of them.

"The amount of sugar which most children consume nowadays is" and there are three answers, "much too much, a little too much, and about right." There isn't room for someone to say that it is not enough, or it is a possibility that should be considered.

Another question: "Television advertising for sugared products during children's programming interferes with what children should know in order to choose a nutritious diet."

"Television commercials for sugared products on children's programming help professional nutritionists to do their job."

And finally, "Television advertising during children's programming encourages eating patterns that include too much sugar in the diet." It would appear to me that there is some effort in this document to lead the witness, to lead the members of the the Society for Nutrition Education down a primrose path. And as members of SNE, some of my colleagues and I have expressed a concern about the nature of this survey.

Mr. Synder: If you are correct, you will have a perfect right to challenge that survey in the rulemaking proceeding. If you believe that the survey was not conducted correctly, that should be an issue that should be investigated. The rulemaking proceeding is large enough to consider that issue.

Dr. Alfano: I know that the Society of Dentistry for Children was contacted about doing a similar survey, and I assume many other groups were as well. I would echo Dr. Schiff's concern about the rush to enter into these proceedings. It seems to me that a survey of people in the field is not the kind of information you need. You need data, you need research, and perhaps you should postpone this thing until some of this data is available.

Mr. Synder: We certainly welcome data, and I believe that there will be data, and I think that everybody will know on November 24 how much data there is. And then we all can make more informed judgments.

Dr. Schiff: Recently, the California Supreme Court, if I remember correctly, had a case in which something happened to a young lady immediately following a television program which was aired at a time of availability of children. The Supreme Court threw that case out, based on the fact that whatever is going on on television was not intended to incite the viewer. I know it is an entirely different issue. But the fact was that something happened on television which children had followed. What you are saying is children follow television advertisement suggestions. It is the same kind of concept.

Mr. Synder: That case did not involve commerical advertising. It involved television programming, a field with which the Federal Trade Commission has nothing to do whatsoever. The Supreme Court did not reach a decision on it; the lower court judge did, and I imagine someday that issue will be fully addressed by the Supreme Court. But there is a distinction between advertising and program content. Commercial speech does have first Admendment protections, and I think that is the intent of your question. That is true. However, the Supreme Court in the Virginia Board case made it clear that false advertising or deceptive advertising was not protected. It is not protected speech. The First Amendment can't be raised. And we believe that any action that we would take ultimately, if we did take an action, would be based on deception or falsity, or on fairness, and therefore it would make an exception to the rule.

Dr. Bahn: There is a scientific question that you did not enunciate, one that is worthwhile. Since the introduction of sweetened breakfast cereals, has there been an increase in caries in children in the United States?

Mr. Synder: I suppose that is one way to look at the question. I suppose there is another way as well, and that is the way that you have been talking about here, which is to look at the role of the product and the characteristics of the product in producing caries. I don't know the answer to your question, but maybe someone else does.

Dr. Bahn: When I was younger, if you wanted to reward a child, you gave him a piece of candy. And we had caries under those circumstances. That was the villain. Now the villain seems to be pre-sweetened cereals. Is it really the villain?

Mr. Synder: Oh, I see. You mean your concern is that we are singling out pre-sweetened cereals.

Dr. Bahn: Or something else.

Mr. Synder: The question is as broad as sugared products. I am not suggesting that pre-sweetened cereals are causing more problems than other products. I don't know that. I am just saying that the entire range of products includes pre-sweetened cereals.

Dr. Bahn: Since this advertising has come up, has there been increase in the disease in the United States.

Mr. Synder: Well, we would have to compare a time period from the time before television to now. I would imagine caries figures are available. I imagine there would be other controls that would have to be looked at.

Dr. Mackay: When was the Federal Trade Commission created?

Mr. Synder: 1914.

Dr. Mackay: When was the Federal Communications Commission created?

Mr. Synder: 1924, when we only had radio.

Dr. Mackay: Well, Life Savers started in about 1908 and has been advertising continuously and heavily since 1908. With newspapers carrying advertising, we used newspapers; with magazines, we used magazines; when radio came in, which had an enormous psychological impact, we used radio very, very heavily. When television came, obviously we used television.

Why TV? Why has it taken since 1914 to recognize the problem? Why doesn't it just say radio advertising, magazine advertising, newspaper advertising, word-of-mouth advertising?

Why sugar? If there is an issue here, it is that there shouldn't be advertising on television to children; that television by its nature has a particular combination of oral and visual inputs that are persuasive. What we are objecting to is the persuasiveness of that particular medium, and that it is wrong to persuade children, I think that is the point Dr. Choate has made many times. That is, apart from the substances about which you are trying to persuade them, it has got nothing to do with the fact that it is sugar.

Therefore, the question is, why sugar? Isn't sugar somehow being made the scapegoat? It is just possible that someone has said, "We have got to make a case to make it believable that there is something wrong about television. What can we pick on."

What are they advertising to children? Sugar. Therefore, you pick on sugar because it is the best handle you have for making your point. Maybe it wouldn't be quite as persuasive if you tried to talk about it was bad to persuade children on toys, or bad to persuade children not to stick their fingers into an electric plug, because it is still persuasion, and if you are going to be consistent, it is the persuasion that is bad, not what you are persuading about.

And if it is going to be sugar — I will even concede sugar — why do we pick caries of all things? I mean sugar has had its day. Claims have been made that it caused obesity, sugar caused diabetes; sugar has caused heart disease and caries. Why do you pick on caries? Is it just because the heart disease thing has sort of faded? Is it because the diabetes thing has faded. Is it just that caries is the only thing left?

My questions are: Why TV? Why sugar? Why caries?

Mr. Synder: First, why TV in this proceeding? Because TV happens to be the medium that is used, almost to the exclusion of the others, in regard to the advertising to children. There is advertising in comic books to children. That is being looked into, but not as part of this proceeding.

Why sugar? Because of the concerns that have been raised — and I think by your discussions in the conference — there seems to be at least a credible viewpoint that there are problems perhaps associated with sugar. And if that is true, our concern at the FTC is what the advertising has to do with that role. If there is a problem in the way it is consumed, the federal statute under which we operate says that should be disclosed to the intended consumer, who is the child.

Why only caries? That has been the focus of my talk, but concerns have also been raised which will be addressed in the proceeding about the effects of sugar on other health diseases, such as obesity, diabetes and heart disease.

Sugar is not the only issue in the proceeding; I highlighted that. There is the whole question of the fairness of advertising to young children of any product, assuming it is shown that they cannot understand the sales message.

And finally, why not pick a lot of other products? The statute is broad enough that the Commission has picked adult products where there had to be disclosures so that the product could be used safely and so that people would not suffer injury.

So that is of concern to the Commission.

You may know the FCC also has an investigation under way into children's advertising. Over the years, we had liaison with the FCC. They have a responsibility principally in regard to children's programming. They are concerned about the amount of children's advertising, and in the past they have taken action, which although formerly not done by them, has led to industry groups lowering the number of ads that have been on television. They could probably do more things. But our concern is with the advertising to children and that is in our mandate.

Mr. Kelly: You stated that the purpose of the hearings is to seek the truth, and you, as a lawyer, must certainly know that the answers you receive can very much be determined by the questions you ask. I was troubled by the fact that you said that the hearings are trying to find the effect of sugar on dental caries.

Well, I would say that is somewhat parallel to saying what is the effect of the automobile on the death rate in this country, how do cigarettes affect lung cancer in this counrty, or are you still beating your wife? The possible answers are limited. You are not asking a broader question of what is the role of cereals in nutrition in our society, or what are the implications of candy to children. These are enormously broader and have far more possibilities than your questions offer the opportunity to answer.

Are you seeking total truth or selective truth?

I would ask whether you aren't just exploring what is politically tolerable and probably politically motivated. What actions are being taken right now on advertising of alcohol? What actions are being taken on advertising of tobacco?

And I won't be content with saying we have them off television, because that plays right back into the political motivation. That seems to be politically acceptable, but not scientifically acceptable.

Mr. Synder: The issues in regard to sugar should not be limited by my statement of them. Anyone who wishes to comment and frame the issues as he thinks they should be framed in a rulemaking proceeding should do so.

The Commission's rulemaking announcement placed many, many questions as examples; we want a full range of issues. My framing of the issues will not be important; the evidence that comes in, and what that ultimately shows will be decisive.

Second, in regard to alcohol and tobacco, giving you my personal views, the regulation of the tobacco advertising is regulated in my division. I don't think that there is anything wrong with asking the question: do cigarettes cause lung cancer? And I don't think that there is any reason that we shouldn't be looking hard at cigarette advertising, and we are doing do. We have required the warnings to be in the print advertising since early 1970. We don't have any control over the package of the cigarette; that is regulated by Congress. But we are monitoring cigarette advertising. We have been in a fight for the last two years to get data from the cigarette companies in regard to the effects of their advertising.

I can't quarrel with you about alcohol advertising either. That is an issue with which the Commission has not had as much investigational experience, but you may know that we are now conducting a joint research project with three other government agencies that seeks to find out the advertising themes that are in alcohol advertising.

I appreciate your concern, but I don't think that there are political implications in this. Any action the Commission takes ultimately has to be based on deception or unfairness, which is going to be reviewed by a Court of Appeals, and if the record is not there for deception or unfairness, it won't stand up.

XIII. FOODS AND FOOD PROCESSING

Ray G. Kelly, Chairman

SEQUENTIAL STEPS FROM IDEA TO MARKET: LEGAL IMPLICATIONS OF NONCARIOGENIC AND ANTICARIOGENIC PRODUCT DEVELOPMENT

David H. Hickman, J.D.

The attempted regulatory road map may appear to some more like a Monopoly board with many spaces marked "stop, do not pass," and few, indeed, that even intimate the existence of Boardwalk or Park Place. Any legal discussion of the steps from concept to marketing of a product for which special claims of noncariogenic or anticariogenic properties are to be made will contain many caveats and warning signs, but they are not intended to discourage. Rather, they are provided to offer some assurance that there may be identifiable paths through the mass of legal requirements and regulations which, if followed carefully, can lead to the results that are desired.

As to a second possibly unwelcome message that might be derived from these remarks, I was less sanguine that I could offer solace. Nevertheless I am compelled to observe that if you move forward with a project in the area of discussion with the purpose of successful marketing and with the intent that the project advance at every stage as smoothly as possible, then inevitably you shall spend considerable time in the company of lawyers.

In fact, it approaches misrepresentation to seek to lay out in a single time span considerations that relate to every phase of product development from the conception of the idea to marketing. It would be a more accurate reflection of the lawyers' proper role in the process, if I had been permitted a few opening remarks at the outset of this program and then appeared after every second speaker to give a progress report on how the legal hurdles had been cleared.

In the beginning, there is a product concept. It is an undertaking to develop and promote a product which has some special benefit in terms of dental health. In the course of development, that concept will be refined by the judgment of individuals with many different professional trainings and viewpoints — in particular, management, science and law. It is imperative that everyone who will have an ulitmate influence on the project participate in the decision-making process from the earliest stages, because initial elections among options will have significant ramifications for the project throughout the years of its development. Management, for example, will at the outset have to make such critical decisions as whether to venture into the operation of a drug establishment, with the ensuing required compliance with drug good manufacturing practices, which are significantly different from those applied to foods. The technical staff will have to evaluate myriad questions, including the feasibility of producing a particular product with a specific ingredient and the possibility that other product ingredients or processing itself may adversely affect the properties of that ingredient. Scientific consultants must evaluate the likelihood that a given ingredient in a projected delivery system can be clinically demonstrated to accomplish the desired effect. Each of these evaluations will have to be made against the background of the applicable legal requirements. Finally, those who will be responsible for the promotion of the ultimate product, and must persuade the consumer that it is in fact useful and benefical to him, must evaluate the kinds of statements they will need to be able to make to accomplish that objective.

This final category of participants may be the most important to the early decision-making process, because it will largely be the claims that are made for the product which will determine the regulatory hurdles that it must surmount.

A product will be regulated not so much for what it inherently is, as for what is said about it. It is largely within the power of the promoter to make it a food, a drug, a cosmetic, a combination of any of those, or all three.

At this point, it becomes important to consider some legal learning. Inescapably, at the most fundamental level, the course of the product development project is governed by a statute and by the intent of the Congress that enacted that statute.

The Federal Food, Drug and Cosmetic Act contains definitions of a food, a drug and a cosmetic. Section 201 (f) of the Act states that food means "(1) articles used for food or drink for man or other animals, (2) chewing gum, and (3) articles used for components of any such article."

The definition of a drug, found in Section 201 (g) of the Act, is considerably more complex. It includes articles listed in the United States Pharmacopoeia and the National Formulary as well as in the homeopathic pharmacopoeia. It includes articles intended for use in the diagnosis, cure, mitigation, treatment or prevention of disease — including, of course, dental disease, of which dental caries is one example. It also includes "articles (other than food) intended to affect the structure or any function of the body of man or other animals."

A cosmetic is any article that is intended to be rubbed, poured, sprinkled, or sprayed on, introduced into, or otherwise applied to the human body or any part thereof, for cleansing, beautifying, promoting attractiveness, or altering the appearance.

The significant feature of these definitions is that they all make reference to the "intended" use of an article. It is the intended use of the article, as determined by the claims made for it, and not necessarily its inherent nature, which will determine its legal status under the Act.

Moreover, it is quite clear that the Congress which enacted this statute recognized and sanctioned that result. A 1943 Senate report accompanying the legislation contains the following discussion:

> The use to which the product is to be put will determine the category under which it will fall. If it is used only as a food, it will fall under the definition food and none other. If it contains nutritive ingredients and is sold for drug use only, as clearly shown by the labeling and advertising, it will come within the definition of a drug but not that of a food. If it is sold to be used both as a food and for the prevention of disease, it would satisfy both definitions and be subject to the substantive requirements for both. The manufacturer of the article, through his representations in connection with its sale, can determine the use to which the article is to be put. For example, the manufacturer of a laxative which is medicated candy or chewing gum, can bring his product within the definition of a drug and escape that of food by representing the article fairly and unequivocally as a drug product.

The law and the legislative history, are quite clear that intended use will control classification. What is not so clear is how various statements that might be made about a product will be interpreted by the regulatory authorities with respect to intent.

There are some apparent lines of demarcation. A statement that a product will prevent tooth decay — that it is anticariogenic — will most certainly be treated as a drug claim. It is a statement that the product is useful in the prevention or mitigation of a disease.

Similarly, it is accepted on the basis of long-standing administrative interpretation at the Food and Drug Administration that a food product which is noncariogenic may be described by the phrase "does not promote tooth decay." Deviations from this standard language may be viewed skeptically by the agency, and fairly recent internal documents circulated at the FDA have even questioned whether the synonymous, single word statement of this proposition — "noncariogenic" — should not be considered as transforming the production into a drug. A contrary view was suggested in the preamble to the final order on labeling of special dietary foods published by the FDA on September 22. Responding to objections against a requirement that products promoted as useful to dental health and labeled as "sugarless" carry an express disclaimer of reduced caloric value, FDA suggested that this crepe labeling could be avoided by the use of product benefit descriptive language which was more narrowly focused — like "noncariogenic."

Finally, statements about "whiter, brighter teeth," are certainly cosmetic, so long as the content in which they are made has reference to the appearance of the teeth, and not their health.

Having emphasized the importance of claims, it is necessary to express the caveat that the mechanism of action of ingredients may also be considered in determining regulatory classification. At one extreme, it is apparent that a potent prescription drug may not be transformed into a food simply because only food claims are made for it. Other provisions of the law, dealing with adulteration and the required approval of food additives, can be brought into play by the agency to prevent such manipulations.

Other situations fall much closer to the borderline between foods and drugs and attorneys in the private sector and those at the FDA might view them quite differently. One example of such a situation is the use of a food ingredient which, rather than substituting for a cariogenic ingredient in a product, neutralizes or counteracts the cariogenic potential of that ingredient. There are suggestions that FDA will consider any measure other than simple substitution to render a product a drug. Perhaps the better reasoning would lead one to conclude that any action which renders an individual product itself noncariogenic, whether by substitution of ingredients or manipulation of ingredients, falls within the category of food production and that only those products whose activity occurs exogenously, at the surface of the tooth, or systemically, should be classified as drugs.

An early decision as to the kind of product intended to be marketed is critical, because the regulatory requirements for the marketing of a food and a drug are quite different, as are the timetables that might be projected between product concept and inital marketing. For present purposes, cosmetics will be left aside, as they appear to be peripheral to the primary interests under consideration.

One decision that may be reached is to market a food product that will be promoted for its noncariogenic properties, which will be accomplished by the substitution in the food of an ingredient not associated with caries production for one that is associated with caries production.

At the outset, it must be determined whether it is presently permissible to use that ingredient in a food for the particular intended technical function. Under the Federal Food, Drug and Cosmetic Act, it is illegal to employ a food additive unless its use has been approved by the FDA. That does not mean that in every instance food ingredients must have a specific prior approval by the Food and Drug Administration, since the definition of a "food additive" in the Act excludes those substances which are generally recognized by qualified experts as safe for their intended purpose — the so-called GRAS (generally recognized as safe) substances.

After the passage of the Food Additives Amendment in 1958, Food and Drug Administration published a list of those items which it had concluded to be GRAS. In addition, over the years, manufacturers undertook the use of many food ingredients, without discussion with the FDA, on an independent conclusion of general recognition of safety, based on available literature and on scientific opinion.

The FDA recently has been seeking very narrowly to limit, if not to eliminate those situations in which a manufacturer can move forward with a new use of a food ingredient on his own determination of GRAS status. For the last decade, the agency has been reviewing the safety of those ingredients which it has blessed, as well as those whose use had been undertaken independently. An extensive survey of industry use of these ingredients was undertaken by the National Academy of Sciences-National Research Council. The literature concerning their safety was collected by independent contractors. Daily diet studies were made, on the basis of which the exposure of various classes of consumers to these ingredients was projected. Finally, all of these data were provided to the Select Committee on GRAS Substances (SCOGS) at the Federated American Societies for Experimental Biology (FASEB), which has been providing comprehensive safety evaluations to the Food and Drug Administration.

On the basis of these evaluations, the FDA has been making specific regulatory proposals with respect to each of these ingredients. Some have been affirmed as GRAS; some have been affirmed as GRAS with specified limitations on use; some have been placed on interim food additive status while further safety testing is undertaken; and some have been regulated as food additives.

It is important that in each of these types of regulation, FDA has generally spelled out the specific food categories of use, the technological functions, and the specific levels of use which have been evaluated in reaching the GRAS determination. Even in the most liberal category—GRAS affirmation—the agency has cautioned that a manufacturer undertakes a use significantly different than those reflected in the regulation at his peril.

It is implicit in this regulatory scheme that the FDA is making safety determinations based on projected human exposure to ingredients as compared with available safety data. Clearly, any decision about whether an ingredient may be employed without prior consultation with the FDA, or whether an amendment of a GRAS regulation should be sought, or a GRAS affirmation petition filed, cannot be reached without a careful evaluation of the potential increased human exposure to the ingredient if the proposed product were indeed to become commercially successful.

If there are not available data on which to base or urge a GRAS determination, then a food additive petition will have to be filed. Initially, extensive animal safety testing will have to be undertaken, which can be both time consuming and expensive. It will require short term and long term toxicity testing, in several species. It is unlikely today that a petition could be approved without at least some investigation of the mutagenic potential of the ingredient, and its carcinogenic potential.

It is important to recognize that so long as this testing is being conducted, and so long as the petition is pending, it is not legal to employ the ingredient in food production. The exception to this prohibition is a provision in the Food, Drug, and Cosmetic Act which requires the Commissioner of the Food and Drug Administration to promulgate regulations for investigational use of food additives by qualified experts prior to their approval, where he concludes that use to be consistent with the public health.

FDA has never promulgated human investigation regulations under this provision. It would not be unreasonable to expect, however, that a program for investigational use submitted to the agency which in general outline followed the requirements for the use of investigational new drugs, might meet with agency approval.

Consideration of this possibility is important in dealing with a substance which must receive food additive approval, because in addition to demonstrating its safety for use, it will be necessary to accumulate some evidence that the ingredient will accomplish the purpose for which it will be promoted.

Both the Food and Drug Administration and the Federal Trade Commission take a keen interest in the accuracy of any special benefit claims made for a new food product. In fact, the Federal Trade Commission has enunciated a doctrine which holds it to be a violation of the FTC Act not to have accumulated information which provides the reasonable basis for the making of a claim in advance of the time at which the claim is made. That the claim might subsequently be shown to be accurate is no defense. The Federal Food, Drug and Cosmetic Act prohibits the making of false and misleading statements in labeling.

It is not clear what kinds and quantities of data would be necessary to meet these legal standards in the case of a food product promoted on the basis that it does not promote tooth decay. Indeed, there are those at the FDA who have taken the position that there are not presently adequate data to support this claim for currently promoted products utilizing traditional ingredients. Implicit acknowledgment of this category of products can be gleaned, however, from the final order on the labeling of special dietary foods.

The product development process for a noncariogenic food, then, is one which will clearly cover an extended time span. It is not possible to overstate the need for periodic review of progress on the project, particularly involving scientific and legal advisers. Minor modifications in protocols, for example, may substantially affect the scientific sufficiency of the results. Failure adequately to monitor for scientific and legal sufficiency the work being done can result in years of wasted effort.

If it is concluded that the product to be marketed will be a drug, wholly different legal requirements are applicable. As with the foods, there are two categories of drug ingredients to be considered. The statutory definition of a "new drug" exempts those ingredients which are generally recognized as safe and effective (GRAS and GRAE) for use under the conditions prescribed, recommended, or suggested in their labeling by experts qualified by scientific training and experience to make that determination. These are so-called "old drugs."

For drug products there is a statutory requirement that effectiveness — the fact that they work—be demonstrated as part of the approval or judgmental process. Demonstration of effectiveness is required to be shown by controlled clinical studies. The question of the difficulties attendant upon the conduct of such studies is the subject of another presentation, and will not be detailed here. It is noteworthy, however, that a Food and Drug Administration Advisory Committee has recommended to the FDA that, at least in the context of studies proposed to be undertaken on chewing gum products, the use of a sugar product as a control was unethical, and the FDA concurred in this conclusion. Among the other various problems to be faced are the presence of fluoride in water supplies, and the general difficulty of attempting to enforce a strictly controlled dietary regimen, or even obtaining accurate recording and reporting of dietary habits.

With respect to old drugs, there is underway at the FDA a program similar to the GRAS review, in which advisory panels are reviewing the available data on the safety and effectiveness of over-the-counter drugs and making recommendations to the FDA as to their future regulatory status. Ultimately, FDA is publishing monographs governing the status of broad classes of OTC products. As you are undoubtedly aware, one of these advisory panels has dental products within its jurisdiction.

A number of ingredients that have not previously been widely used in this country have been submitted to that panel for its review. A primary difficulty that they have encountered is based on the unwillingness of FDA as a general proposition to accept human experience in populations in other countries in support of the use of a product in this country, and its reluctance to accord clinical investigations conducted in other parts of the world the same weight as is accorded clinical investigations conducted domestically.

It is apparently FDA's position that when this review has been completed, the world of GRAS and GRAE will have been defined, and any new ingredients will have to receive agency sanction either through a monograph amendment or under an NDA prior to marketing.

If the ingredient under consideration meets the definition of a new drug, and it should be emphasized that "new" in this context is not limited to a newly discovered ingredient, but includes new uses of old ingredients, the filing of an investigational new drug application will be required. As with food ingredients, extensive acute and chronic toxicity testing in animals is required. This testing can be done prior to the filing of the IND (investigational new drugs).

The regulations governing the IND process and new drug applications are indeed extensive, and, by their reporting requirements, give the FDA a significant authority over the project being conducted. While the agency does not have to approve protocols for clinical tests, they must be submitted for review and can be disapproved.

A significant consideration in the review of a potential drug product is whether it is one that will be restricted to sale by prescription, or permitted to be available over-the-counter. Essentially, the resolution of this question will turn on whether adequate directions for use can be written to permit the consumer safely and effectively to use the product. Obviously, this also has implications for the form and manner in which the product will be offered to the consumer. For example, if the delivery system for the drug is to be a food, and a single dose of the drug achieves the maximum necessary effect, it would not be desirable to deliver the drug in a food which is likely to be consumed *ad libitum*. Similarly, it would not be desirable to introduce the drug into a wide variety of foods which constitute part of the average daily diet, as again unnecessary multiple dosing might occur regularly.

Similar practical questions, with significant legal implications, would occur in the context of determining the classes of foods in which a noncariogenic ingredient was to be utilized. Both the FDA and the FTC might reasonably take the view that there was deception involved in the heavy promotion of a product as noncariogenic, when significant numbers of other products in the same category, without modification, did not exhibit a significant cariogenic potential, or where general use of the product category was not thought to be a significant contributory factor to the problem of dental caries.

Once a product has been shown to be safe and useful, be it a food or a drug, the problem of labeling must be addressed. In most instances, there are specific regulations which state precisely what must be said about the product, and where on the product package that information must be located. In the case of foods which are to be promoted as "sugarless," "sugar free" or the like, an additional labeling requirement was added by the recently published special dietary labeling regulations. If any of these terms is used in labeling, it must be accompanied each time it is used by a statement to the effect that the product is not a reduced or low calorie product, or to the effect that the usefulness of the product is only in the prevention of tooth decay.

Product labeling must be reviewed carefully against legal requirements. Many of the applicable requirements are highly technical, but even small deviations from the requirements can result in product seizure, which can be devastating at the time of a significant promotional rollout.

Advertising and all promotional materials also must be reviewed constantly and carefully. Precise attention to all of the necessary details in product development and labeling which insure that a product will be treated as a food can be completely undone by statements made in advertising which could permit the FDA to treat the product as a drug.

In short, there is no phase of the product development process, from concept to market and beyond, which does not contain potential legal pitfalls. The objective of the process is too important, however, to shirk the course simply because it may be difficult, or because it will necessarily involve extended exposure to lawyers.

DISCUSSION

Mr. Choate: Does the announced target (audience) of an advertisement influence the judgment whether it is accurate or deceptive?

Mr. Hickman: That is a question to be resolved in pending proceedings at the Federal Trade Commission. Certainly the FTC has suggested that this is a relevant consideration. It is currently the subject of considerable debate, and part of the purpose of the children's advertising proceeding is to answer that question.

Mr. Choate: Has there been no precedent as to where this will fall?

Mr. Hickman: Individual cases have investigated the question of whether particular advertising campaigns were, for example, deceptive to a youthful audience. Whether, when you look at those cases, you can decide that a different standard is being applied, I am not sure. I think probably we would have differing views.

Dr. Mackay: You have touched very nicely on the complications or on the use of the word "non-cariogenic." Practically, however, in thinking about the food supply, it is almost scientifically indisputable that the practical steps to be implemented mean decreasing the present level of cariogenicity of many food products. This will therefore bring the question of "less cariogenic," rather than non-cariogenic, as an intermediate step. Would you care to comment on what is involved in the use of that term? Is it possible?

Mr. Hickman: I don't think there is any legal brick wall that stands before the use of the words "less cariogenic." I do think that you are going to face even greater complications than I tried to describe for a non-cariogenic product in establishing two things: First, and this is probably the lesser, in demonstrating that your product is non-cariogenic in a way that is significant within its product category, and second, and I suspect the more difficult problem, in setting a context in the food supply against which you can single out a number of products and say it is important to make them non-cariogenic. Those are going to be difficulties in terms of persuading the Agency about what you want to do. I am concerned about dealing with the Agency in the context of a single product about which I want to make statements as to reduced cariogenicity, because I can see them looking at the total food supply and the total tooth decay problem saying, "That product is not significant enough. We are concerned about economic deception here."

Mr. Kelly: Would you comment on applying the rules recently issued for reduced-calorie foods and low-calorie foods to this same matter of cariogenicity? The Food and Drug Administration has decreed that a low-calorie food must be 40 calories or less per serving, whatever a serving may be, and a reduced-calorie food has to have a ⅓ calorie reduction from the food for which it would normally substitute.

Mr. Hickman: I think it would be inaccurate to say that a consensus has been reached in that area, but at least in a couple of years of hearings, you had most of the available viewpoints presented. You had a lot of issues beaten out hard enough and long enough that the Agency was willing to say, "Well, this is a reasonable kind of rule, this is a reasonable place to stop." People on the other side, the people who were in the industry presentations, may not agree with that, but you are in a range. Even though they are not very clear, you may have some better guidelines there, and something closer to a consensus about what the standards are and what the measurements are, than you do in the area of dental caries at the present time.

Dr. Schiff: I understood that there was a chewing gum product which went the regular IND route, and then the dental advisory group of the IND regulatory agency decided that they would not consider this as a drug, but as a food. Therefore they did not make a judgment and they turned it over to the food regulatory agency. However, the food regulatory agency does not have a dental advisory group, and the agency then returned it for advice and judgment to the same group in the Food and Drug Administration which had previously tossed it to the foods bureau because they said it wasn't a drug.

Do you foresee having separate regulatory expert agencies in the food as well as the drug agency, or is it always going to be that one group who is going to make all the judgments?

Mr. Hickman: I don't think that situation will change unless the market situation changes radically, because you don't have enough food products to warrant bringing in that kind of advisory panel to determine how you are going to go through this investigational process for a food additive, for example, although clearly you might want to have some less stringent requirements. Until you can persuade the Agency to publish something different, you are going to have to live against the backdrop of the IND requirement. As to whether the Agency is going to stay as a single unit or get broken up, I have no idea.

Dr. Smith: When we get into comparative claims, and the lower calorie regulations are a good analogy, what happens if you are really successful with your lower calorie product and the original goes out of business? What is the standard then?

Mr. Hickman: Theoretically, you have got to be lower than something to be "lower." And if that something doesn't exist anymore, then you are not really offering a product benefit.

Dr. Smith: But you have got a good product out there. Now what?

Mr. Hickman: You are now the product class.

Dr. Smith: You are the product class? So you have got to take that claim off, it no longer holds. So the guy comes back with his higher calorie, and beats your pants off. Is that the idea? It is hypothetical, but it is interesting.

Dr. Chilton: You mentioned something that was very important in the concept of clinical trials on non-cariogenic agents: that the dental advisory committee to the Food and Drug Administration has stated that use as a control group of children who ingest sugar or chew sugar gum or suck sugar-containing lozenges is unethical, and this has been accepted by the Food and Drug Administration.

The question of the legal meaning of "unethical" arises because if a study is done where there is not a stand-up comparison with something that is a known cariogenic agent, as most of us feel — although it is not universal — about sugar, there can be many theoretical objections to the design of the trial. So that we are in a bit of a quandary because it is unethical to do a Vipeholm sort of study, where we have a direct comparison with sugar, and yet if this is not done, the design can be called into question.

Does the legal meaning of "unethical" mean that it cannot be done, or if there is well-informed consent which has been approved by the human experimentation committees of the universities or whatever group is performing this study, and the patients and their parents are fully informed that some of the participants in the study will be using a sugar-containing agent, and that in their ordinary lifestyle they are indeed eating sugar in various forms, is this still considered unethical? Is it illegal? What is it?

Mr. Hickman: When we talk about the legal meaning of "unethical," we are really not talking about something that is defined in the Food and Drug Act or is a part of the Food and Drug Act. Before you finished the question, I was going to try and toss it back in your lap, and say that really when you are talking about ethics, you are talking more about what your institutional review committees are willing to accept and what the scientific community has to say about the reasonableness of doing something than you are about legal requirements as imposed by the Food and Drug Act or the Agency. You do get back into legal problems, and your legal problems are going to go back to your institution, and the institutional advice you get from your counsel about some critical questions, e.g., what is informed consent, what is adequate disclosure? He is going to be making a lot of those judgments on the basis of what he thinks is going to happen if one of the people in that study comes out with no teeth and sues you because of it.

The law comes into the ethics in the following questions. Can I sustain this in a courtroom as a reasonable judgment to have been made by someone in the scientific/medical community? Can I sustain what we have told the participants in writing and what they have agreed to as being adequately informative and adequate consent? In the legal sense, it gets down to some very pragmatic problems.

Dr. Chilton: But if on advice of university counsel this is considered to be something which is defensible if suit is brought, is the use of a sugar-containing product out, so far as the Food and Drug Administration is concerned?

Mr. Hickman: If you were to get that approved, it went through fine, and you came up with a study that showed me a comparison of a sugar product and a non-sugar product, and I took it down to FDA and they tried to reject it because it was unethical, I think we would have a good argument.

That rule or that ethical determination has caused some curious problems for them because, as I suggested, there are people there who don't accept the fact that the products traditionally on the market today have been adequately shown to be non-cariogenic. I would have said that was in the area of debate until the publication of this regulation two weeks ago. They have been forced into a position of putting that controversy aside — the technicalities in that controversy about how good the studies were or were not, because they have been forced into a position where they have to use those products as a standard.

Dr. Chilton: Outside of this country, I raised the same point, and many of the countries do not have the same sort of administrative set-up that we have in the Food and Drug Administration. The Dunlop Committee in Britain has much more status, and not as many suits are brought against them. But other countries subscribe in general to what they call the Helsinki Agreements. And inquiring what they specifically meant, the statement was made to me: "Well, it has to come up in terms of a suit, and then a decision will be made."

Now, there are all kinds of agreements and arrangements. Is there any legal status that you know of, or "legal substance," to the so-called Helsinki Agreements so far as testing of drug or food additive products in this country?

Mr. Hickman: I am not going to answer that directly. It is very complicated. You couldn't walk into a courtroom and say, "That violated the Helsinki Agreements, therefore I have a right to a monetary recovery on a tort theory." You certainly could walk in and take that in as evidence of what is the accepted standard of behavior internationally. It is evidentiary.

Question: If I were to remove half of the sugar in a product, what claims could I make for that product?

Mr. Hickman: On the basis of what I have heard here in the last 24 hours, it is not apparent to me that there is any kind of consensus that merely taking 50% of the sugar out of that product is going to result in (a) a 50% caries reduction, or (b) any caries reduction, depending on how the product is used, when it is used, which of the theories and variations I may accept as to how this whole process works.

And in order to get to that product concept, I have to get some kind of consensus, not unanimity, but some reasonable position on the medicine of this problem that I can present to an agency and explain what I am doing and why it works.

The second problem I would have with that product is in not making comparable serving comparisons. I would say you needed to talk about the same weight of another product as in that product. It is just like the difference between a doughnut and an English muffin. While your unit is a serving size, at that point the Agency would force you down to a weight comparison.

Mr. Kelly: What happens if I add an additive to the base material to offset or neutralize or counteract suspected cariogenic properties of the main ingredient? What if I take an approved additive such as phosphate and add that to sucrose, assuming that I can demonstrate that I can neutralize the effects of the sucrose there? What is the FDA rationale in dealing with that situation?

Mr. Hickman: I am not sure there is a rationale, and I probably would come to the answer to that from the other direction; the "does not promote tooth decay" non-cariogenic claim reasonably could have been classified as a drug claim, as a claim that was made about the mitigation of disease. Really, it is an historical anomaly in some respects that this dividing line was created.

At least at some levels at the Agency there is an interest in keeping that as a very narrow exception. Two years ago there were people in the Agency who wanted to make that a drug claim.

That problem resulted in a memorandum from the Office of the Director for Compliance to those committees saying, "This is not within your purview." But it was that same memorandum that said, "If they call it non-cariogenic, that sounds more like a drug." As I tried to suggest, a reasonable dividing line, if you are going to have a division between foods and drugs on that basis, is that when you take a product and you make that product non-cariogenic — and I don't care whether you substitute, or whether you manipulate it, put something else in to counteract the sugar — that product itself is non-cariogenic and should be able to be promoted as such. It is only when you go beyond that and start trying to deliver something into the system, either dealing with the tooth at its surface or systemically, that you are getting into an area that might more appropriately be considered drug.

LIMITATIONS OF FOOD CARIOGENICITY TESTING METHODOLOGIES

George K. Stookey, Ph.D. and James L. McDonald, Jr., Ph.D.

From the point of view of a person involved in research, there are two major problems which face us in attempting to deal with the cariogenicity of foods. The first problem is the dilemma of trying to determine which food items are truly cariogenic, and the second problem logically follows in that once such foods are so identified, how can we identify suitable measures which will reduce their cariogenicity?

It may or may not be obvious to all of us here today that the ideal solution to this research problem is simply not possible. Ideally these answers would be obtained from carefully designed and well-controlled clinical dental caries investigations. However, it is neither possible nor practical to utilize such procedures. For example, even if you could get a large group of several hundred persons to ingest a given food item on a regular basis for the required period of two to three years, what would you use as the control regimen? What foods would you provide to the control subjects as a substitute for the test food? How do you know that the substituted foods are not equally, or even more, cariogenic than the test food? From a moral or ethical consideration, how can we justify providing experimental substances to subjects when there is a reasonable liklihood that the results may indicate that they were in fact harmful to the health of the participants? Therefore, controlled clinical investigations are not possible.

As alternatives to clinical investigations, a wide variety of laboratory and animal research methodologies have been suggested and utilized to obtain information about the cariogenicity of various foodstuffs and to identify additives or other manufacturing procedures which will reduce this problem. While each of these types of alternative methodologies provides a considerable amount of useful information regarding the cariogenic potential of foodstuffs, there is all too frequently a tendency in all of us to forget or overlook their deficiencies.

For the purpose of this discussion we have categorized the various types of studies into eight general areas. No attempt has been made to review each methodology developed by any given group of investigators or to the numerous modifications of each methodology subsequently reported by other groups. Rather, we will examine the general types of studies.

I. Chemical Analyses

a. Sucrose content The first type of investigation of the cariogenicity of foods is that which merely involves the chemical analysis of the food. In particular, a commonly suggested procedure is to analyze various food items for their "sugar" content, or perhaps their content of sucrose, fructose or glucose. While this information is indeed useful in our collection of information regarding the cariogenic potential of foods, it is often misused or misinterpreted. No doubt most of us have seen listings of foods with their sugar or sucrose content and the implication or outright erroneous assumption that the sucrose content of a food is a direct index of its cariogenicity. However, a review of the literature leaves little doubt that the relative amount of sugar in a food is by no means a direct measure of the cariogenicity or cariogenic potential of that food. This is not to say that fermentable carbohydrates are not involved or related to the caries process — it is merely that sugar content, in and of itself, is not the only factor involved.

b. Inherent pH Still other types of analytical data have been utilized in this regard, e.g., the inherent pH. Low pH foods (particularly soft drinks and candies) have long been suspect in the eyes of the dental profession. These types of foods do produce marked erosion in animals in a relatively short period of time. However, the role of erosion and erosion-producing food substances in the actual process of human caries has not been established. Further, the consideration of the inherent pH of a food without consideration of other factors, such as the rate of oral clearance or oral retention or the buffering capacity of saliva, may lead to erroneous implications. The few clinical studies of soft drinks do not appear to suggest a highly cariogenic potential associated with these products.

c. Carbohydrate content Of course the total fermentable carbohydrate content of foods reflects their potential acid production. However, in the last decade, the greater caries potential of sucrose than starch has been amply demonstrated. Thus the total carbohydrate content of foods of itself is probably not of great predictive value with regard to cariogenicity.

d. Protein and fat content Both fats and proteins have been suggested on occasion to possess anti-caries activity. However, obviously diets high in fat or protein are correspondingly lower in fermentable carbohydrates. Thus it is almost impossible to determine whether any potential caries reduction can be attributed to the increase in fat or protein or to the reduction in carbohydrate.

II. Physico-chemical Properties of Foods

a. Oral retention/clearance A variety of methods have been tested to compare the retentiveness of foods on the teeth. These include measurements of sugar released into saliva, food washed from teeth, and *in vitro* adhesiveness of foods. Collectively, these studies indicate that different foods have a broad range of retentiveness. In general, liquid foodstuffs are cleared most rapidly, whereas solid, sticky foodstuffs show higher intraoral retentive properties. Moreover, the Vipeholm' human caries study showed a definite relationship between the ingestion of sticky, solid, sucrose-containing foods and a high caries rate. In summary, the retention of foodstuffs in the mouth appears related to their cariogenic potential; however, retention in and of itself is not the principal determinant of cariogenicity.

b. Buffering capacity Theoretically, the presence of inherent buffers in food substances should neutralize acids produced during fermentation, thereby helping to protect against dental caries. Moreover, Katz[2] found that the major factor in dried breakfast cereals which correlated fairly well with their cariogenic potential in rats was their ability to neutralize acids. However, the addition of various buffering agents to diets in animals has not always resulted in significant caries reductions. The buffering capacity of foods does not appear to be the major determinant of their cariogenicity.

III. Acid Production in Saliva

Foods have been compared with regard to their cariogenic potential on the basis of studying acid production of these foods when incubated in saliva. Many of these tests probably had little meaning because they were conducted in closed systems where the inherent buffering capacity of some foods allowed acid production to continue over long time periods, thereby giving a greater final acid formation. Of course, a high starch content would provide a food a high acid-forming capacity. Whether this is of great significance in caries production is debatable. Of course certain acid foods are already at a level of acidity which would inhibit fermentation by the oral flora. So acid production from foods incubated with saliva is one, but only one, of the determinants of cariogenicity.

IV. Enamel Decalcification by Fermenting Foods

Taking the experimental method just discussed one step further, the amount of enamel decalcification produced by fermenting foods can be measured. Results indicate that the amount of decalcification is not always related to the amount of acid produced in saliva. For example, certain wholemeal products produce more acid but result in less decalcification than refined flours. Thus, apparently some foodstuffs contain enamel-protective substances.

V. Plaque Studies

a. In vitro 1. The *in vitro* study of plaque formation and growth on teeth, with wires and glass slides, has been utilized frequently to screen substances having potential anti-plaque capabilities. The amount of plaque formed can be evaluated either by weight or by visual observation. However, the use of these methods to study the cariogenic potential of specific foodstuffs has been limited primarily to the study of various sugars. Their use for studying plaque formation from other food items is difficult because of problems in basic study design. Major deficiencies of these tests include the use of a single microorganism (rather than mixed oral flora) and the growth of plaque on artifical substrates rather than enamel with consideration of the role of dental pellicle. However, such tests provide information concerning the potential of a given food for supporting plaque formation.

2. *In vitro* studies of acid production in plaque are possible and have generally involved holding homogenized plaque samples on glass pH electrodes and plotting the pH changes related to various substrates introduced into the system. Such studies have not been widely utilized to study acid production from commonly ingested foodstuffs.

b. **In vivo** A number of workers have measured pH changes in the plaque of subjects following the ingestion of different food items. Most recently, the pH telemetry work conducted by Mühlemann and co-workers[3] has become an important tool for assessing pH changes in both dental plaque and oral fluid in response to various food items. The construction and use of telemetric partial prostheses has been described in detail.[4] This methodology has provided detailed information on pH changes in plaque with regard to the acidogenicity of foods. However, this technique also has some deficiencies. For example, the procedure typically involves three or four selected subjects (with no consideration of the variability in plaque responses between subjects). The subjects are typically adults rather than more caries-prone children whose plaque composition and responses typically differ from that of adults. Further, it remains to be seen how well these pH changes correlate with human caries.

VI. In Vitro Caries

A variety of different *in vitro* caries methodologies have been developed to study the caries process. These methods include the traditional "artifical mouth" as well as Bibby's "Orofax,"[5] and caries-like lesions produced using acid gels.[6] Collectively, these methods attempt to simulate many of the conditions existing in the oral cavity during the carious process, while at the same time attempting to control other extraneous factors. Although some of the findings with these methods seem to parallel findings in rat caries studies, certainly more correlations with *in vivo* studies are needed before these methodologies can be considered reliable caries predictors.

VII. In Vivo Caries

Studies have been conducted in which blocks of enamel positioned on removable dental appliances are worn in the mouth. Following the desired time intervals, the amount of demineralization occurring is measured by changes in enamel hardness. Primarily sugars have been tested using this method. More recently the von der Fehr method[7] for studying the initiation of caries-like changes in the enamel surface *in vivo* has been utilized. Here, using much shorter experimental periods than in human clinical trials, subjective changes in the optical properties of enamel are plotted under 15X magnification.

Such studies have not been used widely for testing food cariogenicity. Moreover, they are subject to the same types of limitiations as are full scale human clinical studies: ethical considerations, the selection of an appropriate control group, etc. Again, the correlation of such findings with human data is sorely needed.

VIII. Animal Models

The use of animal models in research testing of food cariogenicity obviously allows a much broader base of experimentation than is possible in human subjects. Rodents and primates have been the models most successfully used in this regard to date.

In the case of rodents (primarily rats), their small size, rapid breeding cycle, general hardiness, and the rapidity with which they become affected with dental caries all contribute to making them a very productive animal model. Moreover, their relatively low cost allows their use in sufficient numbers to generate statistically reliable data. In addition, the sulcal and smooth surface lesions produced in rats resemble their counterparts in humans very closely. Unfortunately, the rat caries model has several inherent weaknesses, particularly with regard to predicting the cariogenicity of human food items. First of all, the small size is a disadvantage in that periodic *in vivo* examination for caries is impractical and the animals must be sacrificed before the caries examination. Moreover, the eating habits of rats who may go to the feed dish 50 or more times a day do not closely resemble the eating habits of humans. Finally, the microbial composition, salivary composition, flow rate, buffering capacity and environmental pH of rats all may differ significantly from that of humans.

Probably nothing has pointed out these weaknesses much more dramatically than did the anti-caries work with phosphates largely conducted in 1960. Here, almost every phosphate imaginable was found to reduce rat caries when added to the diet. In contrast, phosphates as food additives in humans have generally been unsuccessful in reducing dental caries. Very few specific human foods — with the possible exception of dried breakfast cereals — have been extensively studied in the rodent caries model. In general, the studies of breakfast cereals in rats have shown a marked lack of positive correlation between sugar content and cariogenicity.

The greater size of primates does allow the conduct of clinical examinations analogous to those in man, and, of course, one is less reluctant to extrapolate data from primates to man. However, because of the difficulty in obtaining primates, their appreciable cost, and the lengthy experimental time period required, the usefulness of this species in studying the cariogenicity of specific food items has been limited.

Summary

There are a variety of methodologies for studying the cariogenicity of foods, but none of them is particularly meaningful. The use of these various tests does provide a lot of useful information — information regarding the cariogenic potential of various foods.

Among the major objectives of this American Dental Association Program on the Cariogenicity of Foods are the critical review of various methodologies and the development of guidelines, or the identification of preferred methodologies, for use in determining the cariogenic potential of foods. It may be hoped that the results of these tests will have significant impact on both industry and the scientific community in our collective efforts to improve dental health.

VI. PROSPECTS FOR ADDITIVES AFFECTING CARIOGENICITY

Ray G. Kelly, Chairman

PROSPECTS FOR NEW ADDITIVES AFFECTING CARIOGENICITY

Ferdinand Zienty, Ph.D.

A fairly diversified research and development effort is in various stages of progress to define new additives for prospective use in food products with reduced cariogenic potential. Most of this research is being done in the United States and Europe. Although much of it is supported by industrial organizations, a growing proportion is sponsored by U.S. federal government agencies. The effort appears to be directed toward development of food additives with a relatively large volume potential, such as bulking agents, sugar alcohols, phosphates and natural and artificial sweeteners.

Major considerations in development of new additives are regulatory requirements for gaining approval of a food additive petition or a New Drug Application (NDA), the time required to complete product development to commercialization, and the total cost. All of these factors have been evolutionary in the quantitative sense, affected by the changing regulatory environment.

Prospects for development of new food additives are uncertain as only two new chemical entity direct food additives have been approved in the United States since 1969. These are the antioxidant TBHQ,[1] closely related to butylated hydroxyanisole and butylated hydroxytoluene, approved for food use in 1972; and the sweetener, aspartame,[2] approved for specified uses in 1974, but its order was stayed on December 4, 1975.[3] A number of direct food additive petitions have been filed in this period and subsequently withdrawn. Few filings have been made in the past several years of petitions on new direct food additives, indicating general discouragement with the likelihood of commercialization.

Certain base-line toxicology studies will be needed on any new food additive. These include metabolism studies; long-term chronic toxicity studies in two animal species, including a lifetime study designed to detect carcinogenic potential in rodents; three generation reproduction studies; mutagenicity and teratogenicity studies; skin and eye irritation studies; and allergenic tests.

In addition, special tests may be required, contingent on the chemical structure and properties of the product and its behavior under conditions encountered in formulation, manufacture and use of the consumer products for which it is intended. If metabolites are found or if conversion or reaction products are formed in food formulations, these must be isolated, identified and subjected to comprehensive toxicological study to establish safety. No specific protocol can be designed to cover possible safety requirements on all potential food additive candidates, as the detailed testing can vary greatly form case to case.

Depending on the chemistry of the product, use level and overall volume potential, human clinical work may be required to measure tolerance, allergenic properties and functional performance. Age group effects need to be considered as young children and the aged have reduced tolerance for many products including foods. As toxicology work proceeds, one should expect that many unscheduled tests would be added to the program for developing a satisfactory food additive petition.

Methods of analysis will be needed both for biochemical studies and for analysis in food formulations. Stability tests in food products will be required under processing, storage and use conditions.

To develop a new food additive from idea to commercialization requires the following sequence of work. We should expect a program of several years' duration to be necessary to identify a candidate food additive product that someone wants to commit to for commercialization. The exercise of sorting out the final prospective candidate undoubtedly will require some preliminary acute and short-term toxicity studies. Some process development work and manufacturing cost estimate work will be necessary to establish that a realisitc cost performance opportunity has been identified before the expensive toxicology work is started. While the five-year safety testing program is in progress, and if results look favorable, additional process development, pilot plant and cost studies will be done to prepare for future manufacture of the product. Preliminary engineering may be done to validate these findings and estimate probable capital requirements.

During this time, application research will be done on the product forms of the additive and the food product forms in which it will be used. This will include formulation, flavoring, and preference panel tests.

Assuming that all toxicology and pathology tests show no adverse effects, preparation can start on the petition requesting issuance of a regulation for the use of the new product as a direct additive in foods, under specified conditions and limitations. The petition is filed. Issuance of a regulation may be expected to take from several to many months if everything is in order with the petition and the supporting data. More often than not, the petition is found to be deficient resulting in the need to do more work. If that petition is incomplete and far from the standards expected, it may be withdrawn without prejudice and refiled later, when accumulated test data are available. The time for prospective issuance may thus be extended to several years. Litigation resulting from objections filed by third party individuals or organizations may cause further extensive delays. As there is so little experience with issuance of regulations on new chemical entity direct food additives since 1969, it might be fair to say we do not know all of today's requirements to achieve approval in the United States.

Averaging total effort against approvals on only two direct food additives in the period 1970 to 1978 suggests a cost well in excess of $10 million per additive and a time investment of eight to ten years. To recover the research and development cost to achieve clearance on one new product requires gross profit of $1 million per year for ten years. Assuming that a regulation is issued, then a commitment needs to be made to build a manufacturing facility. Construction and start-up of a new plant will require three to four years. Chart 1 summarizes the development of a new food additive from concept to commercialization.

When a drug claim is desired for the use of a new additive, the formulated consumer product to be marketed must satisfy therapeutic efficacy requirements in addition to the extensive safety requirements for the active component. This includes multi-stage testing on humans and finally involves controlled, well-designed clinical studies in sufficiently large numbers of people to be statistically significant for measurement of efficacy and any side effects. In cases of anti-caries agents, it is not ethically acceptable to set up an untreated control group to measure differences in anti-caries performance. Therefore it is difficult to design clinical studies to show product performance of the type readily demonstrated in rats. In the United States, one new chemical entity drug product requires about 13 years from first compound screening to first commercialization. The cost is estimated at $20-40 million.[4–6] Prospects are not good for development of a new drug with supportable anti-caries claims.

Current status of several products under development for use in foods with reduced cariogenic potential is described briefly.

TABLE 1. New Food Additive Development

Year	
0	Recognition of function Optimization *via* synthesis
2	Selection of preferred candidate(s) Short-term toxicology Process development, cost, application studies
4	Decision to try for commercialization of surviving candidate Start intensive safety studies Process development, pilot plant, engineering, application
7-9	Complete toxicology Prepare petition, file
8-10	Regulation issued Capital appropriation Start plant construction
11-14	Start marketing Cost $10 million exclusive of capital

Phosphates Several studies in rats fed a diet high in sucrose demonstrated reduced incidence of dental caries when dibasic calcium phosphate dihydrate (DCPD) was incorporated. Although three clinical studies confirm the findings in rats, the amount of work apparently is not yet sufficient to support the rigorous requirements of a New Drug Application. Therefore no drug claims can be made. As DCPD is generally recognized as safe[7] (GRAS) it could be used in a variety of food products with potential benfits to the consumer. Prospects are poor for development of new phosphates not currently approved for use in foods.

Sugar alcohols Mannitol and sorbitol have been used widely as replacements for sucrose in formulation of specialty foods. Xylitol is under development in the United States after considerable experience with it in Finland and Switzerland. It is as sweet as sucrose and can be used like sugar in many formulations requiring a bulk product to provide texture. It is currently approved in the United States for special dietary use, but a proposal to withdraw this regulation was published in 1971.[8] Long-term chronic toxicity tests completed in Great Britain in 1978 are under study.

Bulking agents Several interesting product concepts have been examined with the goal of developing bulking agents that might be used as replacements for part or all of the sucrose in some food formulations. These include esters of sorbitol with approved food acids,[9] glucosyl sorbitol,[10] and hydrogenated hydrolyzed starch. None of these have achieved food additive status as bulking agents in the United States. Hydrogenated hydrolyzed starch is under development in Sweden and Switzerland.

New sweeteners Aspartame was approved in 1974 as a nutrient sweetener for use in a number of food products.[2, 11] The following year the food additive regulation was stayed[3] pending resolution of questions on safety tests. Several representative toxicology studies run in support of the safety of aspartame are now being validated.[12] If these reviews are satisfactory, a Board of Inquiry is to be convened to consider merits of objections raised by two individuals. Reinstatement of the stayed regulation is not likely to occur before 1979. Future approvals for uses not specified in the 1974 regulation will require filing of petitions. It is interesting to reflect that about 95 toxicology studies had been run on aspartame through 1977.

Two new sweeteners with interesting properties are under development in Western Germany. Acetosulfam,[13] 130 times as sweet as sugar, is a cyclic sulfonamide related to saccharin. The second sweetener, a thiophene analog of saccharin,[14] is about 1,000 times as sweet as sugar. Both have stability similar to saccharin's under use conditions. Toxicological studies are said to be in progress. Both appear to be years away from commercialization in West Germany or from approval for use in the United States.

Dihydrochalcone sweeteners have been under development in the United States for many years.[15a, 15b] However, it does not appear they are near approval for use or near commercialization. More recently, work was started on derivatives of dihydrochalcone sweeteners.[15c] Since these studies are in a very early stage it is difficult to assess prospects for success.

D-tryptophane and D-phenylalanine have been suggested as potential sweeteners.[16] Very little toxicology has been done on these unnatural amino acids as yet, probably because they are not as promising commercially as sweeteners with a much higher sweetness performance. Natural sweeteners[17] such as the ones extracted from the miracle fruit[18] or serendipity berry have some interesting properties. Development to commercialization appears to face formidable problems.

In summary, the 8-10 years of work and $10+ million in cost to achieve regulatory approval are not affordable for any low volume new product. Prospects for commitment of an effective level of research support may be somewhat better for new products with large market potential. However, achievement of regulatory approval for products like new bulking agents will be very difficult since the prospect of massive yearly consumption will raise many special questions concerning safety. The prospects are much better for formulation of attractive food products with reduced cariogenic potential using components already approved.

REFERENCES

1. *Code of Federal Regulations* (CFR), Title 21, 172.185.
2. *CFR* 21, 172.804.
3. *Federal Register* 40:56907, 1975.
4. *Chemical Week*, May 10, 1978, p. 59.
5. Sarett, L.H. *Chemtech*, January 1975, p. 20.
6. The Pharmaceutical Industry, C.M. Lindsay, ed. John Wiley & Sons, 1978, p. 91.
7. *CFR* 21, 182.1217 and 182.5217.
8. *Federal Register* 36:20306, 1971.
9. A food additive petition filed in 1972 on polydextrose, sorbitol modified, polymerized with tartaric or citric acid for use as a bulking agent was withdrawn on October 18, 1973.
10. Layton, R.M. and Vlazny, J.C. *Food Prod. Dev.*: March 1978, p. 53.

11a. Mazur, R.H., in "Symposium Sweeteners," G.C. Inglett, ed., Westport, CT, AVI, 1974, p. 159.

11b. Beck, C.I., *Inbid.*, p. 164.

12. Bost, R.G. and Ripper, A., "Sweeteners and Dental Caries," *Feeding, Weight and Obesity Abstracts*, Sp. supp: p. 269, 1978.
13. Clauss, K. and Jensen, H. *Angew. Chem.* (Intl. Ed.,) 12:869, 1973.
14. German Patent Specification 2, 534, 689 (Filed August 2, 1975, published March 25, 1976).

15a. Horowitz, R.M. and Gentili, B. "Sweeteners and Dental Caries," *Feeding, Weight and Obesity Abstracts*, Sp. Supp: 291, 1978.

15b. Gumbman, M.R. *et al. Ibid*, p. 301.

15c. Crosby, G.A. *et al. Ibid*, p. 341.

16. Solms, J., Vuataz, L. and Egli, F.H. *Experientia* 21:692, 1965.
17. Inglett, G.C. in "Symposium Sweeteners" G.C. Inglett, ed. Westport, CT, AVI, 1974, p. 216.
18. Denial of GRAS affirmation on miracle fruit, berries, concentrates and extracts. Federal Register 42:26467, 1977

IMPLICATIONS FOR NEW PRODUCT DEVELOPMENT

Paul F. Hopper, Ph.D.

We continue to see headlines denouncing processed foods, and especially those with significant sugar content, as a major contributor to dental caries. The way the stories read, the sugared goodies, and these alone, are singled out as the culprit in the "rampant caries" that is so eloquently described by the media, and spawned by inexact science and biased extrapolation.

Can sugar contribute to caries? Of course it can. It is an important source of nutrition for *Streptococcus mutans* and other microorganisms implicated in plaque formation, a key precursor to caries. If we eat sticky sweet foods, especially between meals; if we are neglectful of good dental hygiene and fail to brush our teeth after every meal; if we allow plaque to build with only infrequent visits to the dentist—we are inviting trouble. One might say, "We'll get what we deserve."

But let's take a closer look at what we've just described. If we made absolutely no change in total dietary sugar, but changed the food form and the consumption pattern, we would have a different outcome. Let's put that sugar into a nonsticky form—perhaps even incorporate it in a fibrous matrix. Let's consume this new form primarily at mealtime. Let's further descipline ourselves to brush after every meal. And finally, let's be sure we have frequent checkups at the dentist with a good professional tooth cleaning. What now are the prospects for caries? Indeed, they are very slim, if not nonexistent; so, if we believe this, sugar is no more a contributor to caries than is a more complex form of carbohydrate.

This may be an ideal world we are describing, but it is an important focus for the food scientist to develop, for otherwise he will find himself making the wrong decisions, for the wrong reasons.

Perhaps this a good time to step back and to become philosophical for a moment—again to open our eyes and our ears to the realities of the world—and not to the drum beat of its ill-informed biases.

Why does man eat? For some, the instant answer to this question is a stoical response based on the need to fuel our human furnaces. They would put a period there, and say there is no other role but to provide those nutrients essential to the healthy functioning of the body. They might not even agree to adding "the body *and* the mind" as taken from a simplistic physiological point of view.

But it doesn't end there. Man eats for psychological reasons as well. Man does need those hedonic values in food—the pleasure of the taste and smell; the attractiveness of its color and form; the satiation of both thirst and appetite; the stimulation and the relaxation that only food can bring. Man is not just a biological furnace—he is a complex entity with many needs.

Finally, man eats for social reasons. Food serves as an important focal point for human interaction between individuals and groups of individuals. Whether it be the coffee break, or the bowling team banquet, or the festive family dinner, food brings people together—unites them and gives them a sense of belonging. It serves to perpetuate tradition and the social values inherent therein. Within ethnic groups it serves as a distinguishing form of identity. It helps to stabilize society.

We cannot ignore all of these roles that food must serve. As much as we might wish to, from a dental science point of view, we cannot eliminate all food forms that present some form of risk of caries. I, for one, don't want to be a part of that society that so regiments my life that I have only those choices to make that some bureaucratic function has decided is best for me.

I suggest that this is a risk far greater to society than the possible, but not established, benefit of a somewhat lower caries rate.

The preference for sweetness is an inborn trait, as Dr. Morley Kare of the Monell Chemical Senses Center of the University of Pensylvania has established so well. Very few individuals in our society do not enjoy sweet things. Many foods are more enjoyable when they are sweetened, and this includes many fruits, which in themselves contain sugar. Who doesn't smack his lips when he sprinkles a spoonful of sugar on his strawberries or sniffs the aromatic sweetness of the freshly baked pie? What Thanksgiving dinner would be complete without cranberry sauce or jelly, each prepared with sugar?

Nutritionally, sugar provides energy, and it makes other foods with important nutrients taste better. In short, it has an important role in both our heritage and in our innovational product science and technology.

If sugar, therefore, does to some degree contribute to caries, should we ban its use? That would be absurd. Should we regulate it to death? Probably not. It is a pretty dense individual, devoid of normal sensory perception, who doesn't know when something he eats or drinks tastes sweet. The need for special labeling would be an insult to the average person's intelligence.

The question we really want to ask is "How can we minimize the risk of dental caries when we eat sweet things?" The best insurance against caries is good oral hygiene. There is no substitute. No amount of change in the diet is going to compensate for poor hygiene.

The second and related factor of importance is a good educational program. People should know that in addition to a good brushing after every meal, they should consume sticky foods primarily at meal time. Ample liquid consumption is also important to help "flush" the teeth.

Not only should they be taught these basic factors, but it should be part of a comprehensive nutrition education program. It is an old saw that says..."eat a variety of foods, and eat them in moderation." There are some important aspects of that advice that will go a long way toward calming the waters of the emotional storm generated by those who like the idea of banning foods.

Good nutrition is not achieved by seeking out only those foods that have a high nutrient density, nor is it achieved by fortifying a given food with every vitamin and mineral known to man. Good nutrition is achieved first and formost by the balanced selection of foods from every food group—and I am not necessarily advocating the four food group approach over any other sound classification. Secondly, it is achieved by limiting the total consumption from these food groups to the total number of calories we need as individuals to maintain reasonable weight. There is plenty of room in such a nutrition program to indulge ourselves occasionally with some foods that are strictly hedonic in nature.

To return now to our food scientist sitting before the glowing embers of his fireside, dreaming of new and interesting foods with which to please the consumer's palate, we begin to see the outline of a new concept in new product development that could be helpful in our quest for good dental health. It may not be as scientifically earth shaking as Kekule's vision of the benzene ring, but it may be worth sharing.

Studies with various phosphates, both in animal and in human testing, show a marked effect in certain kinds of food systems. We are learning more about controlling dental erosion as an important part of the caries prevention process. There are, therefore, at least two mechanisms for intervention—compounds that neutralize erosive chemicals, whether in the food or beverage itself or generated inside the oral cavity; and, compounds which destroy or inhibit the microorganisms that are responsible for plaque formation. Phosphates are examples of certain of these compounds. Certainly there are more antidotes in the world—and we should encourage the search, whether in the industrial world or in the academic environment.

We must be fully cognizant of the problems confronting the food scientist. Any additive which in controlled animal studies is shown to be effective against erosion or caries must also be acceptable as a food additive. The full gamut of toxicological tests must be passed successfully. With today's comprehensive and demanding protocols, this can be a highly uncertain process requiring the expenditure of perhaps more than a million dollars and three to five years of time.

In addition , the additive must be compatible with the food systems in which it is placed. It must not impart objectionable taste or texture; it must not interfere with functionality; if used in clear liquid, it cannot cause cloudiness; if used in a sweet system, it cannot impart bitterness; it must be economical; and it must not impair nutritional value. As you can see, the parameters of acceptability are many—not many substances can meet these demands.

In addition to anti-caries additives, the food technologist has the option of substituting ingredients to make a product less cariogenic. The traditional pattern is to place part or all of the simple sugar in a product with a non-nutritive sweetener or with a sugar alcohol such as sorbitol, mannitol or xylitol. We may find that even saccharin has been eliminated as an option. New questions have been raised about the toxicology of the sugar alcohols, and they may be in jeopardy. The one bright hope for new sweeteners—aspartame—has been sidetracked for four years waiting for the Food and Drug Administration to convene a scientific Board of Inquiry. These are certainly not promising prospects encouraging the food scientist to follow this option. What else can be done? Perhaps we can examine practices that help animals to maintain good teeth. Certainly the bone, and its man-made counterparts such as dog biscuits, provide the abrasive matrix that helps to keep the tooth surface free of plaque. Can we develop food systems that operate as edible toothbrushes? Why not?

This might be especially useful when applied to snack type foods consumed primarily between meals.

What about a better understanding of the role of saliva flow in maintaining good dental health? Is it possible to build into selected food systems saliva stimulating properties that help to "flood" the teeth with protective secretions?

Finally, what about the possibility of a dental "Gatorade" for the future?—a refreshing beverage to be swallowed after a gooey, sticky snack, one that will not only flush the teeth, but will contain inhibiting ingredients for added insurance.

The challenge is enormous, but the prospects are exciting. Careful research is needed as is a responsive regulatory climate. We must begin to communicate factually and responsibly with the consuming public. I repeat, there is an urgent need to do a better job of providing sound nutrition education that can bring about good dietary practices—practices that take into account the multiple roles that food must play in satisfying the needs of man. We should get off the "BAN IT" bandwagon and begin to teach the positive elements of good dental hygiene!

DISCUSSION

Dr. Smith: Are we far enough along in our investigation of methods to identify a very small number of potential methods? Is it possible to achieve a consensus that says any foodstuff which lowers the pH in the mouth is a candidate for further investigation, and any which does not lower the pH in the mouth can be ignored as a potential cariogenic food?

If we can get to that stage on a consensus basis, then perhaps we can dwell on other kinds of methodology to evaluate the degree of cariogenicity of the food. Is it possible to narrow down the options we have in methodology?

Dr. McDonald: Among the variety of methods that have been tested, some have been shown to be more reliable indicators. Two methods seem to stand out. The plaque pH responses at the enamel-plaque interface, and ability to lower the pH at that particular site are very relevant in the caries process. The animal models are very appropriate for most intents and purposes for which they have been used. A combination of these two might be appropriate to screen foodstuffs in animal models and determine plaque pH response.

Dr. Smith: Would you then recommend initiating studies with the screening for plaque pH drops, and then just going further into the animal model later on to determine the degree of this cariogenicity?

Dr. McDonald: As a point of departure, I think that would be reasonable.

Dr. Edgar: Dr. McDonald classified our method as an *in vitro* method. The measurement is certainly *in vitro,* but we should really classify it as an *in vivo* method because the plaque is metabolizing in the mouth. It is only removed from the mouth for measurement purposes.

Dr. McDonald: I agree. Your technique seems to lie somewhere between *in vitro* and *in vivo*.

Dr. Edgar: In five tests of foods with which I have been associated, in which the von der Fehr technique was used, our tentative conclusion is that this technique is not appropriate for testing relative cariogenicity between foodstuffs. It may be useful in testing anti-cariogenicity properties of treatments or regimes, but not in trying to rank foods for cariogenicity.

Dr. Shory: What is your industry doing to try to help to educate the public about the proper time for eating these confections, these sweet foods? Only the dairy industry has done anything educational. Is Industry ready to take some of its advertising time and promotion to do something about this?

Dr. Hopper: Any nutrition education program is not the sole responsibility of a specific company or industry. If we are going to be effective in marshaling the resources that this country has at its disposal to bring sound nutritional educational practices to the public in a form it can understand, to motivate it to make appropriate dietary choices, it has to be a collaborative effort. It has to be government and industry and the public sectors of society working together. We have suggested a way in which we might be able to approach this in testimony for the Richmond Committee; it was called "Suggestion of a Nutrition Education Council," patterned after a council that is now in its third year: one that has proven to be a very, very successful approach to thorny problems that society is facing.

The Food Safety Council was begun about 2½ years ago, and it is composed of a board of trustees made up of government people, academics, consumer activists, and industry people. There is no pressure group or private industry group that can control such an activity. They are approaching the questions of food safety from a highly methodical, logical point of view, and have just completed the first activity, which is the development of a scientific product.

Dr. Daniels: Is there a consensus with the opinion that Dr. McDonald gave in response to Dr. Smith's question: if pH doesn't go down there won't be a cariogenic response? May we have a show of hands?
(There was a show of hands.)

Dr. Bibby: The conditions under which the test is taken will have to be evaluated critically, however.

Dr. Hefferren: This is a rather unusual way to achieve a scientific consensus, and I am not sure what it means. You have to be careful in how you define these terms. I don't want you to be rushed into "if plaque doesn't do this," or "the pH doesn't do that," or "whatever doesn't do that," with the idea that forever you are safe. That is very dangerous.

Dr. Bibby: The simplest test would be to mix some saliva in a modeling test tube and take a measurement from that. Salivary pH does parallel plaque pH to some extent. You don't need to go to the human subject to test that. If a thing won't ferment, it won't cause caries.

Mr. Kelly: While it may be unscientific, would those people raise their hands who disagree then with Dr. Daniels' question?

Let the record show that one hand was raised in opposition and more than 20 on the other side.

Dr. Hefferren: When you look for criteria to measure cariogenicity potential, there is a parallel to a student characterizing an unknown compound. He usually makes a solid derivative. If the melting point agrees with literature values, fine. If he makes two derivatives that agree with literature values, that's better. Depending on the importance of the unknown, a number of additional confirmatory tests can be done. Test selection depends upon the importance of the situation. It is dangerous to rely on one test. If you want a consensus on a place to start, the plaque test seems to be a good place. To say that the plaque test is absolute and self sufficient at this point, however, is a little dangerous.

Dr. Kabara: We know at least one instance in which a compound was tested by Mühlemann as being negative, and in animal studies was definitely positive. It is premature, in our ignorance, to have that kind of a consensus, and I agree with Dr. Hefferren that a majority vote doesn't make it true.

Dr. Ciancio: Dr. Hopper said we are looking for a dental "Gatorade." After testifying in the saccharin hearings in Washington, and facing the fact that people do want sweeteners, we initiated a few small studies on subjects in the age range of 17 to 21. We had the subjects simply rinse their mouths with a 10% sucrose solution, and we recorded the pH of saliva and, more importantly, the pH of gingival crevicular fluid, with an antimony microelectrode. We found that the saliva pH and the gingival crevicular fluid pH did decrease to about 4.5 when a 10% sucrose rinse was given.

Looking for the "Gatorade," then we had the subjects rinse with two commercially available mouthrinses, because we live in the real world where it is difficult to get an NDA (New Drug Application), so we examined two different commercial products and let the subjects rinse with those with 10% sucrose added to the mouthrinse. And surprisingly, by adding these so-called anti-plaque or therapeutic agents to the mouthrinses—commercial products—the pH now went to about 5.8 to 6.

So perhaps we can stay with sugars to a certain extent. To talk about eliminating them from the diet is correct, but we are going to be living with them for a long time. We should begin to look at other alternatives, and I propose that one alternative is to consider commercial anti-plaque agents or anti-bacterial agents, which are acceptable to FDA, to see if there is some effect these might have on the concomitant administration of sucrose, in a candy bar or anything else.

Dr. Katz: Dr. Hopper, if we define education as the occurrence of a behavioral change, it seems to me that there is some contradiction between the definition of the roles of foods that you mentioned and the possibility of achieving significant public education in good nutrition. It is going to be a very, very long proposition. It may take more than one generation. The same is true for good oral hygiene education, and there is good evidence. We don't have the manpower, and we don't know how to reach people to achieve good results. Trying to solve the problem of cariogenicity by means of education is avoiding the issue.

Dr. Hopper: The problem is an enormous one, but I am not one to give up very easily. There is enough interest in the whole subject of nutrition at present, so that we can more effectively motivate the public than ever before.

If we join forces, and if our messages reinforce each other, and if we use all of the communication tools and skills available to us in promoting products, in promoting those messages that are important, I think that we do have a chance of success. I agree with you, it is going to be long-term, it is going to require a coordinated effort, and I think we need a lot of good will in the process, too.

Dr. Katz: What else can industry do?

Dr. Hopper: First, industry can provide foods that have less cariogenicity in themselves, perhaps by replacing the simple sugars with other sweeteners or bulking agents; by designing the mechanics of the food, e.g., marketing a beverage that would flow through the mouth and be appealing, but yet would help to change the pH in a beneficial way. Anything that we might do to improve remineralization of the surfaces through additives would be positive steps.

There are significant problems in finding new things that are going to be acceptable with sufficiently high probability to warrant the long-time investment. Therefore, I continue to believe in education as a route. I know it is going to be long and hard. But in the meantime, all of these other suggestions are possibilities.

Dr. Katz: All of us want education, and many of us are in the field of education. The examples of smoking, alcohol, drugs, automobile accidents, etc., show that the route of education is probably the least fruitful of all the possible routes.

Dr. Cornell: Dr. Zienty, with your timetable, it is obvious that essentially no patent protection would be available by the time development is finished. Furthermore, a small corporation has essentially no chance of putting this type of thing through the regulatory agencies.

Dr. Zienty: Ordinarily, we would like to have a patent position in a product when we commit such large resources. If we file and obtain an initial patent at the beginning of the process, which is likely, there won't be very much of the life of the patent available by the time the product becomes commercial. In the case of new drug products, if the current revision of the statute is adopted, there may be a different situation with respect to the equity that the sponsoring company has in the drug product. The patent may expire by the time you finally get the drug product on the market, but you would still have five years from approval of the regulation, or the new drug application, for an exclusive use. Now, whether this finally survives in the revision of the stature remains to be seen. It is a problem and it has to be a consideration.

On the other side of that is the fact that those in industry who have basic positions in raw materials or manufacturing capability would tend to choose products that fit out own special skills, a patent is not absolutely essential for survival.

With respect to smaller companies, you are quite correct; it is becoming less likely that a small company will be able to afford the process of innovation in food additive products, as has happened in the drug field. Only the large drug houses are capable of introducing innovative chemical entity drugs. This has, of course, led to a much lower number of new entity drug introductions.

Mr. Jorgensen: If you design these new products which lower cariogenicity, how are you going to educate the public when you can't promote them or advertise them?

Dr. Hopper: I have been assuming that we would go through the claim substantiation route with whatever legalities are necessary, an IND-NDA (Investigative New Drug-New Drug Application). Thus, if we had something that was effective, we could talk about it as a caries-inhibiting or anti-caries kind of a product. There is a gray area of labeling claim support, e.g., this does not promote caries, or some statement of that kind, which probably is going to be acceptable in the regulatory climate. That, in itself, is a form of communication — this is a product that is less of a risk of caries for you than one that does not carry the label.

If we are really going to be effective, we have got to proceed to something substantiated in clinical trials after the animal tests. That is out most effective form of communication: that this new type of product is going to be considerably better for you in terms of overall potential for caries production.

But if the labeling interpretation that says "Does not promote caries" is a viable one, without having to go through three-year clinical trials and INDs, then we have a step in that direction already.

Dr. Shory: You say we need a coordinated effort in education. Do you think the industry is prepared to modify its advertising to be supportive rather than contradictory of this view? For example, would you market one of these nice, luscious, sweet, exotic snacks, and then tell children that they should not be eaten between meals?

Dr. Hopper: I can't answer for the advertising community. Anything that we do in terms of nutrition education, if indeed we believe that to be the appropriate route, should be part of the communication with the public.

Dr. Shaw: Does some documentation exist to support the enthusiasm that oral hygiene on a community-wide basis would be effective in preventing dental caries extensively.

Dr. Hopper: I will be glad to furnish eight or ten studies, that show DMF scores to have come down.

Dr. Newbrun: Dr. Hopper made the point that he was opposed to regulation, and that we could really solve dental caries if we just had (1) good dental hygiene, and (2) good education.

Nutritional education largely has been unsuccessful in reducing caries. I cited the King study, and there are the studies of Plasschaert and König in The Netherlands, and there are some surveys in Sweden. Here, for example, they asked mothers whether they would do anything about their children's eating habits. Did they know what foods were related to caries? Yes, they knew, but they weren't willing to change their children's habits.

So I can't share your optimism that education per se is going to solve the problem.

You said you could cite eight or 10 studies in which oral hygiene has reduced dental caries. If you exclude studies on fluoride dentifrices, and you exclude studies where the oral hygiene was done by a dental nurse or a dental hygienist who did the flossing, if there are eight or 10 studies in which oral hygiene was performed by the child, I don't know those studies in which caries has been reduced. Certainly periodontal disease can be reduced or periodontal indices controlled.

Dr. Hopper: With your exclusions I would not be able to cite that many studies. I included all kinds of dental assists.

Dr. Newbrun: You made the point of economics and costs to industry. I think we have to look at the economics and cost to society. I am not sure that the cost of the Scandanavian programs where children were treated every two weeks is economical on a nationwide basis in this country. If you exclude those studies, we are left with oral hygiene as it is practiced in the United States, and I think then we have to come to the conclusion that that has not reduced caries effectively.

Dr. Hopper: But I think you will agree that technically it is possible. In practice, we have not yet achieved it.

Dr. Purvis: Conceding that nutrition education may not be a solution to the entire problem, I seek Dr. Hopper's comment on the approach in which we tend to emphasize the label and advertising as being the regulatory focus and not being a method of education. We recognize that the label is not a good tool for nutrition education.

I would like to see a shift in focus to the other areas of nutrition education, where information is available but it is not accessed as much as it should be. I refer to the trade association information.

We have a prevailing problem of credibility here, and this must be overcome. We have to learn to trust each other, but this information is factual. In professional communications it is a real accomplishment if a medical school makes the concession to put two or three hours of nutrition in its curriculum.

The public service television approach to nutrition education has not been adequately utilized.

Dr. Hopper: Certainly, I have to agree that the label itself is not a good education tool. At best, it can provide a limited amount of information. If the information on the label is placed into a positive program, a program that will reach the educators themselves, the people who are teaching, physicians or our dentists or our children, that is an important group to be reached.

There has been a very slow response in building good nutrition programs into the medical school curriculum, and I suspect that that is true in the dental school curriculum as well. Many more people are devoting research dollars to the role of nutrition in good dental health. That is a positive thing, and as soon as we get our professional people appropriately educated, we can do a better job of educating the masses. Documentaries, educational films, public service broadcasting programs, all are going to be helpful. But I don't believe that it is going to be effective unless we marshal the resources not just of government, and not just industry, not just the academic world, but all together, working in the same direction to effect a societal change.

Hit and miss, interruptive programs are not going to do the job. But we have good communication tools and resources and we are not using them appropriately, but we need to start with our professionals and be sure that they have the right baseline.

Dr. Madsen: I want to talk a little bit about nutrition education from the standpoint of someone who faces the problem of teaching dental students, and therefore teaching students how to teach their patients, about food cariogenicity in the context of total nutrition. We can't consider these separately. When you work with an individual patient or communities or groups of people, you have to consider the overall nutrition pattern.

Before publication of Shannon's analysis of sugar in food products I did not have analytical values for how much sugar was in the various products in order to calculate the total consumption per day. We must consider cardiovascular disease, obesity, diabetes, to the extent they are related, if we are going to build a prudent, ideal diet. That information must made available to educate people.

From the standpoint of nutrition education, we really need this information made available. Dr. Hopper, I appreciate your enthusiasm for developing new products, and I don't want to diminish that, but I think we need to label foods so that we can work with patients

Dr. Hopper: You are dealing with a very important part of what I was suggesting in terms of developing a comprehensive coordinated nutrition education program. You cannot tailor each and every food to be the absolutes of 15% protein, 30% fat, and 55% carbohydrate. Each one of them doesn't have to have the same profile. How we select foods that have different values is important. One is a high-protein food, one a high-carbohydrate food, another one a high-fat food. How we blend them all together determines nutrition, not the individual profile of an individual product.

How to use a given food in a dietary regimen is the important piece of information that we must give. Percentages of sugar and percentages of protein are a very uninformative way of conveying nutritional information to the consuming public. That is going to be an important part of the future nutrition education program, to show the absolute intake of various of these nutrients, food macronutrients as well as micronutrients in a dietary regimen, and how to balance them.

Dr. Ciancio: In medical and dental schools throughout the country, from the recent survey we have done, it turns out that education of the practitioner of tomorrow, the dentist or the physician or the dental auxiliary or the paramedic or paradental personnel, nutritional education is completely lacking in the majority of schools. Why? We don't have enough trained people who know enough about nutrition.

This is the general state of the art of nutrition information and education in this country. We need a massive campaign of education of the practitioners as well as the scientists before we can begin to reach the answers to the questions we are asking. We can speculate, and we can look at sucrose and look at pH and complain about the different tests, but as an academic person, I can see the dilemma of the manufacturer. He asked us for advice, and we don't have the answers yet. We have to begin to coordinate efforts between education and industry in developing more knowledge about nutrition and nutritional guidance; this would be a big accomplishment of this conference.

I hope we don't forget that plaque is also related to periodontal disease. Although we are talking about caries today, the foods with which we are concerned may also affect the plaque that produces periodontal disease.

Dr. Glass: Earlier, somebody mentioned that there was a shortage of nutritionists who were interested in dentistry, and that nutrition teaching in dental schools was not what it should be. Having taught on dental faculties for a number of years, I would have to agree that the curriculum of the dental school is in large measure determined by organized dentistry—the American Dental Association and affiliated groups. In the past, the accreditation groups have counted the number of fillings that students place when they practice in a clinic, and they count the number of times they have cleaned patients' teeth, they count the number of dentures that they make, etc., and how many hours they spend in school, but little, if any, time has been devoted to a requirement that adequate courses in nutrition be taught. This could be changed virtually overnight if the accreditation bodies saw fit to require that every accredited dental school had an adequate course in nutrition.

Dr. Choate: Several comments this morning seem curiously evasive of what is really going on in food merchandising today. Mr. Hickman really hit the nail on the head when he said that if you really want to have impact, and if you really want to guide your company though the legal and regulatory jungle, you have to establish at the very beginning how you are going to sell this food, because only then can you start to shape the ingredient so that it will meet the description later to go out over the air or in print.

I am also amazed at the number of persons who have chatted with me about how you regard the horrors of advertising of foods today, particularly on the air to children, mentioning that there is a tremendous pressure from the marketing end of your companies to keep the sugar content high. It seems to me we ought to be able to wed your concern with cavities with Mr. Hickman's early advice, and that is to invite you and your companies to start to think early about how we can market a food without touting its sugaredness, its sweetness, its sucrose content.

I would remind you that if you think the sucrose content of foods advertised to children is high, the sucrose content of the messages is much, much higher. You need only watch TV to find the 30-second ad that touts sweetness 13 times in 30 seconds. Then you start to realize what pressure there is on those who develop foods to devise an even sweeter one. Until we change this pressure, no amount of public education is going to suffice because the moderate TV-watching child today sees 4,200 minutes of food advertising a year and 65% are based on a sweetness characteristic.

Dr. Alfano: In the traditional sense in oral hygiene there are some problems in terms of controlling dental caries, but I think that we need not include all of the Dr. Newbrun caveats.

For example, Lindhe and Axelsson specifically evaluated the effects of hygiene exclusive of fluoride, and noted a significant improvement, irrespective of any fluoride treatment. That is important: it can work if it is well practiced.

As to the cost effectiveness to the individual, I would refer to an editorial by Richard Ranney which appeared in the *Virginia State Dental Association Journal* a few years ago: this program is definitely cost effective. Perhaps one of the problems is the way we dentists perceive the provision of prophylactic services to our patients. We perceive it as twice a year, performed by a dental hygienist, at a cost varying from $25 to $40 per visit. The services provided in the Lindhe-Axelsson studies were much less expensive, being essentially coronal polishing. Ranny speaks to this issue in his editorial. Perhaps it is time to reconsider what this professional care should be, away from two visits a year perhaps to 12 visits a year at $5 each, which becomes considerably more cost effective.

Dr. Katz: In dental caries — even acknowledging that there are many questions to answer — what is probably most important is the contact of the food with the teeth, and not necessarily the nutritional impact upon organisms. In that context the presence of sugar in foods and the risk to the teeth should be evaluated.

Dr. DePaolo: We had one of the two federally-funded programs to implement nutrition in the dental school environment at the Medical College of Virginia. Two things became apparent after about four years of program development. One is that the professional — the student as well as the dentist in continuing education — is educable. With aggressive behavior and visibility you can in fact get a lot of nutrition education programs implemented in a curriculum.

Furthermore, one of the specific recommendations of the National Curriculum Survey done about two years ago, was to include courses on clinical nutrition in dental schools. The climate is becoming more favorable for nutrition and nutrition education to be provided to those who ultimately will have most beneficial influence on the consumer, and that is the dental population.

Dr. Moss: I was concerned when some of the comments were made that it really doesn't help to give nutritional counseling to parents, and that toothbrushing doesn't help. I think we miss the boat when we start talking that way.

Good educational programs are indeed working all over the United States, and we do have the opportunity to raise a generation of cavity-free children, even today with our present diet. Home care starting at birth, so it becomes a cultural habit; good fluoride systemically and topically; routine dental visits; good diet counseling; and sealants indeed are working around the United States today. We should not say that these educational programs aren't working. I think we have to educate people and dentists in the whole scope of what is available today.

Dr. Newbrun: I emphasized that I am quite convinced that oral hygiene is absolutely essential for the maintenance of a healthy peridontium. My point in terms of oral hygiene as practiced in the United States, even in experimentally controlled deplaquing studies, for example, Alice Horowitz's study in Connecticut and Steve Silverstein's study in Oakland, have shown that daily supervised deplaquing studies conducted in the schools did not reduce the caries increments. This is very disappointing; I would be delighted if the data had been different, but it hasn't.

Obviously, as a teacher of preventive dentistry, I think it is absolutely important to teach future dentists and dental students and dental hygiene students principles of good nutrition, and to teach their patients these principles. But as a scientist I have to look at hard, experimentally controlled situations where it has been demonstrated that dietary advice is effective on a community basis. I am sure that Dr. Nizel and other individuals who spend a lot of time on it and who are convinced of it, and can convince their patients, have some success. But I think one has to look at the overall public health picture, and that is where we just don't have the data to sustain it, and I wish it were otherwise.

I would like to comment about Dr. Alfano's notion, that we should change the way dental practice is conducted; instead of two visits a year, we should have 12 visits a year. The studies in Sweden and Denmark indicated that when you go from the prophylaxis every two weeks to once a month, you do not get the same caries reduction. And it has been shown that some of this very high caries reduction is the result of extreme enthusiasm and effectiveness of some of the dental nurses, and that other nurses who were not as enthusiastic did not get the same results.

I think one also has to be realistic. There are very real problems in getting organized dentistry, the American Dental Association and the various state boards, to accept this form of treatment by dental auxiliaries. I think these are real problems, and we should face them.

Dr. Moss: If we single out one preventive measure alone and try to say that toothbrushing doesn't help, we lose sight of what we have available today. And I think in combination, toothbrushing, fluoride treatment, and all the other things today can work, and are indeed working.

Dr. Daniels: Is it realistic to think that no matter what anyone does, you are going to get people to drastically decrease something that is hedonistic? Dr. Newbrun showed yesterday that there is a plateau that can be reached for dental caries, and that further studies that are carried out, once you reach that plateau, are ludicrous. I would agree with that.

But Dr. Navia has suggested for years that the plateau might occur somewhere around 3, 4, or 5%, at least in his animal model. We have heard that in a particular diet, at 3.5% he was able to reach maximum.

Dr. Newbrun believes that plateau to probably be somewhere between 5 and 15%. If the plateau for sucrose is near 5%, discussions of trying to reduce sucrose to that level have to consider: Is dental caries as important as the national economics and world food economics involved? I think we had better find out (1) whether the cure Dr. Newbrun presented is real or representative, and (2) where is the plateau, and is all of this discussion meaningful, or should we be attacking dental caries from an entirely different point of view?

Dr. Schemmel: In relation to the 3% sucrose or sugar in the diet, that plateau was reached when there was a high dietary carbohydrate level. Indeed, that plateau for sucrose in the diet, in all probability, could be elevated if there were other constituents in the diet such as protein or fat, or even some anticariogenic types of materials.

Dr. Sintes: So to the effectiveness of supervised toothbrushing, Zinner *et al.* have evidence that toothbrushing alone with plain deionized water reduces the microbial count and reduces or maintains the DMF, with no statistical difference from the baseline.

Nutrition counseling should be given by people who know not only facts about human nutrition, but are also prepared in behavior modification. The problem with providing nutrition counseling by dentists who have had a course in dental school is the fact that they don't know enough. Therefore, they provide a service that does not work. Having dental auxiliaries in our practices and having public health personnel surrounding practices, and having nutritionists surrounding our practices, I would say that if you would get these services from people who are prepared to provide them, the dental profession would benefit more.

Dr. Ciancio: Things are not as grim as we might think. The DMF has been going down since 1970. Part of that is probably a reflection of better public health education and fluoride in the country.

And, if you look at the *Journal of the American Society of Dentistry for Children*, articles appearing there are saying that the problem facing educators in pediatric dentistry today is that although they are seeing caries, they are not seeing it to the depth that they have seen it before. A problem faced in our own dental school is that we don't have children now with large areas of caries in their teeth that we can use to teach our students how to take care of badly broken-down teeth. It is not happening as much in the fluoridated areas today. So the picture is not so grim. The teaching problem we have today is that we do not have enough of these horrible cases of dental caries.

XIV. SCIENTIFIC AND REGULATORY REVIEW

Bernard Conway, J. D., Chairman

REGULATION IN SCIENCE

Walter E. Wisniewski, J. D.

The American Dental Association does not attempt to regulate products; it does not attempt to regulate therapeutic materials; nor does it attempt to regulate materials and devices. How it really sees its function in these scientific areas is as more of a public instrument. I don't want to have us confused with the government. I see the government more as a public burden; we see ourselves more as a public instrument.

We believe very seriously that dentists should have knowledge about the types of products that they recommend to their patients. In that regard, the American Dental Association has established programs. The most notable two are in the areas of the Council on Dental Materials and Devices and the Council on Dental Therapeutics. You are all familiar with some of the workings of those two Councils; basically those two Councils are trying to establish standards sufficient so that products and materials and therapeutic agents can be measured. And to the extent that they are measured and they prove not harmful to the public, the Councils will allow those types of products to carry a seal of acceptance, which is to be distinguished from approvals or disapprovals.

We concern ourselves to some extent with some of the legal implications in these activities. I am not going to go into that in great detail. Some of the concerns that we have, of course, are really involved with the Federal Trade Commission, that is, the Antitrust Section, Section 5 of the Federal Trade Commission Act, and the Sherman Antitrust Act, Section 2.

We have to be very careful that the standards that are set are universal, they are scientifically credible, and that all products may be measured fairly against those, so that we avoid any boycott type of problem, either factually or creating the appearance of doing that.

It has been suggested that the American Dental Association may have a role to play in establishing some standards in foods. I think that it is a mission that the Association should study very carefully. It is something that both the dentists and the public could utilize to the extent that we do involve ourselves in such activities. Of course, lawyers, being meddlers by nature, will have to take a look at what type of program it is, but I think that it is safe for me to say that we could commit ourselves if the program was properly established, with standards of measurement validly established to promote to the public and to others.

SUGAR, ORAL HEALTH AND REGULATION: A STRATEGY FOR PREVENTION OF ORAL DISEASE

Sanford A. Miller, Ph.D.

Among the many hedonic qualities of food, sweet taste is by far the most compelling. Beginning in fetal life, the developing child responds favorably to sweet material in the amniotic fluid. After birth, it is this taste modality to which a neonate responds most positively and strongly. For no other flavor modality does this response occur. During childhood and adolescence the dominance of this taste drive continues. However, after puberty the drive diminishes and in non-addicted or conditioned adults, this drive is balanced by the desire for a more varied hedonic pattern which, in theory, should lead to a more balanced caloric intake. It has been claimed, however, that in our society unlimited access to sugars of various kinds has led to a conditioned response in which the sustained high intakes of sugars have led to several health problems, the best defined being dental caries.

Although cane sugar, the dominant form consumed in the world today, is of relatively recent origin, the desire and drive for sweet substances has existed probably before *homo sapiens* evolved. The use of honey, dates, figs and other products having high concentrations of sugar and thus providing an intense sweet taste has been known from prehistoric times. However, the rarity of these products made them too precious to be used routinely by the common man. Thus, early in the history of man, the use of sweet substances was associated with pleasure and status, that is, recognition of position and success.

It was not until the introduction of cane sugar, spreading slowly from India to the West, that the capacity for satisfaction of the sweet taste became attainable for most of society. Even more importantly, the discovery of the sugar beet as a source of sugar in the 18th century made available for the first time a capacity for producing sugar sufficient to satisfy world needs. The availability of an inexpensive source of sugar and the movement toward urbanization has accelerated the process of increasing sugar consumption. Sugar still has a status connotation which, when combined with the high degree of acceptability of this taste, has made the regulation of sugar intake difficult.

For many reasons, sugar--pure sucrose--is not considered by nutritionists to be an acceptable food. Generally, the argument is made that this substance does not satisfy any nutritional need other than supplying calories, a need better fulfilled by many other foods having better nutritional patterns. Without regard for the merits of this argument, there are other reasons for considering the elimination of the intake of this group of substances. Chief among these is the fact that sugars are an important component of the etiology of dental caries and, to a lesser extent, other oral diseases.

Dental caries is a disease of considerable antiquity. Lesions have been identified in the teeth of ancient man and in Egyptian mummies, and have been a feature of oral health in virtually every period of man's history. The prevalence of this disease appears to increase with civilization, urbanization and affluence--processes which also tend to result in increases in the intake of simple sugars from a variety of sources. The association between caries incidence and intake of sugar has long been recognized. Aristotle was said to have questioned the damaged teeth produced by ripened soft figs, that is, fruit consumed at a time when these fruits are most sweet. While it is true that the evidence linking simple sugar intake and dental caries is largely presumptive and inferred from epidemiological evidence and animal experiments, it is, in my opinion, unequivocal. Almost uniformly the data demonstrate that the incidence of dental caries is related to the frequency of consumption of simple sugars. When this observation is added to the fact that dental caries is the public health problem of greatest frequency in this country and in the Western world in general, one may ask, "Why has not the FDA or other federal regulatory agencies moved to protect the public from this hazard?"

There are, I believe, several reasons for this lack of action on the part of regulatory agencies. First, there is little clear perception among regulatory agencies that dental caries represents a disease process of some significance. For these agencies to respond there must be a clear perception of a present or future danger threatening life or providing a significant reduction in function. For many people, dental caries does not fulfill these requirements. It is described by many as "holes in teeth" easily correctable at best and prosthetically replaceable at worst. Second, dental caries is not seen as a classical toxic response and thus not normally used as evidence for the regulation of substances added or present in foods. The Select Committee on Gras Substances committee of the Federation of American Societies for Experimental Biology concluded that, indeed, modification of tooth enamel and tooth structure was as much a pathological event of note as any other tissue change. Moreover these changes fall within the definition of toxicity that include any adverse effect of chemicals that directly or indirectly affect human health. Parenthetically, one might add that, for most toxicologists and pathologists, the mouth is an obstacle that gets in the way of their examination of other structures. Nevertheless, it is clear, I believe, that neither of these two beliefs is correct. Dental caries *is* a disease process of concern, particularly in a society in which more acute infectious processes are coming under control. In addition, it can be considered a toxic response, as it does result in a loss of function and a change in tissue morphology. For these reasons, in my opinion, dental caries is a process deserving of consideration in the regulatory decisions of the Food and Drug Administration and other similar agencies.

Accepting this argument, is dental caries a hazard of sufficient threat to warrant immediate and detailed attention by regulatory agencies? There are several reasons to believe that it is. Not only is dental caries a process that affects virtually all members of our society, but it falls within an area in which public health measures can have some effect. This is true because at least one major component of the disease process, the substrate for cariogenic organisms, is a substance whose intake can be controlled by a change in diet. More importantly perhaps, dental caries represents a functional toxic effect that may be included in the list of performance characteristics associated with modern considerations of safety. With the increase in life span, American society is becoming less concerned with maintenance of life and more concerned with quality of life. Everyone expects to live to be a hundred. The concern of most people is *how* they will live to be a hundred. Thus, while the classical toxicologist is concerned with quantifiable, statistically analyzable events (such as death) to estimate hazard, the public, in its estimate of hazard, is interested equally in functions such as behavior, disease resistance, physical performance and phenomena such as dental caries. This concern is underlined by the fact that in a series of food labeling hearings that have recently been conducted around the country by the Food and Drug Administration, the U. S. Department of Agriculture and the Federal Trade Commission, the subject of sugar toxicity was raised by virtually every consumer witness to appear before the committee. This occurred in the context of both full ingredient labeling as well as in considerations of nutritional labeling. The important aspect of this observation is that, in the former case (full ingredient labeling), the concern was over the toxicity of sugar while in the latter (nutritional labeling), the concern was over sugar as a contributor to nutritional disease. While several potentially dangerous effects of sugar were mentioned during the course of these discussions, it was the effect on dental caries experience that was the most common reason given for such labeling needs. It has become a widely held belief in American culture that consumption of sugar leads automatically to dental caries. It should be noted that, while this belief always refers to added sucrose, a considerable number of people include *all* sugars, including those normally present in food, among those that contribute to the caries process. It seems clear that dental caries is not only a public health problem of sufficient magnitude to justify FDA consideration, but, more importantly, it represents an area of important concern to the American people, one in which action is being demanded.

Given the need for regulation, what are the methods by which such regulation can be implemented? There are two principal pathways available to FDA. First, it can restrict the use of the sugars for which an association with dental caries can be made. Even while recognizing that most of the sugar intake occurs as a result of consuming foods in which sugar is a natural constituent, still it may be argued that any reduction in sugar intake is desirable. Because a significant portion of the caries substrate is supplied as added sugar, it is reasonable to assume that such action in restricting use of sugar would result in a measurable decrease in caries incidence if the access to sugar in general could be controlled. However, in my opinion, this action is not feasible and certainly not warranted by the danger offered to the public health by the consumption of sugar. Even though caries is a problem of public health significance, it is not life-threatening. The use of a restriction in use should be limited to present, imminent dangers and should represent a final effort in the regulation of substances affecting health and safety. More importantly, for social reasons a regulatory restriction is not reasonable. As noted, the desire for satisfaction of the sweet taste is a fundamental physiological urge. Moreover, it represents an important component of the social structure by which society organizes and maintains itself. Such a restriction would be observed more in the breech than in the observance, resulting in such ludicrous situations as candy bar smuggling and Mafia gumballs. We don't need another great experiment such as prohibition. Finally, I do not believe that the Congress itself would permit such an action, even if some agency was crazy enough to demand it.

A second more reasonable and feasible option open to the FDA is labeling. This regulatory approach was recognized as a powerful tool early in the history of the Food and Drug Act in this country. It has been used for the past seventy years in several ways but most recently has been proposed as a way of providing for public safety in those areas where immediate danger did not exist and the implication of choices was clear to the consuming public. The relationship of dental caries and sugar intake is probably one of the best examples of a public health problem associated with the consumption of a specific substance for which the consumer might make a choice without resulting in death or severe threat to life. Thus, it is a particularly appropriate subject for the use of labeling. Labeling seems to be a viable alternative to regulatory restriction in the effort to reduce the risk of dental caries. It gives to the consumer an option of accepting the risk implied by the label information or deciding to use the information to make a dietary change. It is important to note, however, that such a system has little chance of success *if* the consumer has no knowledge of the options suggested by the label information. Thus, an information or education program must be an inherent component in any use of labeling as a regulatory strategy in the control of dental disease.

Having made the decision to label, there still remain several questions fundamental to the implementation of this policy. What should be on the label? and should a warning be included in this information?

Traditionally, the function of the label is to provide information with which the consumer can make appropriate choices in the selection of his food supply. Thus, in the case of sugar, the question revolves around the point of what information is required. Indicating only the presence of "sugar" in the product is not sufficient nor is it sufficient to place the sucrose and other sugars in their appropriate position in the list of ingredients in descending order of predominance. For such information to be useful, the *amount* of sugar in the product is essential because only with such data can the consumer decide if the amount they will consume is likely to be excessive or deleterious. Many consumer advocates argue that only *added* sucrose should be quantified on the label, implying in this way that the oral floras are "unnatural" food advocates selectively growing on "refined" sugar only. Because the oral flora are nondiscriminatory in their energy substrate needs, they do not distinguish between sugar put there by man *or* God. Thus, any quantitative labeling system must include *total* sugar, both added and naturally present. The matter becomes more complex, however, when one considers the fact that with the mixed flora of the human oral environment, many sugars can serve as substrates for plaque formation and caries initiation. Sucrose, fructose, and glucose have relatively the same capability of serving as substrates while other simple sugars such as xylose appear to be only somewhat less cariogenic. Pragmatically then, any sugar label designed to facilitate reduction in sugar intake to reduce caries incidence must include *all* potential substrates and therefore must include all simple sugars present in the products, i.e., all monosaccharides and disaccharides. Would it be sufficient, one might ask, to report only total simple sugar, or it is necessary to itemize each? We are always struggling between the desire for precision and maximum information on our labels and a danger of an information glut and subsequent overload to the consumer's ability to perceive and comprehend the information available to him. At this moment, we do not have the information base on which to make such a decision.

A further dimension in this issue of total sugar labeling is the use of a label warning as part of the information package. Such warnings have been used sparingly in the food regulatory history of FDA. They have usually been associated with substances that represent at least a presumptive danger to life. It has been proposed, however, that this provision of the law be extended to include warnings useful in understanding the potential risks associated with a product, irrespective of the nature of the threat involved. On this basis, it has been proposed that such warnings be included in the labeling requirements for sugar in foods--the nature of the statement to warn against the hazards to the teeth of consuming a particular product. Without debating the need or advisability of such an action, it must be pointed out that during the labeling hearings, there was widespread but certainly not unanimous sentiment for such labeling. In fact, only for sodium and sugar was such a desire expressed, again confirming the concern of the consumer over these substances.

In any case, several major problems are associated with the implementation of this policy. A caries warning can be based on either the *total* sugar content of the product (not only on added sucrose as some advocates desire), or on the measured, objective evaluation of the cariogenicity of the individual food product.

As you are well aware, caries is a complex disease of multiple etiology involving not only the provision of appropriate substrate, but the nature of the oral flora, the oral environment, the susceptibility of the target organ (the tooth) and the physiological state of the host. Even in the question of the substrate, its form, texture, frequency and pattern of consumption are principal contributors to its cariogenic potential. Thus, the total sugar content, while important, is not the sole, or even dominant determinant of cariogenicity. Thus, a warning system based on total sugar content alone is unsatisfactory and clearly of limited value.

The most acceptable system for determining cariogenicity would involve objective assays of cariogenicity for individual foods using human subjects. Several methods have been proposed and are currently under investigation. Given the normal pace of such scientific efforts and the relatively low priority assigned to such activities in the past, and considering the limited funds that have been available for such efforts, it seems likely that the validation of these methods and the determination of their viability and their acceptance by the scientific community will be a long, drawn-out process. It has been predicted, as a matter of fact, that ten years or more will be required to produce such a method. The problem, however, is one of time. The regulatory agencies are under pressure to initiate immediate action in sugar labeling, not only through the action of consumer advocates, but more importantly, as a result of one of the most consistent demands emerging from the food labeling hearings. Congress perceives this, and several bills have been proposed which include such mandatory labeling. This issue also has been raised in several committee hearings and by many members of the Congress. Thus it is clear that the Agency does not have the luxury of time to respond to these issues in the careful, slowly evolving process of traditional scientific evaluation.

For these same reasons, the pressure is also on the scientific community and the dental profession. We need answers and decisions on several issues if a rational labeling policy is to be established. The dental profession, expressed perhaps by American Dental Association action, must state unequivocally its stand on the issue of the necessity of sugar labeling in the prevention of caries and the nature of the information most useful for the dentist's use in counseling his patients. These comments must be clear and detailed, irrespective of which side of the issue they support. The scientific community must provide, in the near future, objective methods of caries evaluation, keeping in mind the necessary balance between the desire for perfection and the time scale for development.

One does not always require a perfect system, simply one that can separate foods into broad categories reflecting potential hazard. If the scientific community cannot do this, then we must know on what basis we can discriminate in caries susceptibility among foods. If we can do this on the basis of sugar content (which I doubt), what levels can be used as division points? All this must be done without the usual "on the one hand and on the other hand" approaches normally produced in such scientific activities. If such a scientific decision cannot be made, then, as recent history has shown, other considerations such as those involved with political, social, and economic issues, will form the basis of the regulatory agencies' decisions, science being relatively downgraded in this process. One may add, parenthetically, that because of the inability of science to provide reasonable answers to matters of safety evaluation based on 20th century science rather than on 19th century tradition, there is developing a trend in regulatory activities to make such decisions on the basis of other non-scientific values. While consideration of politics, social dynamics, and economic impact are essential to regulatory decisions, the decreasing influence of science is disturbing, particularly to someone of my background. It is, I believe, a result of the inability of the scientific community to come to grips with a decision in a way that is useful to a regulator. The possible exception to this is the one that says, "You're wrong" to each action made by someone else.

It is clear that whatever decisions are made, they must include *all* foods, not only processed or formulated products. Certainly, figs, dates, ripe pears, and so on are as much a hazard to oral health as any fabricated product, and thus should be labeled as such. The legal limitations on such actions are not clear and may indeed require additional legislative authority for the Agency.

The control and prevention of dental caries and other aspects of oral disease by limiting the intake of sugars is an important goal of modern public health. It is, I believe, a proper function for the FDA to assist in this effort by exploring the use of appropriate labeling strategies in which information useful to the consumer in making food selection can be presented. When combined with an effective education program, we may be able to affect significantly the incidence of this disease. The pressure from the public and the Congress on the Agency make imperative the rapid development of the information and technology required to implement this policy rationally. To accomplish this, we need the advice and support of the scientific and dental communities, but we need it now. This research must become a high priorioty effort, funded adequately and performed well. If this support, data, and techniques are not forthcoming, the decisions will be made without the appropriate scientific input, the principle effort occuring in response to considerations other than scientific. I am afraid that if events develop in this way it will further weaken the role of the scientist and the health professional in the regulatory process. We need your help; I hope you will provide it.

DISCUSSION

Mr. Jorgensen: Would you be willing to comment on what chance you think aspartame has for having its stay lifted, and what the timing would be for such a decision.

Dr. Miller: You know perfectly well I can't, even if I wanted to; even if I knew. After all, the issue is coming up for discussion. The scientific court of inquiry will meet, and they will make a decision. Even if I weren't in the Agency, I wouldn't want to comment on it, because there really are no absolute decisions on matters of science of this kind. There can't be. And the result is that, if you historically look at such activities, you discover that to a certain extent the tenor of the times tends to determine how important certain borderline pieces of evidence are.

Aspartame is a good example of the times in which we are living.

Dr. Daniels: What would be the most appropriate source for the type of scientific information that you have just called for?

Dr. Miller: Objectively, the data should come from anywhere; that is, we need the data. I don't care where it comes from or where the money comes from to support it. We need it and we need it right away, and this is clear. The existence of this group, by the way, I think is an example of the fact that somehow, somewhere, somebody decided that we ought to be doing some work in this area—that there was a public problem involved.

You also understand that there is an incredible—to put it politely—distrust, suspicion, of work supported by industry funds. It exists, and you know absolutely well that if it comes out in any way favorable to the interests of industry, the comment will be made that the work is not truthful or objective.

As a result of this, I think that you need some kind of laundry. There is no other way to describe it. Some way in which money from industry—from where the support must come, by the way—can be funneled into an institution whose *bona fides* are acceptable to everyone and whose veracity is unchallenged. I suspect that the ADA may be one such institution; there are others as well.

Dr. Schiff: Are you planning to have a separate entity for expertise in dentistry in the food area, or are you going to continue to rely on the drug expertise for the dental area?

Dr. Miller: We are hoping to be able to develop our own expertise in the area. There is a different way of looking at this, and we would like to get some people who are oral biologists, and dentists who are also trained in nutrition, for example, on board.

For a group which regulates a business the size of the food business, the Bureau of Foods has been systematically starved for the last 50 years. In fact, our budget was cut this year. This despite all the intense interest and new initiatives on the part of Congress to increase the responsibilities of the Bureau. And among the initiatives we were developing at a time when we had to put a ceiling on hiring was an increase in dental manpower. What I am saying is that for both industry and the consumer, the best hope for a reasonable food supply and some variety is going to be an effective, scientifically sound, operative Food and Drug Administration. It is in fact your only and best friend up there.

Mr. Cornell: Do you have any ideas on labeling as a "carrot" for the manufacturers? Do you envision that this would be a useful function? In other words, identifying the product and giving the manufacturers an advantage for a particular product over another?

Dr. Miller: Far be it from me to tell anybody how to merchandise their products. If the kind of uneasy feeling concerning sugar persists and develops, and if nutrition education counseling of the kind that we talked is developed, then obviously a product which fulfills the hedonic requirements that people have in foods, and at the same time clearly, by labeling, shows a reduction in a substance over which I am concerned, that is going to certainly offer them a product advantage.

The serving size is one of the problems. This is where industry keeps getting into problems. Nutritional labeling came along, and because of the difficulty of assigning for any particular product the size of a serving, the Agency is taking the rather general view that you could establish your own, as long as it is called reasonable. As a result, as many consumers have pointed out, a can of this size is labeled to contain one serving, because somehow it makes certain nutritional qualities look better, and a can of another size, because it contains a high caloric density, has four servings. The public doesn't accept this.

This is part of the problem. The industry is going to have to do it with restraint and understanding; if they oversell it too much, they are going to simply lose the advantage. I think they have to develop a greater sense of statesmanship. The alternative is going to be a total regulation, and the government will have to tell the industry precisely how to make food, and that would detract.

Dr. Newbrun: Let's say one had several predictability tests, and one had a product, and one of the predictability tests included an animal feeding–some sort of a feeding program. Let us say that the product, if it was fed to the animal once a day or twice a day, gave a low caries score, and yet when fed multiple times a day it gave a high caries score. We know, in fact, the definition of a snack food is the use, and not what the food is. So how could that be resolved in the label, that the inherent cariogenicity depends on the use? You noted the fact that this was not just sucrose content, but form and frequency.

Dr. Miller: You have to build that into your assay which predicts the cariogenicity of the food. You decide beforehand that you are going to make the measurement under these conditions, which might include spaced feeding, it would certainly specify the diet and the other components, and that is the agreed circumstance.

Let me warn some of you who have been in this nutrition business before to consider what happened when no one could agree on protein evaluation assays. We ended up with PER (protein efficiency ratio), which is probably the worst single way, for humans at least, of evaluating the quality of a protein. We are still stuck with it, because even ten years later we still can't get agreement from people on what constitutes a better way of doing it.

Dr. Mackay: Dr. Miller, I was very struck by your reference to the dangers that when industry comes forward with data, it appears to be self-serving, which of course is well known, and the suggestion that the American Dental Association be a good vehicle or conduit for results, or perhaps be asked to provide the results themselves. Can you suggest any other such vehicle?

Dr. Miller: I would rather not. There are institutions in certain universities, there are certain professional organizations that have both consumer and industry representatives, or you can set up your own, so to speak.

Dr. Mackay: I am glad to have you say there are none, because Dr. Smith and I have been trying in effect to tell the American Dental Association that they really are by far the best organization to take this responsibility.

Dr. White: Dr. Miller, can your statement: that if scientific information is not available to sustain a given action, then the decision will be made on another basis, perhaps socioeconomic basis, political basis, then be turned around to say that if science cannot provide evidence that a problem actually exists, then science will be ignored?

Dr. Miller: No it doesn't say that at all. What it says is that science very often is not the initiator in concern over a particular issue. It comes from another sector of society. And unless the scientific community, generally speaking, is willing to say unequivocally that there is no problem, then as long as there is enough wishy-washiness going on in terms of what it might be or could be, then that is the point when the non-scientist grabs that portion of the data they want to support their evidence.

Then it becomes very difficult to get scientific later. Most of the scientific community doesn't believe vitamin C is a serious deficiency disease in our society, and there hasn't been a great deal of pressure from anyone to provide any kind of special activity concerning vitamin C.

I think that there is a great deal of pressure to make FDA less a scientific agency and more a compliance agency, which puts their decisions onto grounds less scientific and more "other." In part, this argument has been made because of the things that I have described. Right now it is not true. And right now, the FDA has to deal with the pressures on it from society, expressed through the Congress as well as more directly. These are appropriate, by the way.

Dr. Mackay: Who at FDA considers the consequence of a move to restrict sugar in the sense of the cosmic reordering of the total dietary? If we are going to take sugar out, how do we replace it, are we having more protein, more fats, more starch? Someone has got to consider the consequence of this, no matter how important or how driving the influence of a certain group, and no matter how compelling their evidence. Someone else has got to take the larger view. Who does it?

Dr. Miller: Well, legally, the Commissioner. Practically, what happens is that for virtually any issue, we prepare for him and for others documents outlining the situation. Inside the Bureau, we develop position papers. They are used ultimately as a way of forming a position, of coming to a decision.

The law does not permit us to make benefit considerations, but we do include, even now in information we send to the Commissioner, economic impact statements and environmental impact statements. We are attempting now in the Bureau to figure out ways of including social impact statements. What will be the impact on society of the efforts we are making? The best example I know is the saccharin situation. The response of the public to the potential saccharin ban was a societal one in the sense that there was a social issue involved about people using it, which wasn't considered. We are attempting to include that in our own evaluations, and at the end we hope to come up with something like this. But we don't have the skills to do it very well. We do a lot of talking about benefit calculation, about risk calculation. We don't really have good strategies for this. How do you determine what the social impact will be? I don't know how yet, but at least we will try.

But in the end, the decision will be made—we will come to some conclusions and present them as options for the Commissioner, indicating one as a preference. And then, I suppose, in the end it will come down to me.

SUMMATION

Dr. Hefferren: About a year ago, we planned an open forum to which we invited people with different points of view and differing backgrounds. We formulated a program along the interests of our expected audience. By and large we achieved our aim. We brought out various points of view and gave you the opportunity to comment on a number of situations related to the cariogenicity of foods.

APPENDIX

COOPERATIVE PROGRAM ON FOODS, NUTRITION, AND DENTAL HEALTH

The recognized differential effects of foods and dietary habits in the development of caries have led to research in caries and to the development of products with a reduced caries-producing potential. However, many difficulties, related primarily to the lack of generally recognized laboratory methods of measurements and the complexities of conducting clinical studies of foods, have discouraged attempts to evaluate foods as to their cariogenicity and to modify that cariogenicity.

Investigative Program Established

Representatives of academe, the food industry, federal agencies, and the Research Institute met in May to establish a cooperative program on foods, nutrition, and dental health. The meeting was the culmination of a series of deliberations, which began with a Workshop on the Cariogenicity of Foods in September 1977. An 11-member ad hoc organizing committee, appointed by John J. Hefferren, Ph.D. director of the Research Institute, presented proposals for comment and discussion to the representatives of 25 organizations, who then agreed to help support the proposed program pending approval by their respective organizations.

The following program objectives were delineated:

to foster improved understanding among the food industry, dental researchers, and regulatory and professional agencies;

to continue the workshop on cariogenicity of foods on an annual basis as one means to discuss problems of general mutual interest in a scientific setting;

to further the development of suitable model systems to measure the various parameters relating food to dental caries, but not to the exclusion of plaque and periodontal studies;

to consider relevant regulatory proposals and actions; and

to foster interaction with and liaison to the ADA.

The ad hoc organizing committee will serve until the second workshop, scheduled for Oct. 5-6, when the program membership will elect an executive committee to assume direction of the work. Technical committees will be established to conduct the necessary collaborative studies relevant to the cariogenicity of foods.

Important Considerations Result of Workshop

The September 1977 workshop and the later small group meetings laid the groundwork for the investigative program. The workshop was attended by persons representing 20 university and academic research groups; 36 manufacturers, processors, and ingredient manufacturers of bakery products, beverages, cereals, candy, chewing gum, confections, and baby-adult foods; 8 trade associations; and professional, regulatory, and investigative organizations (the ADA, American Dietetic Association, National Academy of Science, National Institute for Dental Research, and the U.S. Department of Agriculture).

Scientists at the workshop emphasized many factors that must be considered in planning for future studies and investigations. These points were brought out during the meeting:

Fermentable carbohydrates are related to dental caries.

Carbohydrate containing foods are not equally destructive to the teeth.

There is no direct proportional relationship between the concentration of fermentable carbohydrates including sugar, per se, and frequency or extent of caries.

Frequency of eating is at least as important as the total amount of fermentable carbohydrates consumed.

Food retention and thus rate of clearance from the mouth is an important factor in cariogenic potential.

Food properties such as acid buffering capacity can influence cariogenic potential.

Phosphates can influence the cariogenic potential of foods.

It is difficult to measure the cariogenic potential of an individual food item in the total diet.

There are no generally accepted or recognized methods for indicating the cariogenicity of foods.

Assessment of Cariogenicity

In the earlier meetings, detailed consideration was given to a generally acceptable methodology for assessing cariogenicity. The value, limitations, advantages, and disadvantages of using plaque models, animal models, and *in vitro* models were reviewed and tentative potential experimental approaches were considered.

Plaque pH methods, using human plaque specimens, have been used to give a measure of the acidity produced at the plaque-tooth interface when a food is eaten, but this is a measure of the plaque acidity and not cariogenicity, per se. These methods have been useful for giving comparative or relative, but not absolute, pH values at the site of plaque on the tooth.

Cotton and albino rats have been the preferred animal models, because they are somewhat comparable to man in regard to effects of ecological factors, diet, microorganisms, and are hosts that develop caries. The same physical characteristics of food, chemical composition of the diet, and organoleptic properties that influence caries production in humans have been found to apply to rats. A sophisticated programmed feeding of food and fluid by machine has permitted a study of solid and liquid foods with normal or altered sugar content at regular meal and snack intervals. Although there is a strong potential for the use of animal models in predicting the caries-producing properties of foods, there is no reference point available to judge the results in humans.

Certain *in vitro* models also have been useful in providing information on the potential cariogenicity of foods. One specific use may be to determine whether additives or food processing methods have altered characteristics influencing cariogenicity. These models can provide information about composition, especially of carbohydrates; pH of food mixed with water and saliva; effects of food retention; the effects of the physical form of the food; and the pH buffering capacity of food. In comparison with clinical studies, the models are less expensive, of short duration, require fewer personnel and limited quantities of specialized and sophisticated analytical equipment. Although the data from *in vitro* models are useful, they should be used with caution because they may not be relevant to clinical caries production.

Any effort to undertake clinical trials on the cariogenicity of foods is handicapped by at least three difficulties: the concern and reluctance of committees on human studies to consider clinical trials using refined carbohydrates with the control group, the impossibility of feeding a human on a single substance for an extended time period, and the variability of diet within both test and control groups.

The current status of food modification with the intent of influencing caries reduction was reviewed with regard to proposing appropriate experimental investigations. Interest centers primarily on phosphate compounds; sugar alcohols such as xylitol, mannitol, and sorbitol; and artificial sweeteners.

Regulatory agencies have influenced the course of the utilization of data obtained from studies on the modification of food substances through their interpretation of law and establishment of regulations. It is the intended use, rather than the inherent nature, of a substance that determines whether it is to be considered as a food or as a drug, and the claims made for it determine the intent.

The complexity and interactions of many aspects and factors that influence the cariogenicity potential of foods demand that sound methodology be developed, validated, and recognized. The investigative program has initiated a cooperative effort, with widespread support and extensive expertise, which could bring a better understanding of the relation and effect of food to caries.

The proceedings of the Workshop on the Cariogenicity of Foods will be published through the American Dental Association Research Institute.

Information regarding membership in the program may be obtained from Dr. John J. Hefferren, Director, Research Institute.

Members of Foods and Nutrition Program, Organizing Committee

Donald A. Mackay, PhD. *Chairman*
Life Savers, Inc.
Basil G. Bibby, DMD, PhD
Eastman Dental Center
G. Norris Bollenback, PhD
The Sugar Association, Inc.
William H. Bowen, DDS, PhD
National Institute of Dental Research
Ray G. Kelly
The Sunmark Companies
Juan M. Navia, PhD
University of Alabama
Thomas Schiff, DMD
Monsanto Co.
George K. Stookey, PhD
Indiana University
Alan Thomas, PhD
M&M/Mars
Philip White, ScD
American Medical Association
Walter Wolman, PhD
ADA Health Foundation

ATTENDEES
SECTION B:
THE ROLE OF SUGAR AND OTHER FOOD IN DENTAL CARIES
WHAT CAN INDUSTRY DO?

Mr. Edwin Abeling
Vice President
Research and Development
Peter Paul Cadbury Inc.
Naugatuck, Conn. 06770

Mr. Robert A. Aherne
President
Finn-Cal Products, Inc.
1169 Chess Drive, Suite G
Foster City, Calif. 94404

Michael C. Alfano, D.M.D., Ph.D.
Director, Oral Health
Research Center
Fairleigh Dickinson University
110 Fuller Place
Hackensack, N.J. 07601

Mr. Allan Allured
Manufacturers Confectionery
Publishing Company
175 Rock Road
Glen Rock, N.J. 07452

Ray H. Anderson, Ph.D.
Principal Scientist
Corporate Research
General Mills Research
9000 Plymouth Avenue, N.
Minneapolis, Minn. 55427

William Ayer, D.D.S., Ph.D.
Chief Research Scientist
Division of Behavioral Science
ADA Health Foundation
Research Institute
211 E. Chicago Avenue
Chicago, Ill. 60611

Arthur N. Bahn, Ph.D.
Professor of Microbiology
Department of Biomedical Sciences
School of Dental Medicine
Southern Illinois University
Edwardsville, Ill. 62026

Miss Lisa Bahn
Leo Burnett Agency
Prudential Plaza
Chicago, Ill. 60601

Robert Bauer, Ph.D.
Assistant Secretary
Council on Dental Materials
and Devices
American Dental Association
211 E. Chicago Avenue
Chicago, Ill. 60611

Basil G. Bibby, D.M.D., Ph.D.
Eastman Dental Center
625 Elmwood Avenue
Rochester, N.Y. 14620

G. Norris Bollenback, Ph.D.
Scientific Director
The Sugar Association, Inc.
1511 K Street, N.W.
Washington, D.C. 20005

William H. Bowen, B.D.S., Ph.D.
Assistant Director
National Caries Program
National Institute of Dental Research
Westwood Building
5333 Westbard
Bethesda, Md. 20016

Mr. Walter F. Brightman
Ragold, Inc.
500 N. Michigan Avenue
Suite 250
Chicago, Ill. 60611

Ronald J. Carlotti, Ph.D.
Manager, Nutrition Research
Basic Research
Frito-Lay, Inc.
900 N. Loop 12
Irving, Tex. 75061

Ms. Catharine L. Chamberlin
Legal Assistant
Kirkland & Ellis
1776 K Street, N.W.
Washington, D.C. 20006

Miss An-Shih Cheng
Director
Office of Advertising Review
American Dental Association
211 E. Chicago Avenue
Chicago, Ill. 60611

D.O. Chichester, Ph.D.
Vice President
The Nutrition Foundation, Inc.
489 Fifth Avenue
New York, N.Y. 10017

Mrs. Velma Child
Editorial consultant
Research Institute
American Dental Association
211 E. Chicago Avenue
Chicago, Ill. 60611

Neal W. Chilton, D.D.S.
Research Professor of Oral Medicine
Clinical Research Center
University of Pennsylvania
School of Dental Medicine A-I
4001 Spruce Street
Philadelphia, Pa. 19104

Mr. Robert B. Choate
President
Council on Child Media and
Merchandising
1346 Connecticut, N.W.
Washington, D.C. 20036

Lawrence Chow, Ph.D.
Chief Research Scientist
Division of Chemistry
ADA Research Unit
National Bureau of Standards
Washington, D.C. 20234

Sebastian G. Ciancio, D.D.S.
School of Dentistry, Farber Hall
State University of New York
at Buffalo
Buffalo, N.Y. 14214

Clesteen Clark
Manager, Nutrition Communication
Public Affairs Department
Kellogg Company
235 Porter Street
Battle Creek, Mich. 49016

Fergus M. Clydesdale, Ph.D.
Professor, Department of Food
Science and Nutrition
University of Massachusetts
Amherst, Mass. 01003

Bernard Conway, J.D.
Assistant Executive Director
Legislation and Legal Affairs
American Dental Association
211 E. Chicago Avenue
Chicago, Ill. 60611

William E. Cooley, Ph.D.
The Procter & Gamble Company
Winton Hill Technical center
Cincinnati, Ohio 45224

Mr. John Cornell
Executive Director
Westwood Research Laboratory, Inc.
32nd & Spring Garden Streets
Philadelphia, Pa. 19104

Richard W. Daniels, Ph.D.
Group Director
Nutrition, Health & Product Safety
Standard Brands Incorporated
Betts Avenue
Stamford, Conn. 06904

Mrs. Pat Darchun
Assistant to the Diretor
of Administration
ADA Health Foundation
211 E. Chicago Avenue
Chicago, Ill. 60611

Miss Dana Davis
Assistant Director
Bureau of Dental Health Education
American Dental Association
211 E. Chicago, Ill. 60611

Dominick P. DePaola, D.D.S., Ph.D.
Nutrition Director
Oral Health Research Center
Fairleigh Dickinson University
110 Fuller Place
Hackensack, N.J. 07601

W. Michael Edgar, B.D.S., Ph.D.
Senior Lecturer
Department of Oral Physiology
Dental School
University of Newcastle upon Tyne
Framington Place
Newcastle upon Tyne, England NEZ 4BW

E. Eugene Fisher, Ph.D.
Vice President
Research and Quality Control
William Wrigley, Jr. Company
410 N. Michigan Avenue
Chicago, Ill. 60611

Wilbert Fletke, D.D.S.
1515 Mount Hope Avenue
Lansing, Mich. 48910

Mrs. Susan Flor
Staff Associate
Council on Dental Health
and Health Planning
American Dental Association
211 E. Chicago Avenue
Chicago, Ill. 60611

Mr. Robin Foor
Kellogg Company
235 Porter Street
Battle Creek, Mich. 49016

Victor P. Frattali, Ph.D.
Assistant to Associate Director
for Nutrition & Consumer Sciences
HFF-200
FDA Bureau of Foods
200 C. Street, S.W., Room 1832
Washington, D.C. 20204

Ms. Darlene Fujii
Staff Associate
Council on Dental Health
and Health Planning
American Dental Association
211 E. Chicago Avenue
Chicago, Ill 60611

Wayne Geiselman, Ph.D.
Manager, Clinical Research
Department of Dental Science
American Chicle Division
Warner-Lambert Company
170 Tabor Road
Morris Plains, N.J. 07950

Robert L. Glass, D.M.D., Dr. P.H.
Forsyth Dental Center
140 The Fenway
Boston, Mass. 02115

Mr. John Goetz
Managing Editor
American Dental Association
211 E. Chicago Avenue
Chicago, Ill. 60611

Mr. Peter C. Goulding
Assistant Executive Direcctor
Communications
American Dental Association
211 E. Chicago Avenue
Chicago, Ill. 60611

Mrs. Judith Grumley
Chief, Animal Facility
ADA Health Foundation
Research Institute
211 E. Chicago Avenue
Chicago, Ill. 60611

Timothy S. Hardy, L.L.D.
Attorney, Kirkland & Ellis
1776 K Street, N.W.
Washington, D.C. 20006

Robert W. Harkins, Ph.D.
Vice President, Scientific Affairs
Grocery Manufacturers of America, Inc.
1010 Wisconsin Avenue, N.W., Suite 800
Washington, D.C. 20007

Eugene B. Hayden, Ph.D.
President
Cereal Institute, Inc.
1111 Plaza Drive, Suite 720
Schaumburg, Ill. 60195

John J. Hefferren, Ph.D.
Director
ADA Health Foundation
Research Institute
211 E. Chicago Avenue
Chicago, Ill. 60611

David H. Hickman, L.L.B.
Covington & Burling
888 16th Street, N.W.
Washington, D.C. 20006

Kirk C. Hoerman, D.D.S.
Associate Professor, Department of
Preventive Dentistry
Loyola University
School of Dentistry
2160 S. First Avenue
Maywood, Ill. 60153

John H. Hopper, Ph.D.
Senior Vice President
Scientific Affairs
Kellogg Company
234 Porter Street
Battle Creek, Mich. 49016

Paul F. Hopper, Ph.D.
Corporate Director for Scientific
Affairs
General Foods Corporation
White Plains, N.Y. 10625

James M. Iacono, Ph.D.
Acting Associate Administrator
Human Nutrition Center, SEA
U.S. Department of Agriculture
Administration Building, Room 351-A
Washington, D.C. 20250

Ms. Karen Ilsemann
Bowers Reporting Company
7309 Arlington Blvd.
Falls Church, Va. 22042

Mr. Donald J. Jorgensen
Commercial Development Manager
Specialty Chemicals Division
Monsanto Industrial Chemical Co.
800 N. Lindbergh Blv.
St. Louis, Mo. 63166

John Kabara, Ph.D.
Professor, Department of
Biomechanics
Michigan State University
East Lansing, Mich. 48824

Dr. John Kagan
Consultant
Westwood Research Laboratory, Inc.
1810 Second Ave., Apt. 2C
New York, N.Y. 10028

Robert S. Katz, Ph.D.
Assistant Director
Nutrition Research
National Dairy Council
6300 N. River Road
Rosemont, Ill. 60018

Dr. Simon Katz
Indiana University
School of Dentistry
410 Beauty Avenue
Indianapolis, Ind. 46202

Mr. Ray G. Kelly
Vice President—Development
The Sunmark Companies
8155 New Hampshire Ave.
St. Louis, Mo. 63123

William J. King, Ph.D.
Manager, New Science & Technology
Colgate-Palmolive Company
909 River road
Piscataway, N.J. 08854

Mr. Henry Koehler
Editor, *Oral Research Abstracts*
American Dental Association
211 E. Chicago Avenue
Chicago, Ill. 60611

Mr. Alan Komensky
Secretary
Council on Bylaws and Judicial Affairs
American Dental Association
211 E. Chicago Avenue
Chicago, Ill. 60611

Mr. Ajit Kothari
Senior Product Marketing Manager
Roche Chemical Division
Hoffman-La Roche, Inc.
Nutley, N.J. 07110

Mr. Jack W. Kuiper
Director, Research & Development-Biscuit
Keebler Company
One Hollow Tree Lane
Elmhurst, Ill. 60148

Ms. Karen Lechowich
Coordinator, Council on Practice
American Dietetic Association
430 N. Michigan Ave.
Chicago, Ill. 60611

Ms. Kathy Leisten
Staff Associate
Council on Dental Health and Health Planning
American Dental Association
211 E. Chicago Avenue
Chicago, Ill. 60611

Betty W. Li, Ph.D.
Research Chemist
Nutrition Institute
U.S. Department of Agriculture
Room 225, Building 308-BARC, East
Beltsville, Md. 20705

Harvey W. Lyon, D.D.S., Ph.D.
Secretary
Council on Dental Research
American Dental Association
211 E. Chicago Avenue
Chicago, Ill. 60611

James L. McDonald, Jr., Ph.D.
Indiana University
School of Dentistry
410 Beauty Avenue
Indianapolis, Ind. 46202

Donald A.M. Mackay, Ph.D.
Vice President
Research & Development
Life Savers, Inc.
40 West 57th Street
New York, N.Y. 10019

Kenneth O. Madsen, Ph.D.
Professor
Nutrition & Biochemistry
University of Texas
Health Science Center at Houston
University of Texas Dental Branch
Box 20068
Houston, Texas 77025

Mr. James Marshall
Assistant Secretary
Council on Dental Care Programs
American Dental Association
211 E. Chicago Avenue
Chicago, Ill 60611

H. Eugene Miller, Ph.D.
Senior Research Chemist
Corporate Research
General Mills, Inc.
9000 Plymouth Avenue, N.
Minneapolis, Minn. 55427

Sanford A. Miller, Ph.D.
Director, Bureau of Foods
Food and Drug Administration
200 C Street, S.W.
Washington, D.C. 20204

Miss B. Bayley Milton
Senior Analyst
Bureau of Economic Research
and Statistics
American Dental Association
211 E. Chicago Avenue
Chicago, Ill. 60611

Edgar Mitchell, Ph.D.
Assistant Secretary
Council on Dental Therapeutics
American Dental Association
211 E. Chicago Avenue
Chicago, Ill. 60611

Ms. Barbara Mortensen
Program Specialist
Bureau of Dental Health Education
American Dental Association
211 E. Chicago Avenue
Chicago, Ill. 60611

Stephen J. Moss, D.D.S., M.S.
Professor and Chairman
Department of Pedodontics
Division of Growth & Development
New York University
College of Dentistry
421 First Avenue
New York, N.Y. 10010

Mr. Tommy Muller
Chief, Biostatistics Facility
ADA Health Foundation
Research Institute
211 E. Chicago Avenue
Chicago, Ill. 60611

Mr. George Najarian
Research Assistant
ADA Health Foundation
Research Institute
211 E. Chicago Avenue
Chicago, Ill. 60611

Conrad Naleway, Ph.D.
Director, Division of Chemistry
Council on Dental Therapeutics
American Dental Association
211 E. Chicago Avenue
Chicago, Ill. 60611

Ernest Newbrun, D.M.D., Ph.D.
Professor of Oral Biology
Department of Oral Medicine and
Hospital Dentistry
University of California
San Francisco, Calif. 94143

Mr. S. William Oberg
Materials Development Manager
Bureau of Dental Health Education
American Dental Association
211 E. Chicago Avenue
Chicago, Ill. 660611

Ms. Mary O'Brien
Managing Editor
Food Product Development
Two North Riverside Plaza
Chicago, Ill. 60606

Mr. R.J. Ohlson
Vice President
Research & Development
Mars, Incorporated
1651 Old Meadow Road
McLean, Va. 22102

Mr. Archie B. Forter
Pepsico, Incorporated
Purchase, N.Y. 10577

Mr. Harold P. Preuss
Manager, Regulatory Sciences
The Coca-Cola company
P.O. Drawer 1734
Atlanta, Georgia 30301

George A. Purvis, Ph.D.
Director of Nutrition
Gerber Products Company
445 State Street
Fremont, Mich. 49412

Mr. Barry Ranallo
Program Specialist
Bureau of Dental Health Education
American Dental Association
211 E. Chicago Avenue
Chicago, Ill. 60611

Gur S. Ranhotra, Ph.D.
Group Leader - Nutrition
Research Department
American Institute of Baking
1213 Bakers Way
Manhattan, Kan. 66502

G. Subba Rao, Ph.D.
Chief, Division of Biochemistry
ADA Health Foundation
Research Institute
211 E. Chicago Avenue
Chicago, Ill. 60611

Mrs. Nancy Resnick
Associate Editor, *ADA News*
American Dental Association
211 E. Chicago Avenue
Chicago, Ill. 60611

Dr. Ina Retief
Medical Practitioner
3624 Belle Meade Way
Birmingham, Ala. 35294

D. Hugo Retief, B.D.S., Ph.D.
Senior Scientist
Institute of Dental Research
University of Alabama
University Station
Birmingham, Ala. 35294

Carl Richberg, Ph.D.
Development Scientist
Research Center
Lever Brothers Company, Inc.
45 River Road
Edgewater, N.J. 07020

Ms. Annette Ripper
Manager, Market Development
Aspartame Division
G.D. Searle & Company
Box 1045
Skokie, Ill. 60076

Morton Ross, D.D.S.
Director, Department of
Dental Science
American Chicle Division
Warner-Lambert Company
170 Tabor Road
Morris Plains, N.J. 07950

John T. Rotruck, Ph.D.
Section Head
Nutrition Research
Procter & Gamble
Miami Valley Laboratories
Cincinnati, Ohio 45247

Irving I. Rusoff, Ph.D.
Senior Scientist
Nabisco, Inc.
2111 Route 208
Fairlawn, N.J. 07410

Mr. Zaker I. Sabri
ADA Health Foundation
Research Institute
American Dental Association
211 E. Chicago Avenue
Chicago, Ill. 60611

Miss Karen Schaid
Senior Analyst
Bureau of Economic Research
and Statistics
American Dental Association
211 E. Chicago Avenue
Chicago, Ill 60611

Rachel Schemmel, Ph.D., R.D.
Professor, Department of Food
Science & Human Nutrition
302 Food Science Bldg.
Michigan State University
East Lansing, Mich. 48824

Thomas Schiff, D.M.D.
Head Clinical Dentist
Monsanto Company
800 N. Lindbergh Blvd.
St. Louis, Mo. 63166

Gordon H. Schrotenboer, Ph.D.
Secretary, Council on Dental
Therapeutics
American Dental Association
211 E. Chicago Avenue
Chicago, Ill. 60611

Charles Schoenfeld, D.D.S., Ph.D.
Chief Research Scientist
Clinical Studies
ADA Health Foundation
Research Institute
211 E. Chicago Avenue
Chicago, Ill. 60611

Roger Scholle, D.D.S.
Editor, Journal American Dental
Association
211 E. Chicago Avenue
Chicago, Ill. 60611

Miss Susan Seffrin
Coordinator: Special Programs
Bureau of Dental Health Education
American Dental Association
211 E. Chicago, Avenue
Chicago, Ill. 60611

James H. Shaw, Ph.D.
Professor of Nutrition
Harvard School of Dental Medicine
188 Longwood Avenue
Boston, Mass. 02115

Irving L. Shklair, Ph.D.
Chief, Microbiology Division
Scientific Department
Naval Dental Research Institute
Building 1-H
Great Lakes, Ill. 60088

Naseeb L. Shory, D.D.S.
Bureau of Dental Health
Alabama Department of Public Health
State Office Building
Montgomery, Ala. 36130

Chakwan Siew, Ph.D.
Chief, Toxicology Laboratory
Division of Biochemistry
ADA Foundation
Research Institute
211 E. Chicago Avenue
Chicago, Ill. 60611

Ms. Mona Signer
Assistant Secretary
Council on Dental Health and Health Planning
American Dental Association
211 E. Chicago Ave.
Chicago, Ill. 60611

Jorge L. Sintes, D.M.D., Ph.D.
Scientist, Cariologist
Oral Health Research Center
Fairleigh Dickinson University
110 Fuller Place
Hackensack, N.J. 07601

A. Elizabeth Sloan, Ph.D.
Manager, Nutrition Education & Communication Services
Nutrition Department
General Mills, Inc.
P.O. Box 1113
Minneapolis, Minn. 55440

Mr. Jay Smith
Public Relations Director
National Soft Drink Association
1101 16th Street, N.W.
Washington, D.C. 20036

Robert E. Smith, Ph.D.
Vice President
Research & Development
Foods Division
Grocery Products Group
The Quaker Oats Company
617 W. Main Street
Barrington, Ill. 60010

Mr. Wallace S. Synder
Assistant Director for Advertising Practices
Bureau of Consumer Protection
Federal Trade Commission
Washington, D.C. 20580

Mr. Delmar Stauffer
Assistant Executive Director
Dental Health
American Dental Association
211 E. Chicago Avenue
Chicago, Ill. 60611

Anthony J.Steffek, D.D.S., Ph.D.
Chief, Division of Developmental Biology
ADA Health Foundation
Research Institute
211 E. Chicago Avenue
Chicago, Ill. 60611

Edward J. Stegemann, L.L.D.
General Counsel
Mars, Incorporated
1651 Old Meadow Road
McLean, Va. 22102

Charles D. Stone, Ph.D.
Senior Research Scientist
Scientific Affairs
M & M Mars
High Street
Hackettstown, N.J. 07840

Mr. John Stroz
Research Coordinator
Life Savers, Inc.
40 W. 57th Street
New York, N.Y. 10019

Mr. Reinhardt Thiessen, Jr.
Central Research Manager
General Food Corporation
Technical Center
250 North Street
White Plains, N.Y. 10625

Richard Tiecke, D.D.S.
Assistant Executive Director
Scientific Affairs
American Dental Association
211 E. Chicago Avenue
Chicago, Ill. 60611

Miss Geraldine Udell
Editorial Consultant
Research Institute
American Dental Association
211 E. Chicago Avenue
Chicago, Ill. 60611

Ms. Violeta S. Velasco
Technical Service Representative
Industrial Division
Corn Products Company
Moffett Technical Center
P.O. Box 345
Argo, Ill. 60501

Dr. Theresa Volpe
ITT Continential Baking Co.
P.O. Box 731
Rye, N.Y. 10580

James H. Wallace, Jr., L.L.D.
Attorney, Kirkland & Ellis
1776 K Street, N.W.
Washington, D.C. 20006

Mr. Kris Warren
Assistant Secretay
Council on Dental Heath and Planning
American Dental Association
211 E. Chicago Avenue
Chicago, Ill. 60611

Mr. Richard K. Wickstrom
Chief, Instrument Facility
ADA Health Foundation
Research Institute
211 E. Chicago Avenue
Chicago, Ill. 60611

Mr. Howard Wilkins
Director of Quality Assurances
Standard Brands, Inc.
Curtiss Division
3401 Mt. Prospect Road
Franklin Park, Ill. 60131

Walter E. Wisniewski, J.D.
Associate Counsel
Secretary, Council on Insurance
American Dental Association
211 E. Chicago Avenue
Chicago, Ill. 60611

Philip White, Sc.D.
Director, Department of Foods and Nutrition
American Medical Association
535 N. Dearborn
Chicago, Ill. 60610

Walter Wolman, Ph.D.
Assistant to the Director
ADA Health Foundation
Research Institute
211 E. Chicago Avenue
Chicago, Ill. 60611

Bernard Wolnak, Ph.D.
President, B. Wolnak Associates
75 E. Wacker
Chicago, Ill. 60601

Wayne T. Wozniak, Ph.D.
Research Associate
Division of Biopyhsics
ADA Health Foundation
Research Institute
211 E. Chiago Avenue
Chicago, Ill.60611

Harold Wyckoff, D.D.S.
Assistant Secretary
Council on Dental Materials & Devices
American Dental Association
211 E. Chicago Avenue
Chicago, Ill. 60611

Ferdinand Zienty, Ph.D.
Manager, Research & Development
Food, Feed & Fine Chemicals
Speciality Chemicals Division
Monsanto Company
800 N. Lindbergh Blvd.
St. Louis, Mo. 63166

Barry L. Zoumas. Ph.D.
Director, Research
Hershey Foods Corporation
P.O. Box 54
925 Reese Avenue
Hershey, Pa. 17033

BY COMPANY (Alphabetically)

Cadbury Corporation	Mr. E. Abeling
The Coca-Cola Company	Harold Preuss
Colgate-Palmolive Co.	William J. King
Corn Products Co.	Violeta Velasco
Finn-Cal Products, Inc.	R.A. Aherne
Frito Lay, Inc.	R.J. Carlotti
General Foods Corp.	R. Thiessen
	Paul F. Hopper
General Mills	R.H. Anderson
	H.E. Miller
	A.E. Sloan
Gerber Products Co.	G.A. Purvis
Hershey Foods Corporation	B.L. Zoumas
Hoffman-LaRoche, Inc.	Ajit Kothari
IT Continental Baking Co.	Terry Volpe
Keebler Company	Jack W. Kuiper
Kellogg Company	John Hopper
	Clesteen Clark
	Robin Foor
Lever Brothers, Co.	Carl Richberg
Life Savers, Inc.	Donald A.M. Mackay
	John Stroz
M & M Mars	Charles D. Stone
Monsanto Company	D.J. Jorgensen
	Thomas Schiff
	Ferdinand Zienty
Nabisco, Inc.	I.I. Rusoff
Pepsi Company, Inc.	Archie B. Porter
Procter & Gamble	William E. Cooley
	John Rotruck
The Quaker Oats Co.	R.E. Smith
Ragold, Inc.	W.F. Brightman
G.D. Searle	Annett Ripper
Standard Brands, Inc.	R.W. Daniels
	H. Wilkins
The Sunmark Companies	R.G. Kelly
Warner-Lambert Co.	Norton Ross
	Wayne Geiselmann
William Wrigley, Jr., Co.	E. Eugene Fisher

BY TRADE ASSOCIATIONS

American Institute of Baking	Gur S. Ranhotra
National Dairy Council	Robert S. Katz
National Soft Drink Assoc.	Jay Smith
The Sugar Association	G.N. Bollenback
Cereal Institute	E.B. Hayden
Grocery Manufacturers of America, Inc.	R.W. Harkins

ACADEMIA

Alabama, University of	D.H. Retief
Alabama Department of Public Health	Naseeb L. Shory
American Academy of Pedodontics New York University, College of Dentistry	Stephen J. Moss
California, University of	Ernest Newbrun
Council on Child Media & Merchandising	Robert B. Choate
Eastman Dental Center	Basil G. Bibby
Fairleigh Dickinson University	J. Sintes
	M.C. Alfano
	D.P. DePaola
Food & Drug Administration	Sanford Miller
	Victor P. Frattali
Forsyth Dental Center	Robert L. Glass
Harvard University	James H. Shaw
Illinois University, Southern	Arthur N. Bahn
Indiana University	Simon Katz
	James McDonald
Loyola University	Kirk C. Hoerman
Massachusetts, University of	F.M. Clydesdale
Michigan State University	John Kabara
	Rachel Schemmel
National Institute of Dental Research	William H. Bowen
Naval Dental Research Institute	Irving Shklair
Newcastle, University of	W. Michael Edgar
The Nutrition Foundation	D.O. Chichester
Pennsylvania, University of	Neal W. Chilton
Texas, University of	Kenneth A. Madsen
U.S. Department of Agriculture	Betty W. Li
	James M. Iacono

PROFESSIONAL ORGANIZATIONS

ADA Health Foundation, Research Institute	William Ayer Judy Grumley John J. Hefferren Tommy Muller George Najarian G. Subba Rao Zaker Sabri Charles Shoenfeld Chakwan Siew Anthony Steffek Richard Wickstrom Walter Wolman Wayne T. Wozniak
ADA Health Foundation, Research Institute, Editorial Consultants	Velma Child Geraldine Udell
ADA Health Foundation, Administration	Pat Darchun
ADA Research Unit, Washington	L. Chow
ADA Bureau of Dental Health Education	Dana Davis Barb Mortensen S. William Oberg Barry Ranallo Susan Seffrin
ADA Bureau of Economic Research and Statistics	E. Bayley Milton Karen Schaid
ADA Bureau of Public Information	Peter C. Goulding
ADA Council on Dental Care Programs	James Marshall
ADA Council on Dental Health and Health Planning	Wilbert Fletke, Council member Susan Flor Darlene Fujii Kathy Leisten Mona Signer Kris Warren
ADA Council on Dental Materials and Devices	Robert Bauer Harold Wyckoff
ADA Council on Dental Research	Harvey Lyon
ADA Council on Dental Therapeutics	S.G. Ciancio, Council member Gordon H. Schrotenboer Edgar Mitchell Conrad A. Naleway
ADA Council on Insurance	Walter E. Wisniewski
ADA Council on Bylaws and Judicial Affairs	Alan M. Komensky
ADA Council on Legislation	Bernard Conway
ADA Editorial Office	John B. Goetz

	Henry Koehler
	Nancy Resnick
	Roger Scholle
ADA Health Affairs	Delmar Stauffer
ADA Office of Advertising Review	An-Shih Cheng
ADA Scientific Affairs	Richard W. Tiecke
ADA Department of Foods and Nutrition	Philip White
American Dietetic Association	Karen Lechowich

BY INDIVIDUALS

Edward J. Stegemann	Mars Incorporated
Karen Ilsemann	Bowers Reporting Co.
Mary O'Brien	Food Product Development
David H. Hickman	Covington & Burling
Allan Allured	Manufacturers Confectionery Publ. Co.
Lisa Bahn	Leo Burnett Agency
C.H. Chamberlain	Kirkland & Ellis
J.H. Wallace	
Timothy S. Hardy	

CONSULTING LAB

Bernard Wolnak Associates	Bernard Wolnak
Westwood Research Labs Inc.	John Cornell
	John Kagan

FOODS, NUTRITION AND DENTAL HEALTH

SUBJECT INDEX

AUTHOR INDEX